Your Child's Health

The Parents' One-Stop Reference Guide to: Symptoms
Emergencies
Common Illnesses
Behavior Problems
Healthy Development

Your Child's Health

Barton D. Schmitt, M.D., F.A.A.P.

*Director of the Sleep Disorder Clinic, Enuresis-Encopresis Clinic,
and After-Hours Call Center, The Children's Hospital of Denver
Professor of Pediatrics, University of Colorado School of Medicine*

BANTAM BOOKS

YOUR CHILD'S HEALTH

THE PARENTS' ONE-STOP REFERENCE GUIDE TO: SYMPTOMS, EMERGENCIES, COMMON ILLNESSES, BEHAVIOR PROBLEMS, AND HEALTHY DEVELOPMENT, REVISED EDITION

PUBLISHING HISTORY
A Bantam Book / September 1987
Revised edition published September 1991
Second revision published December 2005

Published by Bantam Dell
A Division of Random House, Inc.
New York, New York

Book design by Maura Fadden Rosenthal/Mspace •

Library of Congress Cataloging in Publication Data is on file with the publisher

ISBN-13: 978-0-553-38369-0
ISBN-10: 0-553-38369-8

Printed in the United States of America
Published simultaneously in Canada

www.bantamdell.com

BVG 10 9 8 7 6 5 4 3 2 1

This book is dedicated to the inner strength of families:

To my parents, for believing in me.

To Mary, for her enduring love and encouragement.

To Dave, Elaine, Becky, and Mike, for everything they taught me about
    fractured femurs, sea urchins, wolf spiders, pill-swallowing, suturing
    on the kitchen table, strep cultures in the furnace room, hypothermia,
    and having fun.

To Lauren, Megan, Dylan, Ethan, Graham, Griffin, Gavin, and Juliana—the
    best grandkids one could ever ask for. They keep us active and hopeful.
    They affirm that life can be beautiful.

Contents

II. Trauma (Injuries)

III. New Baby Care

Normal Newborns   93

IV. Health Promotion: Keeping Your Child Healthy

VI. Common Symptoms and Illnesses

VII. Glossary

Essential Topics for Each Age

Prenatal:
- Breast-feeding, 150
- Formula-feeding, 156
- Circumcision decision, 113
- Newborn equipment, 118
- Car safety seats, 216
- Sibling rivalry, 126

Newborn:
- Normal newborn's appearance, 103
- Newborn rashes and birthmarks, 108
- Newborn skin care, 111
- Jaundice, newborn, 135
- Sleep position for young infants, 125
- First weeks at home, 97
- Sick newborn: subtle symptoms, 130

2 Weeks:
- Crying baby, 253
- Sleep problems, prevention, 257
- Pacifiers, 367
- Spitting up, 138

2 Months:
- Immunizations, 225

- Immunization reactions, 226
- Diaper rash, 133

4 Months:
- Sick infant: judging the severity, 131
- Working mother, 407
- Solid foods, 167
- Overeating, prevention, 201

6 Months:
- Developmental stimulation, 211
- Sleep problems, prevention, 261
- Fever, 427
- Temperature, how to measure, 433

8 Months:
- Life-threatening 911 symptoms, 5
- Emergency symptoms, 6
- Teething, 573
- Baby bottle tooth decay, prevention, 192

10 Months:
- Infections, prevention of, 222
- Injury prevention, 215
- Poisoning, 55

Introduction

Dear Parents, Stepparents, Grandparents, and Other Caregivers,

After 40 years of working with families, this is what I know: You want your child to have a better start in life than you did. You're ready to sacrifice for your child. You want to fill your child's heart with love. You want to teach your child to be self-disciplined, self-reliant, and responsible for his or her actions. You want to teach your child to be thoughtful, kind, honest, generous, and respectful toward you and others. You want your child to know that every life is precious and that the highest moral value is helping the less fortunate among us. If this be so, you are an active member of the universal family of those who care for our children.

While our hopes for our children are similar, family structures have changed and become more diverse in our country, since the first edition of this book was published in 1987. There are foster parents who shelter our abused and abandoned children. There are adoptive parents who reach out to children from faraway shores. There are traditional, biological mom and dad families, but in these times over 60 percent of mothers work outside the home. Finally, there are the single parents who raise over 25 percent of our children while working full-time. Just so you know, the rest of us stand in awe of what you do.

These guidelines were written to help you provide better health care, nurturing, and protection for your child. I've emphasized the common illnesses, injuries, and behavior problems that befall the majority of children. When possible, I've stressed the healthy lifestyles and preventive measures you can take to keep your child physically and psychologically healthy. When appropriate, I've cautioned you about the limitations of surgery and drugs. The table of contents, cross-references in the text, and the index have been organized and interwoven so you can find needed advice quickly. And finally, the topics are covered in depth, so you can find answers to almost all of your questions in one book.

To help you use this book, information relating to each of the topics or diseases is organized in the following way:

Symptoms and Characteristics
- What are the symptoms?
- What does it look like?
- What's normal?

Causes—Is it caused by virus, bacteria, allergy, injury, heredity, stress, or some other factor? Is it contagious?

Expected Course—How long will it last? How bad will it get? What are the possible complications?

Guidelines for Calling Your Child's Physician
- How can you recognize serious symptoms and emergencies?
- Should you call 911?
- Should you call the doctor immediately?
- Can you safely wait to call during office hours?
- Can your child safely be treated at home without a call?

Home Care Recommendations
- What first aid measures can you take for emergencies?
- For nonemergencies, what can you do to make your child comfortable?
- How can you prevent similar infections or injuries in the future?
- How can you speed recovery?
- What are the nuts and bolts of home care?
- How can you improve your child's behavior?

Your desire to be better informed about child rearing and childhood illnesses is universal. These guidelines are meant to supplement the health education provided by your child's physician. Most parents also receive ongoing health advice from friends, relatives, newspapers, magazines, the Internet, radio, and television. Unfortunately, information from the media or nonprofessionals may be confusing, conflicting, or downright alarming. One of the main purposes of this book is to help bridge the information gap with accurate, up-to-date, and straightforward health facts and advice. The guidelines for when to call your child's physician have been tested by thousands of physicians and nurses across the country who use my book *Pediatric Telephone Protocols* in their offices.

One sound rule of child rearing is: Don't do anything for your child that he can do for himself (such as feeding or dressing). The same advice can easily be applied to parents with regard to health care decision-making. You are an important member of your child's health care team and you can do more on your own than you think. You have innate common sense and you know your child better than anyone else. Observe your child's symptoms. Use this book as your reference and make informed decisions. As your ability to differentiate (triage) between serious and nonserious illnesses and injuries increases, so will your confidence. The common illnesses and behavior of childhood will come into perspective as something you can competently manage. You will become a smart consumer of health care services, and in the process you'll teach your child that their body is a powerful structure that can defeat most infections and heal most injuries on its own. Don't underestimate your abilities.

Best wishes for enjoyable and successful parenting during these exciting years.

—BARTON D. SCHMITT, M.D.
Medical Director of the After-Hours Call Center,
Sleep Disorders Clinic, Enuresis-Encopresis Clinic,
and attending physician at The Children's Hospital,
Denver, Colorado

Acknowledgments

I am immeasurably indebted to my original pediatric and parent reviewers for their careful examination of my text for accuracy, safety, objectivity, clarity, and completeness. Their efforts were extraordinary and their feedback invaluable.

Pediatric Review Board
Joseph H. Banks, M.D., Columbus, Ohio
John M. Benbow, M.D., Concord, North Carolina
Daniel D. Broughton, M.D., Rochester, Minnesota
Rosemary D. Casey, M.D., Philadelphia, Pennsylvania
David M. Christopher, M.D., Renton, Washington
Jessie R. Groothuis, M.D., La Jolla, California
Robin L. Hansen, M.D., Sacramento, California
David L. Kerns, M.D., San Jose, California
Bruce J. McIntosh, M.D., Jacksonville, Florida
Robert D. Mauro, M.D., Denver, Colorado
Cajsa J. Schumacher, M.D., Albany, New York
Daniel R. Terwelp, M.D., Austin, Texas
Wallace C. White, M.D., Denver, Colorado

Parent Review Board
Lynnette Baer, Bowmar, Colorado
Elizabeth T. Berk, Concord, Massachusetts
Gayle N. Ebel, Bowmar, Colorado
Candy Ergen, Bowmar, Colorado
Nancy Gary, Child Psychologist, Denver, Colorado
Doris L. Klein, Child Life Worker, Denver, Colorado
Carol J. Markley, Bowmar, Colorado
Christina Podolak, Bowmar, Colorado
Sara Rotbart, Denver, Colorado
Mary C. Schmitt, Bowmar, Colorado
Lynne M. Weaver, Littleton, Colorado

Sandra Wilday, Bowmar, Colorado
Marjorie S. Wise, Englewood, Colorado

My appreciation and admiration to the following pediatric subspecialists and pediatric surgeons who have graciously helped me with specific topics and ongoing questions in their areas of expertise:

General Pediatrics:	Drs. Robert Mauro, Robert Brayden, Steven Poole, Allison Kempe, Stephen Berman, Candice Johnson, and Karen Dodd
Adolescent Medicine:	Drs. David Kaplan and Eric Sigel
Emergency Pediatrics:	Drs. Joan Bothner, David Thompson, Mark Roback, Louis Hampers, and Michael Clemmens
Infectious Disease:	Drs. James Todd, Mary Glode, Harley Rotbart, Mark Abzug, Christine Nyquist, and Brian Lauer
Dermatology:	Drs. William Weston and Joseph Morelli
Allergy:	Drs. James Shira, Allen Bock, David Pearlman, and Dan Atkins
Psychology:	Drs. Edward Christophersen, Jeffrey Dolgan, and Nancy Gary
Neonatology:	Drs. Jacinto Hernandez, Susan Niermeyer, and Elizabeth Thilo
Breast-Feeding:	Drs. Marianne Neifert, Joy Seacat, and Lisbeth Gabrielski
Cardiology:	Drs. James Wiggins, Robert Wolfe, and Henry Sondheimer
Pulmonology:	Drs. Jeffrey Wagener and Frank Accurso
Gastroenterology:	Drs. Arnold Silverman, Ronald Sokol, Judy Sondheimer, and Nancy Krebs
Neurology:	Dr. Paul Moe
Car Safety Seats:	Theresa Rapstine, R.N., TCH Pediatric Trauma Institute
Endocrinology:	Dr. Michael Kappy
Ear, Nose, and Throat:	Dr. Kenny Chan
Ophthalmology:	Drs. Robert King and Robert Sargent
Dentistry:	Drs. William Mueller and Stephen Wilson
Urology:	Dr. Martin Koyle
Orthopedics:	Drs. Robert Eilert and Frank Chang

I'm immeasurably grateful to Dr. Bob Mauro for his comprehensive review. His keen intellect and sound clinical judgment have left their mark on this third edition. My special thanks to Toni Burbank, my editor and advocate at Bantam Dell. Her intelligence, experience, and support are everything an author could ask for. Thanks also to Trish Cozart, medical editor at Clinical Reference Systems. Her excellent assistance with the *Pediatric Advisor* is also reflected in this update. Finally, my deep gratitude goes out to the many physicians, nurses, students, and parents who have shared ideas and questions with me over the last 40 years—especially my wonderful colleagues who practice medicine in the Mile-High City.

The Reader's Responsibility

The contents of this book have been carefully reviewed for accuracy.

If you have any questions as to the correct diagnosis or proper treatment for your child, call your child's physician for help.

If you feel your child's condition has become serious, don't be reluctant to recontact your physician. Trust your intuition; you know your child better than anyone else.

The author and publisher disclaim responsibility for any harmful consequences resulting from the misinterpretation or misapplication of information or advice contained in these guidelines.

I. Emergencies

EMERGENCY TELEPHONE CALLS

Life-Threatening Emergencies

Dial 911 (Emergency Medical Services). In larger cities, this call will dispatch an emergency vehicle staffed by a rescue squad and based at the nearest fire department. In smaller towns and counties, the operator will connect you with an emergency ambulance service. The direct number for this service is usually found on the first page of your telephone directory. In areas that use 911, children should be taught to dial this number for crises. Increasingly, 911 is being linked to a computer system ("enhanced 911") that can determine the address of the incoming call even if the caller can't speak.

Non-Life-Threatening Emergencies

Call Your Child's Physician. If you don't have a physician, call the nearest emergency room. Always call in first, rather than simply going to an emergency room. Your physician may provide you with critical first aid instructions by phone (e.g., for burns, animal bites, or fractures). Your physician also can help you decide whether a rescue squad should be sent out or if it is safe for you to drive in. In addition, your physician can also tell you if it's safe to be seen in the office or where to take your child for the best emergency care.

Poisoning

If you know the phone number of the nearest Poison Center, call them now. If not, call the National Poison Center hotline at 1-800-222-1222. They will automatically connect you with your local Poison Center.

How to Cut Through Red Tape

When you call in, always state assertively, "This is an emergency." Do not let the answering service or receptionist put you on hold before talking with you. If you are put on hold, hang up and call back immediately.

EMERGENCY TRANSPORTATION

Life-Threatening or Major Emergencies
Call your rescue squad (911) or ambulance service.

Definition of a Life-Threatening Emergency—Children who may need resuscitation en route (for instance, those with severe breathing difficulty, severe choking, or not breathing) require a 911 call. Other potentially life-threatening emergencies are persistent loss of consciousness (coma), continuing seizure, or bleeding that can't be stopped by direct pressure. Children with major trauma or possible neck injury need splinting before transportation.

The Staff of Emergency Vehicles—Emergency vehicles are staffed by EMTs (Emergency Medical Technicians) or Paramedics. EMTs are trained in Basic Life Support: cardiopulmonary resuscitation (CPR), splinting, bandaging, and so on. Paramedics are EMTs with additional training in Advanced Life Support: drawing blood, starting IVs, intubation, recording EKGs, and so on. EMTs receive 160 hours of training and Paramedics receive 1,200 hours. These pre-hospital care specialists are certified by their national associations. While providing emergency care, they are linked by two-way radio to an emergency room physician at their base hospital.

Rescue Squads Versus Ambulance Services—In larger cities, rescue squads are often available through local fire departments. Usually rescue squads can respond more rapidly than ambulances, and their service is free. After the patient's condition has been stabilized, they will often call an ambulance company for transport to the hospital if it is warranted. In general the police do not transport sick people, so don't call them for medical emergencies.

Non-Life-Threatening Emergencies
Go to the nearest hospital offering emergency services. Try to call your child's physician first.

Definition of Less Severe Emergencies—These concern children who need to be seen as quickly as possible but whose condition is currently stable or at least does not pose a danger of suddenly needing resuscitation. Examples are poisonings, slow bleeding controlled by pressure, severe pain, and seizures that have stopped.

Advantage of Car over an Ambulance—A private car is quicker and less expensive than an ambulance. Another option is to call a taxi.

Driving in to Seek Emergency Care—If you are going by private car, don't leave until you know the exact location of the emergency room you will be going to. It is a good idea to rehearse the drive by the fastest route before an emergency occurs. Keep your sick child in a car safety seat. Try to have a friend or neighbor accompany you and do the driving. Some parents are too shaken by their child's injury to drive safely.

What to Bring with You to the Emergency Room
- Your health insurance card
- Your child's immunization record
- Your pharmacy's telephone number
- Any medicines your child is taking (or a list of drugs and dosages)
- If your child has been poisoned, bring the container.
- If your child has passed blood in the urine, stool, or vomited material, bring a sample for testing.
- Your child's security object or favorite toy

LIFE-THREATENING 911 SYMPTOMS

Every parent should learn how to identify life-threatening symptoms. You need to know in advance when to call 911 rather than trying to reach your doctor, and when it's not safe to try to drive to the hospital. Then you will not make the tragic mistake of attempting to drive your seriously ill child to an emergency room only to have him/her stop breathing or go into shock on the way. If your child ever has any of the following symptoms, call Emergency Medical Services (911) immediately.

Severe Breathing Problems

- Breathing has stopped.
- Your child is choking and unable to breathe or is turning blue.
- Difficulty breathing follows a medicine, food, or bee sting (the concern is for severe allergic reaction or anaphylaxis).

Severe Bleeding

- Blood is pumping or spurting from the wound.
- Blood is pouring out and can't be stopped with direct pressure.

Severe Neck Injury

Try not to move your child until EMS arrives.

Seizure or Convulsion Now (hasn't stopped)

Can't Wake Up

Your child is unconscious (in a coma).

EMERGENCY SYMPTOMS

All the conditions discussed in this chapter are emergencies. The following emergency symptoms, however, are highlighted because they are either difficult to recognize or not considered serious by some parents. If your child has any of the following symptoms, contact your child's physician immediately.

Sick Newborn

If your baby is less than one month old and looks or acts sick in any way, the problem could be serious (e.g., vomiting, cough, poor color).

Severe Lethargy

To be tired during an illness is normal, but if your child stares off into space, won't smile, has no interest in playing, is too weak to cry, is floppy, or is hard to awaken, these are serious symptoms.

Severe Pain

If your child cries when you touch him or move him, this can be a symptom of meningitis. Such children also don't want to be held. Constant screaming or the inability to sleep also points to severe pain.

Can't Walk

If your child has learned to walk and then loses the ability to stand or walk, the most likely reason is that he or she has a serious injury to the legs or an acute problem with balance. If your child walks bent over, holding his abdomen, he probably has a serious abdominal problem such as appendicitis.

Tender Abdomen

Press on your child's belly while he or she is sitting up in your lap and looking at a book. Normally you should be able to press an inch or so in with your fingers in all parts of the belly without resistance. If he pushes your hand away or screams, this is an important finding. If the belly is also bloated and hard, the condition is even more worrisome. (See ABDOMINAL PAIN, page 596.)

Tender Testicle or Scrotum

The sudden onset of pain in the groin area can be due to twisting (torsion) of the testicle. This requires surgery within 8 hours to save the testicle.

Labored Breathing

You should assess your child's breathing after cleaning out the nose and when he is not coughing. If your child is working hard at breathing, has tight croup, or has obvious wheezing, he or she needs to be seen immediately. Other signs of respiratory distress are a rapid breathing rate, bluish lips, or retractions (pulling in between the ribs). (See BREATHING DIFFICULTY, SEVERE, page 36.)

Bluish Lips

Bluish lips, gums, or tongue (cyanosis) can indicate a reduced amount of oxygen in the bloodstream. (See BLUISH LIPS, page 490.)

Drooling

The sudden onset of drooling or spitting, especially associated with difficulty in swallowing, can mean that your child has a serious infection of the tonsils, throat, or epiglottis (top part of the windpipe).

Dehydration

Dehydration means that your child's body fluids are at a low level. Dehydration usually follows severe vomiting and/or diarrhea. Suspect dehydration if your child has not urinated in 8 hours (12 hours if over 1 year old), crying produces no tears, the inside of the mouth is dry rather than moist, or the soft spot in the skull is sunken. Dehydrated children are also tired and weak. If your child is alert and active but not making much urine, he isn't dehydrated. Dehydration requires immediate fluid replacement by mouth or intravenously.

Bulging Soft Spot

If the anterior fontanel is tense and bulging, the brain is under pressure. (See SOFT SPOT, BULGING, page 520.) Since the fontanel normally bulges slightly with crying, assess it when your child is quiet and in an upright position.

Stiff Neck

To test for a stiff neck: With your child lying down, lift his head until the chin touches the middle of the chest. If he is resistant to this, place a toy or other object of interest on his belly so he will have to look down in order to see it. Older children can simply be asked to look at their belly button. A stiff neck can be an early sign of meningitis.

Injured Neck

Any injury to the neck, regardless of symptoms, should be discussed with your physician because of the risk of damage to the spinal cord.

Purple Spots or Dots

Purple or blood-red spots or dots on the skin can be a sign of a serious bloodstream infection. Explained bruises don't count. (See PURPLE SPOTS, page 460.)

Fever Over 105°F

All the preceding symptoms are stronger indicators of serious illness than is the level of fever. All of them can occur with low fevers as well as high ones. Serious infections become a special concern only when the temperature rises above 105°F (40.6°C). In infants a rectal temperature less than 96.8°F (36.0°C) can also be serious.

Suicide Concerns

Because of the marked increase in suicide attempts in adolescence, parents should be alert to any of the following warning signs: preoccupation with thoughts of death or suicide, themes of death in writing or conversation, abrupt withdrawal from friends and family, abrupt loss of interest in favorite pastimes, abrupt decline in schoolwork, reckless risk-taking behavior, depressed mood. Call either the suicide hotline or your child's physician.

Child Abuse Concerns

Call your child's physician or the child abuse hotline if you are afraid you might hurt your child, if someone has injured your child, or if someone has shaken your child. Child abuse has a tendency to escalate, so protect your child by seeking help early. Infants are at the greatest risk for a serious reinjury.

Related Topics

SICK NEWBORN: SUBTLE SYMPTOMS (SEE PAGE 130)
SICK INFANT: JUDGING THE SEVERITY OF ILLNESS (see page 131)

RESUSCITATION (Mouth-to-Mouth Breathing)

If your child has stopped breathing or is gasping for breath (e.g., from choking, croup, carbon monoxide poisoning, drowning, or head trauma), you won't have time to read these guidelines. So read them now. And take an approved CPR (cardiopulmonary resuscitation) or first aid course. You can't learn external cardiac massage purely from reading. Fortunately, more than 90 percent of children who stop breathing still have a pulse and heartbeat (unlike heart attack victims) and they need only artificial respiration to revive them. The steps in mouth-to-mouth breathing are as follows.

Preparation

Rescue Squad—Have someone call a rescue squad (911) immediately. You're going to need help.

Clear the Mouth—Look for any gum, food, foreign object, or loose orthodontic retainer. If present, remove them with your fingers or a

Heimlich maneuver (see CHOKING, page 11). If any liquid is in the mouth, remove it by turning your child on one side and using gravity.

Position the Head—With your child lying faceup, put a folded blanket or towel (½ inch to 2 inches thick) directly under the back of your child's head. Do not put anything under the shoulders or neck. This "sniffing," head-forward position opens the airway and closes the esophagus (thereby keeping air out of the stomach). The jaw and chin can also be pulled forward to open the airway more. (Note: Some adolescents and adults may require slight extension of the neck for optimal breathing.)

Mouth-to-Mouth Breathing

Pinch your child's nostrils closed with one hand and seal the mouth with yours. (In small children, an adult can often seal both the child's nostrils and mouth with his mouth.) Blow air with a steady pressure into your child's lungs until you see the chest rise (the smaller the child, the smaller the volume of your puff). Then remove your mouth and your child will automatically blow the air out without any help (normal recoil of the lungs). During this time, take a breath and refill your lungs. Repeat this at the following rates:

• Under 2 years old: 20 times per minute (once every 3 seconds)
• 2 to 12 years old: 15 times per minute (once every 4 seconds)
• Over 12 years old: 12 times per minute (once every 5 seconds)

Occasionally, take several quite deep breaths to bring plenty of oxygen into your lungs. (Note: If it is impossible to open the victim's mouth, cover the mouth and give mouth-to-nose breathing.) If 4 or 5 breaths don't move the chest, assume the airway is blocked and perform a Heimlich maneuver 10 times in rapid succession (see CHOKING, p. 11).

If the heartbeat and carotid pulse are absent, also perform external cardiac massage if you know how to do it. In general, give 5 heart compressions for every 1 breath (i.e., 1-2-3-4-5-breathe, then repeat).

CHOKING

Choking is the coughing spasm and sputtering that follow getting liquids or solids on the vocal cords or into the airway. Most children choke on liquids that go down the wrong way or mucus from sniffing back nasal secretions. Choking may also follow vomiting. The child's cough reflex will clear the windpipe of aspirated liquid within 30 seconds. Complete blockage occurs when solid food (a grape or a piece of hot dog, for instance) or a foreign object (e.g., a toy) becomes lodged in the voice box. (It can also occur with severe croup.) Under these conditions, the child is unable to breathe, cry, or speak. The child will be in a state of panic, and if the obstruction isn't relieved in 1 or 2 minutes, the child will pass out and may die.

First Aid for Choking

Call the rescue squad (911) immediately in all cases of choking on a solid object. In general, choking on liquids is temporary and harmless. For liquids, call the rescue squad if your child turns blue, becomes limp, or passes out.

Encourage Coughing—As long as your child is breathing and coughing, do nothing except encourage him to cough the material up by himself. Reassure him that it will come out. The main purpose of your child's cough reflex is to clear the windpipe. Don't offer anything to drink unless your child is choking on something dry and flaky. In general, fluids just worsen the problem by taking up some of the space needed for the passage of air.

If Breathing Stops in a Child over 1 Year Old—If the child can't breathe, cough, or make a sound, proceed with the Heimlich maneuver.
- Grasp the child from behind, just below the lower ribs but above the navel, in bear-hug fashion. Make a fist with one hand and fold the other hand over it.
- Give a sudden upward and backward jerk (at 45-degree angle) to try to squeeze all the air out of the chest and pop the lodged object out of the windpipe.
- Repeat this upward abdominal thrust 10 times in rapid succession, until the object comes out.
- If the child is too heavy for you to suspend from your arms, lay him on his back on the floor. Put your hands on both sides of the abdomen, just below the ribs, and apply sudden, strong bursts of upward pressure.

If Breathing Stops in a Child Under 1 Year Old—Give back blows and chest compressions.

- Place him or her facedown in a 60-degree incline over your knees or on your forearm.
- Deliver 5 blows with your hand between the shoulder blades in rapid succession.
- If breathing has not resumed, lay the child on the floor and apply 5 rapid chest compressions over the lower third of the breastbone (sternum) using 2 fingers (called chest thrusts). Alternate back blows and chest thrusts until the object comes out. (Avoid abdominal thrusts and the true Heimlich maneuver in children under 1 because it carries a risk of liver or spleen laceration.)

If the Child Passes Out—Give mouth-to-mouth breathing.

- Quickly open the mouth and look inside to see if there is any object that can be removed with a sweep of your finger (usually there is not). Avoid "blind" sweeps.
- Then begin mouth-to-mouth breathing (page 10). Air can usually be forced past the foreign object temporarily until help arrives.
- If mouth-to-mouth breathing doesn't move the chest, repeat the abdominal thrusts or chest compressions.

Prevention of Choking on Foods and Other Objects

Choking can be life-threatening, so try to prevent its happening. Choking on foods kills as many children each year as accidental poisonings.

- Foods that are likely to be aspirated into the lungs are nuts of any kind, sunflower seeds, orange seeds, cherry pits, watermelon seeds, gum, hard candies, popcorn, raw carrot, raw peas, and raw celery. These hard foods should not be given to children under 4 years of age because back molars are needed to chew them and knowledge is needed to spit them out.
- The soft foods that most commonly cause fatal choking by completely blocking the windpipe are hot dogs, sausage, large pieces of any meat, grapes, gummy candy, and caramels (especially if the child is in a hurry). These dangerous soft foods must be chopped up before serving.
- Warn baby-sitters and older siblings not to share these foods with small children.
- In general, teach your child to chew all foods thoroughly before attempting to swallow them.
- Don't allow your child to fill his cheeks with food like a chipmunk.

- An especially dangerous time is the morning after parties, when some of these foods may be found on the floor by a toddler. Clean up early.
- Choking on a rubber balloon is the leading cause of choking deaths from objects other than foods. Most incidents occur while children are chewing on a deflated balloon and suddenly inhale it. Warn your child never to chew or suck on pieces of rubber balloons. Even teenagers have died from this freak accident. Chewing on an inflated balloon is also dangerous because it could burst. Mylar helium balloons are much safer. Rubber balloons should only be used with strict supervision.
- Don't give a young child a toy with small, detachable parts. In 5 minutes you'll find the missing part in the mouth (if you're lucky).
- Periodically check your child's environment for small objects (anything with a diameter less than 1¼ inches) that your child could choke on. Ask older children to protect younger siblings by checking the carpet for missing small pieces from toys or games.
- Dispose of button batteries carefully.
- Remind people of all ages not to run or play sports with gum or other material in their mouths.

ALLERGIC REACTION, SEVERE
(Anaphylactic Reaction)

Symptoms and Characteristics
- Immediate symptoms within 30 to 60 minutes
- Wheezing, croupy cough, hoarseness, or difficulty breathing
- Tightness in the chest or throat
- Widespread hives, swelling, or itching
- Dizziness or passing out
- Previous allergic reaction to the same item is added evidence.
- Usually caused by a bee sting, drug, or food

First Aid
Call the rescue squad (911) if your child is having difficulty breathing or passes out. Have your child lie down with the feet elevated to prevent

shock. Call your physician immediately if you think the allergic reaction is not severe.

Epinephrine—If you have an anaphylactic kit, give an injection of epinephrine (adrenaline).

- Children 20 to 50 pounds: Auto-inject Epi-Pen Jr.
- Over 50 pounds: Auto-inject Epi-Pen.
- Inject it into the upper outer thigh muscle (giving into the fat tissue is also effective).
- Some parents are hesitant to give their child a shot of epinephrine. If there is any possibility your child is having symptoms of an anaphylactic reaction, give the epinephrine immediately. In addition, if your child has had a life-threatening reaction in the past and now has been reexposed to the same allergic substance (e.g., food or bee sting), give epinephrine *before* your child develops symptoms. There is no harm from giving epinephrine, just from not giving it.

Benadryl—Give an antihistamine by mouth as soon as possible if your child can swallow. Use Benadryl or any antihistamine you have. See the dosage tables (pages 238–240). The regular Benadryl dosage for teens is 50 mg.

Bee Sting Treatment—for Severe Reactions—If a stinger is still present in the wound, remove it. Do this by scraping it off with the edge of a knife blade or credit card rather than squeezing it. Once a reaction has begun, a tourniquet is not helpful, according to the American College of Emergency Physicians.

Transportation—If you can't reach your physician and your child is stable, go to the nearest emergency room (see EMERGENCY TRANSPORTATION, page 4).

Prevention of Severe Allergic Reactions

Children with anaphylactic reactions need to be evaluated later by an allergist. Since the reactions can be fatal, you should keep emergency kits containing epinephrine at home, at school, and in a backpack or fanny pack. (These are available by prescription only.)

All these children must carry a card in pocket or purse listing their name, parent's home and work phone numbers, physician's name, physician's phone number, and type of allergy. Ideally, your child should wear a medical identification necklace or bracelet that records the insect, food, or drug allergy. Some can be found in pharmacies. They can also be ordered from MedicAlert Foundation International, 2323 Colorado Ave., Turlock, CA 95382, at 1-888-633-4298.

BITES: ANIMAL OR HUMAN

The following three types of bites are covered in the next few pages. Go directly to the one that applies to your child.

BITES, WILD ANIMAL (see below)
BITES, PET ANIMAL (see page 16)
BITES, HUMAN (see page 18)

BITES, WILD ANIMAL

There are two basic types of wild-animal bites: rabies-prone bites and safe ones.

Rabies-Prone Bites—Rabies is a fatal disease. Bites or scratches from a bat, skunk, raccoon, fox, coyote, or large wild animal are especially dangerous. These animals can transmit rabies even if they themselves have no symptoms. Squirrels rarely carry rabies.

Safe Wild-Animal Bites—Rodents such as mice, rats, moles, gophers, chipmunks, and rabbits fortunately are considered free of rabies. In the Southwest, prairie dogs can carry plague, and people should not handle them. Campers should avoid placing bedrolls over rodent burrows.

Call Your Child's Physician Immediately If
• The bite was by a rabies-prone wild animal.
• The bite penetrated the skin (even a puncture from one tooth).
• You have other urgent questions.

First Aid for Suspected Rabies Contact
Washing the wound immediately with soap and water for 10 to 15 minutes is critical. If possible, flush the wound thoroughly under a faucet. If the wild

animal is still on the premises, call the police department immediately. If the animal is captured or dead, avoid all contact with it. Saliva from a rabid animal can cause rabies by getting into a cut. In the future, teach your child to avoid direct contact with any wild animal (even healthy ones).

BITES, PET ANIMAL

Most of these bites are from dogs or cats. Bites from domestic animals such as horses can be handled using these guidelines. Small indoor pets (such as gerbils, hamsters, guinea pigs, and white mice) are at no risk for rabies. Dogs and cats are free of rabies in many metropolitan areas. The main risk in pet bites is serious wound infection, not rabies. Cat bites become infected five times more frequently than dog bites. Puncture wounds are more likely to become infected than cuts. Claw wounds are treated the same as bite wounds, since they are contaminated with saliva.

Call Your Child's Physician Immediately If

- The teeth or claws went through the skin (that includes all puncture wounds). Caution: Cat bites of the hand can become infected rapidly and need prompt attention.
- The skin is split open (i.e., a laceration) and probably needs sutures.
- There are superficial cuts *and* the animal seemed to be sick, the attack was unprovoked, or the animal was a stray.
- There are superficial cuts *and* the animal is one without rabies shots. (Exception: a known, healthy, friendly dog who was teased or became frightened.)
- Caution: Most animal bites need to be seen because all of them are prone to wound infection.
- You think your child needs to be seen.

Home Care for Pet-Animal Bites

First Aid for Puncture Wound or Laceration (Deep Cut)—Wash the area with a liquid soap and running water for 10 minutes before going to the physician's office. Scrub the wound enough to make it rebleed a little. Immediate, vigorous flushing under a faucet is the best protection against wound infection. Also check your child's immunization status for tetanus.

Scrapes or Superficial Cuts—For wounds that don't penetrate the skin, wash the area with lots of water and a liquid soap for 5 minutes. You can leave it exposed to the air, or put a dressing on it for 12 hours if it's on an area that easily gets dirty. No antiseptic is necessary.

Observation of the Pet—If there is any possibility of rabies, the pet should be carefully watched for any signs of sickness and isolated from contact with humans for 10 days. If the animal belongs to another family and they are not cooperative, report the incident to the police so they can deal with the problem. Too many pets are left to roam without supervision.

Call Your Child's Physician Later If

- The wound begins to look infected.
- The pain increases after the second day.
- The redness increases after the second day.
- You feel your child is getting worse.

Prevention of Pet-Animal Bites

- Choose a pet that is friendly and tolerates children. Pit bull terriers are extremely dangerous. German shepherds, Dobermans, and St. Bernards are not good dogs for children.
- Teach your dog the commands of "down" and "sit." Teach your child how to give these commands.
- Teach your children not to touch strange animals, break up dogfights, go near a dog that's eating, or touch a sleeping dog.
- Children under 4 years of age should always be supervised around dogs and cats. Never allow them to tease a pet.
- Infants under 1 year of age should never be left alone in a room with a pet. Some have been attacked, possibly due to the pet's jealousy. There are rare reports of a sleeping newborn being smothered by a cat.
- Protect your pet against rabies by yearly rabies shots. The first shot is normally given when your pet is 3 to 4 months old.
- Teach your child not to run from a strange dog. Rapid movement can trigger a dog's predatory instinct.

- Never keep wild animals as pets. For example, ferrets have caused disfiguring bites to the faces of young children.

BITES, HUMAN

Most of these bites occur during fighting. In younger children, the bite is usually deliberate and on the arm or hand. In older children, sometimes a fist is cut when it strikes a tooth. Human bites are more likely to become infected than any animal bite. Bites on the hands are at increased risk of complications.

Call Your Child's Physician Immediately If

- The teeth went through the skin.
- The skin is split open and probably needs sutures.
- You think your child needs to be seen.

Home Care for Human Bites

First Aid for Puncture Wound or Laceration—Wash the area with a liquid soap and running water for 10 minutes before going to the physician's office. Also check your child's immunization status for tetanus.

Scrapes and Superficial Cuts—Wash the area with lots of water and a liquid soap for 5 minutes. You can leave it exposed to the air, or put a bandage on it for 12 hours if it's on an area that easily gets dirty. No antiseptic is necessary.

Children Who Bite—See the guidelines on BITING, page 340.

Call Your Child's Physician Later If

- The wound begins to look infected.
- The pain increases after the second day.
- The redness increases after the second day.
- You feel your child is getting worse.

BITES: INSECT, BEE, OR TICK

The following 4 types of insect bites and stings are covered. A bite involves biting with the insect's mouth parts and removing a drop of blood from the human. A sting involves injecting a venom into the human from the insect's stinger. Go directly to the one that applies to your child.

BEE OR YELLOW JACKET STINGS (see below)
ITCHY INSECT BITES (see page 20)
PAINFUL INSECT BITES (see page 22)
TICK BITES (see page 23)

If your child has difficulty breathing, difficulty swallowing, hives, or other worrisome symptoms within 30 minutes following an insect bite (especially with stings) or has had a previous severe allergic reaction, turn directly to ALLERGIC REACTION, SEVERE, page 13.

BEE OR YELLOW JACKET STINGS

Your child was stung by a honeybee, bumblebee, hornet, paper wasp, or yellow jacket. Over 95 percent of stings are from yellow jackets. These stings cause immediate painful red bumps. While the pain is usually better in 2 hours, the swelling may increase for up to 24 hours. Multiple stings (more than 10) can cause vomiting, diarrhea, a headache, and fever. This is a toxic reaction related to the amount of venom received (i.e., not an allergic reaction). A sting on the tongue can cause swelling that interferes with breathing.

Call Your Child's Physician Immediately If

- Breathing or swallowing is difficult. (Call 911.)
- Hives are present.
- There are 10 or more stings.
- A sting is inside the mouth.
- You think your child needs to be seen.

Home Care

Treatment—If you see a little black dot in the wound, the stinger is still present. (This means your child was stung by a honeybee.) Remove it by scraping it off with the edge of a knife blade or credit card. If only a small fragment remains, don't worry about it. It will come out with normal skin shedding. Then rub each sting with a meat tenderizer/water solution for 10 minutes (exception: sting is near the eye). This will neutralize the venom and relieve the pain. If meat tenderizer is not available, apply an aluminum-based deodorant or a baking soda solution for 20 minutes. For persistent pain, massage with an ice cube for 10 minutes. Give acetaminophen or ibuprofen immediately for relief of pain and burning.

Call Your Child's Physician During Office Hours If

- The swelling continues to spread after 24 hours.
- Swelling of the hand (or foot) spreads past the wrist (or ankle).
- You want the sting looked at.

Prevention of Bee Stings

Some bee stings can be prevented by avoiding gardens, flowers, clover fields, orchards in bloom, perfumes, and going barefoot. Also teach your young children how to identify nests. Insect repellents are not effective against these stinging insects.

ITCHY INSECT BITES

Bites of mosquitoes, chiggers (harvest mites), fleas, and bedbugs usually cause itchy red bumps. The size of the swelling following a mosquito bite means very little. Mosquito bites near the eye always cause massive swelling for 2 days. Clues to a bite's being due to a mosquito are itchiness, a central raised dot in the swelling, bites on surfaces not covered by clothing, summertime, and the child's being an infant. Some mosquito bites in sensitive children form hard lumps that last for months. In contrast to mosquitoes, fleas and bedbugs don't fly; therefore, they crawl under clothing to nibble. Flea bites can turn into little blisters in young children. Some children appeal to these insects more than other children do and repeatedly acquire numerous bites.

Home Care

Treatment—Apply calamine lotion or a baking soda paste. If the itch is severe (as with chiggers), apply nonprescription 1 percent hydrocortisone cream. Oral antihistamines usually do not help local itching.

Another way to reduce the itch is to apply firm, sharp, direct, steady pressure to the bite for 10 seconds. A fingernail, pen cap, or other object can be used.

Encourage your child not to scratch because it increases the itching. Encourage your child not to pick at the bites, as they could become infected.

Call Your Child's Physician Later If
- Itching interferes with sleep.
- The bites become infected due to scratching.
- You think your child needs to be seen.

Prevention of Itchy Insect Bites

Mosquitoes and Chiggers—Many of these bites can be prevented by applying an insect repellent sparingly to the clothing or exposed skin before going outdoors or into the woods. Repellents are essential for infants (especially those less than 1 year of age), because their inability to bat away the pesky critters leaves them helpless targets.

Insect Repellents for Skin: DEET
- DEET is a very effective mosquito repellent. It also repels ticks and other bugs.
- The American Academy of Pediatrics has approved the use of 30 percent DEET or less for all children over 2 months of age.
- Use products containing 30 percent DEET for children and adolescents. This will protect the child for 6 hours. Use products containing 10 percent DEET if you need protection for only 2 hours.
- Breast-feeding women may use DEET. No problems have been reported.
- Don't apply DEET to the hands if the child sucks his thumb or other fingers, to prevent ingestion.
- Apply to exposed areas of skin only. Do not apply to eyes or mouth. Don't put any repellent on areas that are sunburned or have rashes

because DEET is more easily absorbed in these areas. Do not apply to skin that is covered by clothing.

- Warn older children who apply their own repellent that a total of 3 or 4 drops can protect the whole body.
- Remember to wash it off with soap and water when your child returns indoors.
- Caution: DEET can damage clothing made of synthetic fibers, plastics (e.g., eyeglasses), and leather, but it can be safely applied to cotton clothing.

Insect Repellent for Clothing: Permethrin

- Permethrin-containing products (e.g., Duranon, Permanone, and Congo Creek Tick Spray) are highly effective mosquito repellents. They also repel ticks.
- An advantage over using DEET is that they are applied to clothing instead of skin. Apply it to shirt cuffs, pants cuffs, shoes, and hat. You can also put it on other outdoor items (shoes, mosquito screens, sleeping bags).
- Do not apply permethrin to skin, as it will lose effectiveness very quickly.
- Picaridin is a newly approved repellent that is equivalent to 10 percent DEET. It can safely be applied to skin or clothing.

Bedbugs—Beds and baseboards can be sprayed with 1 percent malathion, which can be obtained from any garden supply store. Keep young children away from the area until it dries, because this substance is somewhat poisonous. You may need to call in an exterminator.

Fleas—Usually you will find the fleas on your dog or cat. If the bites started after you moved into a different house or apartment, fleas from the previous owner's pet are the most common cause. Fleas can live in carpeting for several months without a meal. Fleas can often be removed by bringing a dog or cat inside the house for 2 hours to collect the fleas—they prefer the dog or cat to living in the carpet. In either case, apply flea powder or soap to your animal outdoors. Careful vacuuming will usually capture any remaining fleas. Malathion bug spray (see BEDBUGS, above) can be used for persistent cases.

PAINFUL INSECT BITES

Bites of horseflies, deerflies, sandflies, gnats, fire ants, harvester ants, cone-nosed bugs, blister beetles, and centipedes usually cause a painful (sometimes burning) red bump. Within a few hours, fire ant bites change to blisters or pimples.

Home Care

Treatment—Rub the bite area with a cotton ball soaked in meat-tenderizer-and-water solution for 10 minutes (exception: bite is near the eye). This will relieve the pain. If you have no meat tenderizer, use a baking soda solution. Give acetaminophen or ibuprofen for pain relief.

Call Your Child's Physician Later If
- Your child has more than 10 fire ant bites.
- Pain interferes with sleep.
- The bites become infected.
- You think your child needs to be seen.

Prevention of Painful Insect Bites

Apply insect repellent sparingly to exposed parts and clothing. (See precautions on page 21.)

TICK BITES

A tick is a brown bug that attaches to the skin and sucks blood for 3 to 6 days. The bite is usually painless and doesn't itch. Therefore, your child will usually be unaware of its presence. The wood tick (or dog tick), which transmits Rocky Mountain spotted fever and Colorado tick fever, is up to ½ inch in size (the size of a watermelon seed). The deer tick, which transmits Lyme disease, is the size of a pinhead. After feeding on blood, both of these ticks become quite swollen and easy to see.

Lyme Disease—Lyme disease is the disease most frequently spread by a tick bite. About 16,000 cases are reported each year in our country. It's not carried by wood ticks, only by the tiny deer ticks, which are harder to notice. In most states, only 2 percent of ticks carry the disease. But in the New England states, Wisconsin, and Minnesota, up to 50 percent of ticks are infected. Still, even in these high-risk areas, only 1 percent of children bitten by a deer tick develop Lyme disease. For Lyme disease to be transmitted, the tick needs to be attached for at least 18 hours. Within 1 to 3 weeks of the bite, most infected people develop a unique rash where they are bitten. The rash (erythema migrans) consists of a red ring or bull's-eye that expands in size. The rash is neither painful nor itchy. At this stage, Lyme disease is easily treatable with an antibiotic. So watch for the rash, but don't panic. Complications are rare. It's not yet time to give up picnics, hikes, and camping because of this pest.

Home Care

Tick Removal—The simplest and quickest way to remove a wood tick is to pull it off. Use a tweezers to grasp the tick as close to the skin as possible (try to get a grip on its head). Apply a steady upward traction until it releases its grip. Do not twist the tick or jerk it suddenly because these maneuvers can break off the tick's head or mouth parts. Do not squeeze the tweezers to the point of crushing the tick, because the secretions released may spread disease. If you have no tweezers, pull the tick off in the same way, using your fingers, a loop of thread around the jaws, or a needle between the jaws for traction. Tiny deer ticks need to be scraped off with a knife blade or the edge of a credit card.

If the body is removed but the head is left in the skin, it must be removed. Use a sterile needle (as you would to remove a sliver). Then apply antibiotic ointment to the bite once. Dispose of the tick by returning it to nature or flushing it down the toilet. You don't need to save the tick for positive identification by your doctor; he's seen more than his share of them. If you are unsure if it's a dog tick or a deer tick, measure it but don't save it. Don't crush ticks with your hands, since this practice increases your chances of getting a disease. Wash the wound and your hands with soap and water after removal.

A study by Dr. G. R. Needham showed that embedded ticks do not back out when covered with petroleum jelly, fingernail polish, or rubbing alcohol. We used to think that this would block the tick's breathing pores and take its mind off eating. Unfortunately, ticks breathe only a few times per hour. The application of a hot match to the tick failed to cause it to detach, and also carried the risk of inducing the tick to vomit infected secretions into the wound. (Yuck!)

Call Your Child's Physician Later If
• You can't remove the tick.
• The tick's head remains embedded. (Note: If the tick is moving, you got it all out.)
• A fever or rash occurs in the 2 weeks following the bite.

- You think your child has some of the symptoms of Lyme disease (e.g., bull's-eye rash near the bite).
- You think your child needs to be seen.

Prevention of Tick Bites

Ticks like to hide in underbrush and shrubbery. They don't drop out of the trees; they come aboard from ground level. Children and adults who are hiking in tick-infested areas should wear long clothing and tuck the ends of the pants into the socks. Apply an insect repellent to shoes and socks (permethrin products applied to clothing are more effective than DEET products against ticks—see page 22). During the hike, perform tick checks using a buddy system every 4 hours to remove ticks on the clothing or exposed skin. Immediately after the hike or at least once a day, do a bare-skin check. A brisk shower at the end of a hike will also remove any tick that isn't firmly attached. Because the bite is painless and doesn't itch, the child will usually be unaware of its presence. Favorite hiding places for ticks are in the hair, so carefully check the scalp, neck, armpit, and groin. Removing ticks promptly may prevent infection, because transmission of Lyme disease requires at least 24 hours of feeding. Also, the tick is easier to remove before it becomes firmly attached. To prevent the spread of Lyme disease from your dog, wash him with an antitick soap during the spring and summer months. Perform tick checks on him if he accompanies you on a hike. Pull off any that are found.

BITES, MARINE ANIMAL

The following five types of marine bites are covered in the next few pages. Go directly to the one that applies to your child.

Jellyfish or Portuguese Man-of-War Reactions (see page 26)
Venomous Fish Reactions (as from stingray, stonefish, scorpion fish, catfish) (see page 26)
Cuts or Lacerations (as from moray eels, sharks, barracudas) (see page 27)
Sea Urchin Stings (see page 28)
Shocks (e.g., from electric eels) (see page 28)

Clearly, all of these unpleasantries occur in saltwater. But the dangers of the deep are a small price to pay for the rejuvenating qualities of an ocean vacation. Go to a beach with lifeguards and observe all warning signs or flags. Getting caught in a riptide or undertow is the main risk of ocean swimming.

JELLYFISH OR PORTUGUESE MAN-OF-WAR REACTIONS

The jellyfish and Portuguese man-of-war have long, stinging tentacles (the stinging parts are called nematocysts). Fragments of tentacles washed up on the beach after a storm can still cause sharp stings. They produce lines of redness and burning pain. Sometimes they cause generalized symptoms of weakness, dizziness, nausea, and headache. Sea anemones (sea nettles) cause similar local reactions for 24 to 48 hours.

First Aid

- Scrape off any stinging tentacles with the edge of a credit card or knife. Don't scrub the area because that can trigger the nematocysts. Be careful to protect your hands, since the stingers can even penetrate gloves. Rinse the wound with seawater.
- Neutralize the venom with the continuous application of vinegar for 30 minutes. Meat tenderizer is a second-choice agent for deactivating the toxin.
- Apply a 1 percent hydrocortisone cream (no prescription needed) 4 times a day for a few days to reduce itching.

Call a Physician Immediately If

- Any generalized symptoms have occurred.

VENOMOUS FISH REACTIONS

Stings from these creatures cause localized pain and redness. They also commonly cause weakness, sweating, fever, vomiting, muscle cramps, paralysis, or even shock. The stinging fish usually have venom in dorsal spines. The stingray has one or more venomous spines on its tail. Because of its powerful strike, the stingray often also causes a laceration.

First Aid

Fortunately, the venom of all these fish can be destroyed by heat.

- Rinse the area with lots of seawater to dilute the venom.
- Remove any particles of stingray spine left in the wound.
- Soak the affected area in pleasantly hot water (110–114°F or 43–45°C) for 30 minutes. (Caution: do not burn your child.) Hot water breaks down (neutralizes) any venom from a poisonous fish or sea urchin and thus helps to reduce pain.

Call a Physician Immediately If

- Any generalized symptoms have developed.
  For stingrays:
- The skin is split open.
- The barb or spine needs to be removed.

CUTS OR LACERATIONS, MARINE ANIMAL

Some fish cause a bite mark of varying severity without injecting any venom.

Call a Physician Immediately If

- Bleeding won't stop after 10 minutes of direct pressure.
- The skin is split open.
- A puncture wound is present.

First Aid

Wash the area with lots of seawater. Later, wash with soap and water for 10 minutes.

SEA URCHIN STINGS

A sea urchin usually causes localized burning pain if part of a venomous spine breaks off in the skin. If not removed, it may be dissolved by the body or it may cause persistent pain and swelling (a foreign-body reaction).

First Aid

First, stop the flow of venom by pulling out any spine that protrudes from the skin. Also neutralize the venom with a hot water soak (see VENOMOUS FISH REACTIONS, page 26, for details). If any large fragment of a sea urchin barb remains beneath the skin, try to remove it with a sterile needle and tweezers as you would for a splinter. A mild acid such as vinegar can dissolve small pieces of spine that you can't get out. If purplish discoloration remains after the spine is removed, it's merely due to dye from the spine and is unimportant.

SHOCKS, MARINE ANIMAL

Your child may feel shocked, stunned, or partially paralyzed after contact with an electric eel.

First Aid

Reassurance should be offered. Your child will be feeling and acting normal in 20 to 30 minutes. No treatment is necessary except lying down with the feet elevated.

BITES, SNAKE

The following three types of snakebites are covered in the next few pages. Go directly to the one that applies to your child.

SNAKEBITES, POISONOUS (see page 29)
SNAKEBITES, NONPOISONOUS (see page 29)
SNAKEBITES, UNIDENTIFIED (see page 30)

SNAKEBITES, POISONOUS

In the United States the poisonous snakes are rattlers, copperheads, cottonmouths (water moccasins), and coral snakes. Currently about 8,000 people per year in the United States are bitten by a poisonous snake. Of these, about 6 victims die. Over 90 percent of snakebites occur on the leg. In about 30 percent of poisonous snakebites, luckily, no venom is injected (dry bites). If the venom was injected (envenomation), the fang marks will begin to burn, hurt, and swell within 5 minutes. Therefore, begin first aid only if these signs develop.

Call Your Child's Physician Immediately in All Cases

First Aid

Antivenin—The most important treatment for poisonous snakebites is going to a hospital emergency department as rapidly as possible so the child can receive appropriate antivenin and other emergency measures. A tourniquet is not warranted unless the child is more than 2 hours from medical attention. Cutting incisions over the fang marks and applying suction is no longer recommended because it is not effective.

SNAKEBITES, NONPOISONOUS

Most nonpoisonous bites are from garter snakes during attempted capture or from pet snakes. All are harmless.

Home Care for Nonpoisonous Snakebites

Treatment—Usually, the small teeth of a snake leave a scrape that doesn't even puncture the skin. Wash it well with soap and water. A bandage isn't necessary. If the skin is punctured, call in for a tetanus booster if your child hasn't had one in over 5 years.

Call Your Child's Physician Later If

- Your child develops any symptoms in the next 6 hours.

SNAKEBITES, UNIDENTIFIED

Sometimes the snake has disappeared by the time the parent has been notified. In other cases, the snake has been killed but is hard to identify. (If your child needs to be seen by a physician, bring the snake with you after you're certain it is dead.) Most bites are from harmless snakes, and you can assume this to be the case unless the bite mark burns or swells within 5 minutes.

Call Your Child's Physician Immediately If

- One or two puncture (fang) marks are present.
- The bite area burns or hurts.
- The bite area is swollen.
- Blood blisters or purple spots are present in the bite area.
- Your child is acting sick in any way.
- You think your child needs to be seen.

Home Care for Unidentified Snakebites

See HOME CARE FOR NONPOISONOUS SNAKEBITES, page 29.

BITES, SPIDER OR SCORPION

The following five types of bites are covered in the next few pages. Go directly to the one that applies to your child.

SCORPION BITES (see below)
SPIDER BITES, BLACK WIDOW (see page 31)
SPIDER BITES, BROWN RECLUSE (see page 31)
SPIDER BITES, NONDANGEROUS (see page 32)
SPIDER BITES, UNIDENTIFIED (see page 33)

SCORPION BITES

Scorpions belong to the same class as spiders—called the arachnids. They are found in desert areas. About twenty different kinds occur in the southwestern United States. Scorpions have a poisonous stinger in the tail. Over 90 percent of scorpion bites are on the hands. Most of the bites cause symptoms similar to those of black widow spiders, namely, immediate local pain with slight swelling. In the United States, only one scorpion *(Centruroides sculpturatus)* can cause serious or fatal reactions. It is small (1 to 3 inches), uniformly yellow, and without stripes.

Call Your Child's Physician Immediately in All Cases

First Aid
See FIRST AID for black widow spider bites, below.

SPIDER BITES, BLACK WIDOW

The black widow is a shiny, jet-black spider with long legs and a red (or orange) hourglass-shaped marking on its underside. It is about an inch in length, including the legs, and is easy to recognize. The black widow and brown recluse spiders are the only highly venomous spiders in North America. Black widow bites cause immediate local pain and swelling. Because the symptoms begin rapidly, the spider is usually still in the vicinity. Muscle cramps also occur for 6 to 24 hours. They rarely cause death (except in younger children or when the victim is bitten by several spiders).

Call Your Child's Physician Immediately in All Cases

First Aid
Apply an ice cube or ice pack to the bite for 20 minutes to reduce the spread of the venom. Then go to the nearest emergency room or wherever your physician directs you. A tourniquet is not helpful. Antivenin is available for severe bites in young children, and other medicines can relieve muscle pain.

SPIDER BITES, BROWN RECLUSE

The brown recluse is brown, has long legs, and has a dark, violin-shaped marking on its head. It is about ½ inch in length, including the legs, and is difficult to recognize. Brown recluse spider bites cause delayed local pain and blister formation in 4 to 8 hours. The center of the reaction becomes bluish-black and depressed (i.e., crater-like). The skin damage may require grafting. The bites are rarely fatal.

Call Your Child's Physician Immediately in All Cases

First Aid

Wash the bite thoroughly with soap and water. Bring the spider with you if possible. (Brown recluse spiders may be hard to identify.)

SPIDER BITES, NONDANGEROUS

More than fifty types of spiders in the United States can cause local but nondangerous reactions (such as golden garden spiders). The bites are painful and mildly swollen for 1 or 2 days, much like a bee sting. In fact, spiders are probably responsible for many of the single, unexplained, tender bites that occur on children during the night. (Mosquito bites, on the other hand, are usually multiple and itchy rather than painful.) Many people are unduly concerned about the tarantula, a black, hairy spider that is 2 to 3 inches long. The tarantula is not dangerous. Its mild venom also causes a local reaction resembling a bee sting.

Home Care for Nondangerous Spider Bites

Treatment—Wash the bite thoroughly with soap and water. Then rub the area with a cotton ball soaked with a meat tenderizer/water solution for 10 minutes. (Exception: bite is near the eye.) If meat tenderizer is not available, an ice cube applied to the area often helps.

Call Your Child's Physician Later If

- Muscle spasm occurs in the bite area.
- The bite turns into a blister or purple spot.
- A sore occurs that doesn't heal.
- Other new symptoms occur.
- You think your child needs to be seen.

SPIDER BITES, UNIDENTIFIED

Although most of these bites are harmless, an occasional one may be due to a black widow spider.

Call Your Child's Physician Immediately If

- The bite area burns or hurts.
- Muscle spasm occurs in the bite area.
- Your child is acting sick.

Try to capture the spider (dead or alive) in a jar and bring it along to the physician's office. Don't bludgeon it beyond recognition.

Home Care for Unidentified Spider Bites

Treatment—Wash the bite thoroughly with soap and water.

Call Your Child's Physician Later If

- The bite turns into a blister or purple spot.
- A sore occurs that doesn't heal.
- You feel your child is getting worse.

Prevention of Spider Bites

- Don't work in woodpiles, rock piles, rubbish heaps, window wells, or dark corners of outdoor buildings without wearing gloves.
- Spray with insecticides any area where black widow spiders are seen.
- Spiders normally come indoors with the onset of cold weather. Prevent this fall migration into your house by repairing cracks and spraying near outside doors with insecticide.

BLEEDING, SEVERE

This guideline covers arterial (from an artery) bleeding or major venous (from a vein) bleeding. In arterial bleeding, the blood pumps or spurts from the wound with each heartbeat. In major venous bleeding, the blood just runs out of the wound at a steady rate. Arterial bleeding is bright red compared to the darker red of venous bleeding. Minor bleeding (from capillaries), however, can also be bright red. For minor bleeding, see the guidelines on Skin Trauma, page 78, or Nosebleed, page 559.

First Aid for Arterial Bleeding

Apply Direct Pressure—Immediately place several sterile dressings or the first clean cloth at hand (towels, sheets, shirts, or handkerchiefs) over the wound and apply direct pressure. The pressure must be forceful and continuous, often applied with the palm of the hand. Act quickly, because the ongoing blood loss can cause shock.

Rescue Squad—Have someone call a rescue squad (911) immediately while you tend to the bleeding. (See Emergency Transportation, page 4.)

Prevent Shock—Have your child lie down with the feet elevated 10 to 12 inches to prevent symptoms of shock (low blood pressure). If your child is pale and the hands and feet are cold, shock is imminent.

Arterial Tourniquet for Severe Bleeding from the Arm or Leg— A tourniquet is needed only under the following unusual circumstances: the bleeding is arterial; it is from the arm or leg; it cannot be controlled by direct pressure (as with an amputated or mangled limb); and the patient is located at a significant distance from emergency facilities. Again, an arterial tourniquet is a last resort, to be used only when direct pressure fails. A tourniquet should be avoided if at all possible since it can damage the uninjured tissues. Once an arterial tourniquet is applied, it should be released for a few seconds every 10 minutes to reestablish blood flow to the limb. During this time, direct pressure must be used to prevent excessive blood loss. Apply a tourniquet as follows:

- If you have a blood pressure cuff, use it as a tourniquet. The second choice is a tight elastic bandage. If these items are unavailable, use a piece of cloth (such as a bandanna or stocking).
- Tie it around the limb above the wound (usually the upper arm or leg).
- Lay a 4- to 5-inch piece of wood or an eating utensil above the knot and tie the tourniquet again.
- Twist the wooden or metal handle until the tourniquet is tight enough to stop the bleeding.
- Tie the stick in place so it won't unwind before you reach the hospital.

First Aid for Venous Bleeding

Apply Direct Pressure

- Place two or three sterile dressings (or a clean towel or sheet) over the wound immediately.
- Apply direct pressure to the wound for 8 to 10 minutes, using your entire hand. Direct pressure can always stop venous bleeding if it is applied to the right spot.
- Then bandage the dressings tightly in place (an elastic bandage gives excellent compression) and leave them there until arrival at the emergency room.
- If bleeding resumes, reapply direct pressure.

Seek Emergency Care—Call for a rescue squad (911) for major bleeding or if your child is in shock. (See EMERGENCY TRANSPORTATION, page 4.)

Prevent Shock—Have your child lie down with the feet elevated to prevent symptoms of shock. If your child is pale and the hands and feet are cold, shock is imminent. Act quickly.

First Aid for Open Abdominal Wounds

Cover the wound with a sterile dressing. If a knife or other weapon protrudes from the wound, don't remove it before reaching the hospital. This precaution is critical. When it is removed, the cut it leaves could bleed uncontrollably. Call a rescue squad (see EMERGENCY TRANSPORTATION, page 4).

First Aid for Open Chest Wounds

A sucking wound of the chest is one that goes through to the pleural space or lung. It can be recognized by the sound of air being sucked into the chest with each effort to breathe in. This type of wound quickly collapses the lung if it is not treated properly.

First Aid—Seal the opening as quickly as possible. Use several sterile dressings or pieces of clean cloth and lots of adhesive tape or plastic wrap to make it airtight. If possible, apply the seal while your child is breathing out. If one part of the chest bulges out when your child breathes out, there are several broken ribs in that area (flail chest). Have your child lie with the bulging part down, or hold a pillow or towel over it to keep it from bulging. If a knife or other weapon protrudes from the wound, don't remove it before reaching the hospital. When it is removed, the cut it leaves could bleed uncontrollably. Call a rescue squad (see EMERGENCY TRANSPORTATION, page 4).

BREATHING DIFFICULTY, SEVERE

Stopped Breathing, Persistent
- Call a rescue squad (911).
- Begin mouth-to-mouth resuscitation if you know how. (Otherwise, go to the guidelines on RESUSCITATION, page 9.)

Breathing, Very Slow and Weak
- Call a rescue squad (911).

Stopped Breathing, Transient; and Now Normal Breathing
- Call your child's physician immediately or go to the nearest emergency room.
- Note: In an infant, prolonged periods without breathing (apnea), especially if accompanied by turning blue or limpness, should always receive an urgent medical evaluation. On the other hand, breathing pauses of less than 10 seconds (periodic breathing) in infants from birth to 3 months are normal. Occasionally, normal pauses can last for 15 seconds, but check with your physician.

Choking
Turn directly to page 10.

Croup
Turn directly to page 588.

Breathing Fast

Rapid Breathing Rates—The following rates are abnormal:

2 months or younger:	more than 60 per minute
2 to 12 months:	more than 50 per minute
1 to 5 years:	more than 40 per minute
6 to 12 years:	more than 30 per minute
12 years or older:	more than 20 per minute

These rates apply to children who are not crying. The breathing rate normally goes up 10 to 20 breaths per minute in children who are upset or crying. Also, healthy infants occasionally pant and have higher rates. If your infant seems well, recheck the rate while the child is asleep.

Rapid and Labored—Call your child's physician immediately.

Rapid with Wheezing—Call your child's physician immediately.

Rapid with Fever—With fever, the rate of breathing rises by 2 for each degree Fahrenheit of elevation (or by 4 for each degree Centigrade). If the rate is appropriate for the level of fever, all is probably well. In general, rapid respirations are not due to the fever, and these children need to be seen to rule out pneumonia as the cause.

Rapid with Snorting—Clean the nose with warm water or saline drops and a rubber suction bulb. If that doesn't help and the breathing rate remains high, call your child's physician immediately.

Related Topics

BREATH-HOLDING SPELLS (see page 370)
BREATHING, NOISY (see page 581)

BURNS, CHEMICAL

Chemical burns are external burns from alkalis, acids, or other tissue-damaging chemicals splashed on the skin. Most of these accidents cause only first-degree burns, which may peel like a sunburn during the following week. A mild irritation and burning of the scalp has been caused by some home hair permanent solutions. A few of the stronger chemicals may cause deep burns.

First Aid

Remove contaminated clothing and rinse off the burned part of your child's body with clear water for 20 minutes, using the shower or tub. Don't rub the skin during this rinse. Don't apply any burn ointments because washing them off will cause pain. Also, don't apply butter; it only increases the infection rate. If the burned area is large, cover it loosely with a wet clean sheet.

Call Your Child's Physician Immediately If

Call in all cases, after carrying out first aid instructions. The physician will probably need to examine your child if there are any blisters, facial burns, or extensive burns.

Related Topics

EYE, CHEMICAL IN (see page 49)
POISONING (see page 55)

BURNS, THERMAL

Most of these burns are scalds from hot water or hot drinks. A few are from hot ovens, stoves, space heaters, exhaust pipes, grease, hair-curling irons, hair dryers, clothes irons, heating grates, and cigarettes. Usually the burn is first degree (reddened skin without blisters) or second degree (with blisters). Neither of these leave any scars. Second-degree burns take up to 3 weeks to heal. A third-degree burn is deep and leaves areas of black (leathery) or white skin that are numb. During healing a third-degree burn usually needs a skin graft to prevent bad scarring if it is larger than a quarter (1-inch diameter).

First Aid for Thermal Burns

Immediately (don't take time to remove clothing) put the burned part in cold tap water or pour cold water over it for 10 minutes. If you are outdoors, the nearest garden hose will do. If the burn is small, massage it with an ice cube. This will lessen the depth of the burn and relieve pain. Don't apply any butter or ointments.

If the burned area is large, cover it loosely with a clean sheet or plastic wrap. The covering will keep the burn clean and reduce pain until you reach a medical facility.

Call Your Child's Physician Immediately If

- Three or more blisters are present.
- A blister is larger than 1 inch (i.e., won't fit under a Band-Aid).
- The burn is on the face, neck, hands, feet, or genitals.
- Areas of charred or white skin are present.

- It was an electrical burn.
- An explosion caused the burn.
- You think your child needs to be seen.

Home Care for Thermal Burns

Treatment—Wash the area gently with warm water once a day. Avoid soap unless the burn is dirty (reason: soaps can slow healing). Don't open any blisters—the outer skin still protects the burn from infection. For any broken burns (second degree), apply an antibiotic ointment and cover it with a Band-Aid. Change the dressing every other day. Use warm water and 1 or 2 gentle wipes with a wet washcloth to remove any surface debris. For pain, apply cold compresses and give acetaminophen or ibuprofen. Do not apply any butter or burn ointments. Note: Once the blisters break open, the dead skin needs to be removed (debrided) with a fine scissors. Often wiping the thin skin with a wet washcloth will remove it. Otherwise the hidden pockets become an ideal breeding ground for infections.

Call Your Child's Physician Later If
- Any blisters break open.
- The burn starts to look infected.
- Tenderness or redness increases after day 2.
- The burn hasn't healed after 10 days.
- You feel your child is getting worse.

Prevention of Burns
Think about how you can prevent similar accidents in the future.
- Never drink anything hot (such as coffee, tea, or cocoa) while holding a young baby. The baby will grab for it, spill it, and probably get burned.
- On the stove, try to use the back burners and keep handles turned in.
- Once your child can walk, keep hot substances away from the edge of the table or stove (such as a pan of boiling water, a coffeepot, a curling iron, or an iron). The burn from a crockpot usually causes scarring because the contents are sticky and at high temperature.
- Always supervise young children in the bathtub. Don't let a young child touch the faucet handles. He or she may turn on the hot water and be scalded.

- Lower your hot water heater setting to 130°F or to the low-medium setting. Higher settings can cause burns in 2 or 3 seconds. You can test the temperature of your hot water by using a candy or meat thermometer.
- Use cool humidifiers if you have young children, not hot steam vaporizers. A vaporizer can cause severe burns if a child overturns it or puts his or her face too close to it.
- Supervise children around fires, stoves, and heaters of any kind.
- Use flame-resistant sleepwear.
- Give up smoking, or at least dispose of used cigarettes conscientiously. Cigarettes are the most common cause of residential fires.
- Keep cigarette lighters away from children. Even a 2-year-old can ignite one by inverting it and pushing it across the floor.
- Install smoke detectors in your home on every floor. Check them monthly for proper functioning. More people die from smoke inhalation than from burns. Smoke alarms detect smoke long before your nose can.
- Teach your children not to hide if a house fire occurs, but to go outside. Have a fire drill and rehearse it.
- Before placing a child under 1 year old in a car seat, check the seat's temperature. Hot straps or buckles have caused second-degree burns. Whenever you park in direct sunlight, cover the car seat with a towel or sheet.
- Avoid fireworks, or allow older children to use them only with close adult supervision. In addition to burns, fireworks (especially bottle rockets) cause 300 cases of blindness per year.

COMA

A child who is unconscious, cannot be fully awakened, or is very difficult to awaken is in a coma. The causes are many, including substance abuse, drug overdose, poisoning, head injury, encephalitis, and low blood sugar. In all cases, you should contact your child's physician immediately.

Call a Rescue Squad (911) for Assistance and Transportation for All Comatose Children

The following symptoms place your child at greater risk:

• Your child can't be awakened at all.

• The head or neck may be injured.

• A severe allergic reaction to a bee sting or medication is possible.

• Your child is not breathing.

• Breathing is slow or weak.

• Breathing is labored (croup, wheezing, choking, etc.).

• The lips are bluish or dusky.

• Caution: If your child starts to vomit, place him on the side or abdomen.

CONVULSIONS WITH FEVER (Febrile Seizures)

Febrile (fever-related) convulsions are seizures triggered by fever. They are the most common type of convulsion (occurring in 4 percent of children) and in general are harmless. The children are usually between 6 months and 5 years of age. Most first seizures occur by 3 years of age. The average temperature at which they occur is 104°F, although half occur at lower levels of fever. Everyone has a convulsion threshold. For most children the threshold is 106° or 107°F, so they never have a febrile seizure. The fever itself can be caused by an infection in any part of the body, including a simple cold or ear infection.

During a seizure, the child becomes unconscious. The eyes stare or roll upward. The arms and legs become stiff or jerk. Each febrile seizure usually lasts 1 to 10 minutes without any treatment. Most of these children have just 1 febrile seizure in a lifetime. The other 40 percent of children with febrile seizures have 1 to 3 recurrences over the years. Recurrences are more likely if the initial seizure occurred with a low-grade fever (less than 103°F). They usually stop occurring by age 5 or 6. While seeing a seizure is frightening, there is no cause for alarm. The seizure does not cause any brain damage or epilepsy. Occasionally a child will hurt himself during a fall. Only a few children (3 percent) will go on to have seizures without fever (epilepsy) at a later age.

First Aid for Febrile Convulsions

Reduce the Fever—Bringing your child's fever down as quickly as possible may shorten the seizure. Remove most clothing and apply cold washcloths to the forehead and neck. If the seizure persists, sponge the body surface with cool water (but avoid rubbing alcohol, which could cause a coma). As the water evaporates, the temperature will fall. Don't put your child in a bathtub, however; that could be dangerous during the seizure. When the seizure is over and your child is fully awake, give the appropriate dose of acetaminophen or ibuprofen. (For dosage, see tables, pages 238–40). Also encourage cool fluids.

Protect Your Child's Airway—If he has anything in his mouth, clear it with a finger to prevent choking. Place him on his side or abdomen (facedown) to help drain secretions. If he vomits, help clear the mouth. If available, use a suction bulb. If breathing becomes noisy, pull the jaw and chin forward by placing two fingers behind the corner of the jaw on each side (this will automatically bring the tongue forward).

Common Mistakes in First Aid for Convulsions—During the seizure, don't try to restrain your child or stop the seizure movements. Once started, the seizure will run its course no matter what you do. Don't try to resuscitate your child just because breathing stops momentarily for 5 to 10 seconds. Instead, try to clear the airway. Don't try to force anything into your child's mouth. This is unnecessary and can cut the mouth, injure a tooth, cause vomiting, or result in a serious bite of your finger. Don't try to hold the tongue. While children may rarely bite the tongue during a convulsion, they can't "swallow the tongue."

Call Your Child's Physician Immediately If

• The febrile convulsion lasts more than 5 minutes. (Start timing the length of the seizure as soon as it begins.) Call 911 for these.

• In all other cases, after the seizure has stopped.

If you are told to bring your child to your physician's office or the nearest emergency room, try to keep the fever down during transport. Dress your child lightly (weather permitting) and continue applying a cold washcloth to the forehead. (Warning: Prolonged seizures due to persistent fever have been caused by bundling up sick infants during a long drive. A seizure lasting more than 30 minutes can be harmful.)

Home Care for Febrile Convulsions

Oral Fever-Reducing Medicines—If your physician agrees, place your child on acetaminophen or ibuprofen for the next 48 hours (or longer if the fever persists). For dosages, use the tables on pages 238–40.

Fever-Reducing Suppositories—Have some acetaminophen suppositories on hand in case your child ever has another febrile seizure (same dosage as oral medicine). Since your pharmacist may keep these suppositories refrigerated, you may have to ask for them. When your child awakens fully, you can give the other fever-reducing medicine by mouth.

Light Covers or Clothing—Avoid covering your child with more than one blanket. Bundling during sleep can push the temperature up 1 or 2 extra degrees.

Lots of Fluids—Keep your child well hydrated by offering plenty of fluids.

Call Your Child's Physician Later If
- Another seizure occurs.
- The neck becomes stiff. (Note: The inability to touch the chin to the chest is an early symptom of meningitis.)
- Your child becomes confused or delirious.
- Your child becomes difficult to awaken.
- You feel your child is getting worse.

Prevention of Febrile Convulsions

The only way to prevent future convulsions completely is for your child to take an anticonvulsant medicine daily until age 3 or 4. Since anticonvulsants have side effects and febrile seizures are generally harmless, anticonvulsants are rarely prescribed anymore unless your child has other neurologic problems. Your physician will discuss this decision with you.

Febrile convulsions usually occur during the first day of an illness. Although good research is lacking, preventing high fevers may prevent some febrile seizures. If your child has had a seizure in the past, try to control fever more closely than is necessary for children who have not had febrile seizures. Begin acetaminophen or ibuprofen at the first sign of any fever (a rectal temperature over 100.4°F or 38°C) and give it continuously for the first 48 hours of the illness. If your child has a fever at bedtime, awaken her once during the night to give the fever medicine.

Because fever may occur after diphtheria-tetanus-pertussis (DTaP) immunizations, begin acetaminophen or ibuprofen in the physician's office when your child is immunized and continue it for at least 24 hours.

Related Topics

FEVER (see page 427)
DELIRIUM (see page 45)

CONVULSIONS WITHOUT FEVER

During a convulsion (seizure), a child becomes unconscious and falls, the eyes stare or roll upward, the body stiffens, and the arms and legs jerk. Most seizures last less than 5 minutes. Convulsions without fever occur in 0.4 percent of children. If they become recurrent, the child is said to have epilepsy. While the causes are many, the usual one is a small scar in the brain tissue that triggers seizures. Recurrent seizures can usually be controlled with medicines called anticonvulsants.

First Aid for Convulsions Without Fever

Your child should be left on the floor or ground. Move him only if he is in a dangerous place.

Protect Your Child's Airway—See CONVULSIONS WITH FEVER, page 41.

Common Mistakes in First Aid—See CONVULSIONS WITH FEVER, page 41.

Call a Rescue Squad (911) If

- A first seizure lasts more than 5 minutes.
- The seizure in a child with epilepsy lasts more than 10 minutes. (In general, a seizure won't hurt the brain unless it continues for more than 30 minutes.)

Call Your Child's Physician Immediately If

- It's the first one.
- Seizures are occurring frequently.

Home Care for Convulsions Without Fever

Treatment for Previously Diagnosed Convulsions—After the seizure is over, let your child sleep if he wishes. The brain is temporarily exhausted, and there is no point in trying to keep your child awake. Since recurrent seizures are common, work out a plan with your child's physician in advance. Some will want you to give your child an extra dose of anticonvulsants at this time. If you have recently missed giving a dose, giving twice the usual dose now may be in order. If your child has epilepsy, there is no need to bring your child to an emergency room for every seizure.

Precautions—While most sports are safe, be certain your child avoids activities that would be unsafe if he suddenly had a seizure. These include activities involving heights (e.g., climbing a tree or rope), cycling on a highway, or swimming alone. Wind surfing, scuba diving, and hang gliding must also be avoided. Have him take showers instead of baths, and only when someone else is in the house.

Call Your Child's Physician Later If
- Another seizure occurs.
- Your child stays confused or groggy for more than 2 hours.

DELIRIUM

Delirium is the sudden onset of disorientation (talking crazy), strange behavior (acting "wild"), and visual hallucinations (seeing things that aren't there). Judgment and memory are also impaired. Commonly, the child's confused thinking comes and goes (fluctuates). Young children mainly get delirium with fevers over 104°F. It should go away once the fever is lowered. Illegal drugs can cause delirium. So can some cold and cough medicines, especially if two are given together or one is given in too large a dose. Brief delirium can occur when a child awakens in strange surroundings, as on the first night of a vacation. If your child has no fever and has recently sustained head trauma, see the guideline on HEAD TRAUMA, page 72.

Call Your Child's Physician Immediately If
- Your child's temperature is normal or less than 103°F.
- Your child is on any medicine that could cause delirium (like antihistamines).

- Poisoning is a possibility.
- Your child may be using drugs.
- Head trauma recently occurred. (Unobserved head trauma with amnesia should be considered.)
- The neck is stiff.
- Your child is also vomiting.
- Before the delirium, your child was acting very sick.
- Delirium with fever has persisted longer than 30 minutes.

Home Care for Febrile Delirium

Fever-Reducing Therapy—Give your child acetaminophen or ibuprofen. Remove the clothing and apply cold washcloths to the forehead and neck. Sponge the body surface with cool water. If your child shivers, raise the water temperature. Don't put your child in the bathtub, however; that could be dangerous. See FEVER for details, page 427.

Delirium Therapy—Keep the lights on in your child's room. Be sure a familiar person stays with your child at all times until he or she feels better. It's best if you reassure your child by touching and talking to him. Tell him where he is, who you are, and that he will feel better soon.

Call Your Child's Physician Later If
- The delirium lasts for over 30 minutes.
- The delirium is still present after you lower the fever below 103°F.
- The delirium clears up but your child develops other symptoms that worry you.

DROWNING

First Aid
Have someone call a rescue squad (911) immediately. (See EMERGENCY TRANSPORTATION, page 4.)

Resuscitation—Begin mouth-to-mouth breathing as soon as possible. (Review RESUSCITATION, page 9.) This should be started immediately—in the boat, in a life preserver, or at the latest when the rescuer reaches shallow water. It should be continued until the child is brought to a medical facility, since children have survived long submersions (especially in cold water).

Neck Injury—If there is any possibility of a neck injury (for example, a diving accident), protect the neck from any bending or twisting. If the child is still in the water, he or she can be helped to float on the surface until a spine board is applied or until several people can remove him while supporting the head and back as a unit.

Vomiting—Vomiting is common because the stomach is usually filled with water from drowning. If vomiting occurs, quickly turn the child on his or her side, or facedown, and try to keep the water from entering the lungs. The lungs are usually free of water because they are protected by spasm of the vocal cords. Avoid pressure on the stomach during resuscitation because it can trigger vomiting.

Prevention of Drowning

- Never leave a child less than 3 years old unattended in the bathtub or a wading pool. Toddlers can drown in 2 inches of water.
- Never leave a toddler unattended near a 5-gallon industrial bucket with any water inside. If they peer inside, they may fall in and drown because these large buckets don't easily tip over.
- Never leave children who can't swim well unattended near a swimming pool. (More children drown in backyard swimming pools than at beaches or public pools.)
- Never leave children unattended near spas or hot tubs. Risks include entrapment in the outflow vent and overheating, not just drowning.
- Make sure that neighborhood pools are totally fenced off and the gates are kept locked.
- Try to arrange swimming lessons for your child before age 8. (Children are often ready by age 4.)
- Caution children of all ages to check the depth of the water before diving in and to avoid any diving in the shallow end of a pool.
- Caution children not to overbreathe as a way to stay underwater longer. This practice can lead to passing out underwater.
- Caution the accomplished swimmer never to swim alone. Continue to swim with a buddy.

Infant or Toddler "Swimming" Programs

Toddler swimming lessons are very popular, especially in the Sunbelt. The American Academy of Pediatrics is opposed to organized group swimming lessons for children under 3 years of age for the following reasons:

• If your child is pushed or hurried, he can develop a fear of water.

• If he is not being held and happens to go under, he can inhale enough water in the first 10 seconds to cause symptoms of drowning.

• Swallowed pool water can also be dangerous. Excessive ingestion of water can lower the body sodium and cause seizures. Infant programs that encourage submersion of the head for more than a few seconds should be avoided for this reason.

• Even if your child can be taught how to swim, he cannot learn to save himself. Children are not able to understand the basic elements of water safety and cannot be made "water safe" before 4 years of age. Don't allow the ability to dog-paddle give you a false sense of security.

If you want to acquaint your infant or toddler with water, do so in shallow water and concentrate on having fun, not learning how to swim. Infant water programs held in pools should also teach water fun. You can enroll your youngster in true swimming lessons at age 4 or 5. If you have already taught him to enjoy the water, he may learn to swim quickly.

ELECTRIC SHOCK OR LIGHTNING INJURY

Electrocution (death from electricity) usually occurs from contact with high-tension wires that have fallen or which the child has climbed up to. Household current can cause severe electric shock if your child is standing in water at the time contact is made. Electric shock usually stops breathing and the heartbeat. Rapid resuscitation can lead to a full recovery.

First Aid

Breaking Contact—If your child is still in contact with a live wire, turn off the electricity or break contact with the wire. Be sure to use a nonconducting object (such as a wooden pole).

Call a Rescue Squad (911) Immediately—(See EMERGENCY TRANSPORTATION, page 4.)

Resuscitation—Begin mouth-to-mouth breathing as soon as possible if breathing has stopped. (Review RESUSCITATION, page 9.) Often external cardiac massage will also be needed. Take a CPR course in advance.

Prevention of Electric Shock

- Cover all electrical outlets with plastic safety caps.
- Unplug appliances, such as hair dryers and curling irons, when not in use.
- Keep electrical cords away from toddlers who might chew on them. (Note: This accident could burn off part of the lip or the end of the tongue.)
- Teach your child not to turn on lights or electrical appliances while standing on a wet floor or wet ground.
- Teach your child never to touch an electrical appliance, such as a hair dryer or radio, while in a bathtub. (Note: This mistake can result in immediate electrocution if the appliance is plugged into the socket, even with the switch turned to "off.")
- Teach your child to avoid open water, tall trees, high ground, or metal objects (e.g., a shovel) during thunderstorms. Cars and houses are safe.

EYE, CHEMICAL IN

Acids (e.g., toilet bowl cleaners) and alkalis (e.g., drain cleaners) splashed into the eye can severely damage the cornea, the clear part of the eye. However, most chemicals (such as alcohol or hydrocarbons) just cause temporary stinging and superficial irritation. All should be treated as emergencies until your physician or a Poison Center expert tells you otherwise.

First Aid for Chemical in Eye

Immediate and thorough irrigation of the eye with tap water is essential to prevent damage to the cornea. (Do not use antidotes such as vinegar.) This irrigation should be performed at home and as quickly as possible. Have your child lie down or lean back over a sink, and continuously pour lukewarm water into the eye from a pitcher or glass. It is very important to hold the eyelid open or to blink repeatedly during this process. For most chemicals, the eye should be irrigated for 5 minutes; for acids, 10 minutes; and for alkalis, 20 minutes. If one eye is not burned, cover it while irrigating the other. Any chemical particles that can't be flushed away should be wiped away with a moistened cotton swab. Call your physician immediately after irrigating the eye.

Related Topic

For mild irritants like soap or food, see the guideline on RED OR PINKEYE WITHOUT PUS, page 524.

EYE, FOREIGN BODY IN

The most common objects that get in the eye are an eyelash or a piece of dried mucus (sleep). Particulate matter such as sand, dirt, sawdust, or other grit also can be blown into the eyes. The main symptoms are irritation, pain, and tears. Rubbing the eye can lead to the foreign object's scratching the cornea (clear part). See also EYE, CHEMICAL IN, above.

Some parents needlessly worry that the foreign body can get lost behind the eyeball. This is impossible, since the space where the object is hidden is a dead end. The space on the sides and beyond the eyelids goes back ¼ inch and then stops.

First Aid for Glass Fragments on the Eyelids

Have your child bend forward and try to get flakes of glass off the skin by blowing on the closed eyelids. A few pieces can often be removed from the eyelids by touching them with a piece of Scotch tape. Pour water over the eyelids and face to get off any remaining glass. Cover the eyes with a wet washcloth and go to your physician's office. The eye should not be rubbed.

Call Your Child's Physician Immediately If

- Any particle is stuck to the eyeball (especially the cornea).
- Fluid or blood is coming from the eyeball.
- The object hit the eye at high speed (e.g., a particle from striking metal on metal, or from a lawn mower).

- The foreign object is sharp.
- You think your child needs to be seen.

Home Care for Foreign Body in Eye

Treatment for Numerous Particles—If there are numerous particles in the eye (such as dirt or sand), clean around the eye with a wet washcloth first. Then have your child try to open and close the eye repeatedly while submerging that side of the face in a pan of water. If you are at the beach, have your child open and close the eyes underwater to clear sand from the eyes. If your child is too young to cooperate with this, continuously pour lukewarm water into the eye from a pitcher or glass for 5 minutes. The eyelids must be held open during the irrigation and this usually requires the help of another person.

Treatment for Particle in a Corner of the Eye—If the particle is in the corner of the eye, try to get it out with the corner of a piece of cloth, a moistened cotton swab, or a piece of Scotch tape.

Treatment for Particle Under the Lower Lid—If the particle is under the lower eyelid, pull the lower lid out by depressing the cheek, and touch the particle with a moistened cotton swab. If that doesn't work, try pouring water on the speck while holding the lid out.

Treatment for Particle Under the Upper Lid—If the particle can't be seen, it's probably under the upper lid, the most common hiding place. Try having your child open and close the eye several times while it is submerged in a pan or bowl of water. If you have an eye cup, use it. If this fails, pull the upper lid out and draw it over the lower lid while the eye is closed. When the eye is opened, the lower lid may sweep the particle out from under the upper lid, if you're lucky.

Call Your Child's Physician Later If

- This approach does not remove all the foreign material from the eye— i.e., if the sensation of grittiness or pain persists.

  First Aid: While waiting to be seen by the physician, cover the eye with a wet washcloth or bandage it shut to relieve discomfort. If eye movement causes pain, cover both eyes.

- The vision does not return to normal after the eye has been allowed to rest for an hour.

• The foreign object has been removed, but tearing and blinking persist for more than 2 hours.

FROSTBITE

Frostbitten skin is cold, white, painful, tingly, or numb. The most common sites are toes, fingers, tip of the nose, outer ear, or cheeks. The nerves, blood vessels, and skin cells are temporarily frozen. The windchill temperature determines how quickly it occurs. The frostbite is much worse if the skin and clothing are also wet at the time of cold exposure. Touching bare hands to cold metal or volatile products (like gasoline) stored outside during freezing weather can cause immediate frostbite. Frostbite of the cheeks can occur in the summertime when a toddler keeps a Popsicle in his mouth too long. Cold injuries are painful and sometimes dangerous. Severe cold exposure (hypothermia) with shivering and sleepiness is an emergency.

Call Your Child's Physician Immediately If

• Three or more areas are involved.
• A large area is involved.
• The frostbite resulted from severe cold exposure.
• Your child's temperature is less than 95°F (35°C).
• Severe shivering is present.
• Speech is slurred or confused.
• You think your child needs to be seen.

Home Care

Treatment—The main treatment for frostbite is to rewarm the area rapidly with wet heat. Bring your child into a warm room. Place the frostbitten part in very warm water or cover it with warm wet compresses. A bath is often the quickest approach. The water should be very warm (104° to 108°F, or 40° to 42°C) but not hot enough to burn. Immersion in this warm water should continue until a pink flush signals the return of circulation to the frostbitten part (usually 30 minutes). At this point, the numbness should disappear. If your child has lots of frostbite, the last 10 minutes of rewarming is usually quite painful. The rest of your child's body should also be kept warm by plenty of blankets. If there is any pain, give your child acetaminophen or ibuprofen. Offer warm fluids to drink.

Common Mistakes—A common error is to apply snow to the frostbitten area or to massage it; both can cause damage to thawing tissues. Do not rewarm with dry heat, such as a heat lamp or electric heater, because frostbitten skin is easily burned.

Prevention of Frostbite

- Be sure your child dresses in layers for cold weather. The first layer should be thermal underwear, and the outer layer needs to be waterproof. The layers should be loose, not tight. Mittens are warmer than gloves.
- Have your child wear a hat, because over 50 percent of heat loss occurs from the head.
- Set limits on the time spent outdoors when the windchill temperature falls below 0°F.
- Teach your child to recognize the earliest warnings of frostbite. Tell him that the tingling and numbness are reminders that he is not dressed adequately for the weather and needs to go indoors.

Call Your Child's Physician Later If

- The color and sensation don't return to normal after 60 minutes of rewarming.
- The frostbitten part develops blisters.

HEAT REACTIONS

There are three main reactions to an extremely hot environment. All three are caused by excessive loss of water through sweating. They mainly occur in people who are exercising during hot weather. Infants are at added risk because they are less able to sweat with heat stress. For treatment, select the type of heat reaction that pertains to your child. A rectal temperature is more reliable than an oral temperature for these disorders.

Heatstroke or Sunstroke

Hot, flushed skin; high fever (at least 105°F); the absence of sweating; confusion or unconsciousness; and shock (low blood pressure) are present. The onset is usually rapid.

Heat Exhaustion

Cold, pale skin; no fever (temperature less than 100°F); profuse sweating; and dizziness, fainting, or weakness are present. The onset is usually gradual.

Heat Cramps

Severe cramps in the limbs (especially calf or thigh muscles) and abdomen, with no fever, are present.

First Aid for Heatstroke or Sunstroke

- Call a rescue squad (911) immediately.
- Heatstroke can be life-threatening. The high fever is a serious emergency.
- Cool your child off as rapidly as possible. Move him or her to a cool place. Undress your child (except for underwear) so the body surface can give off heat. Place ice packs in the armpits and groin. Sponge your child with cool water (as cold as is tolerable), and fan him. If your child is unconscious, immersion in cold water could be lifesaving. (Note: acetaminophen or ibuprofen is of no help.)
- If your child is conscious, give as much cold water to drink as he or she can tolerate.

First Aid for Heat Exhaustion

- Call your child's physician immediately.
- Put your child in a cool place. Have him or her lie down with the feet elevated.
- Cover your child with cold wet towels.
- Give as much cold water to drink as your child can tolerate until he or she feels better.
- Your physician will probably want to examine your child's state of hydration. After 2 or 3 glasses of water, drive in. Provide unlimited amounts of water in the car.

Home Care for Heat Cramps

Heat cramps are the most common reaction to excessive heat. They are never serious. Give your child as much cold water to drink as he can tolerate until he feels better. Your child will not need to be seen by the physician.

Prevention of Heat Reactions

- When your child is working or exercising in a hot environment, have him or her drink large amounts of cool water. Water is the ideal solution for replacing lost sweat. Very little salt is lost. Special glucose-electrolyte solutions offer no advantage over water unless you are exercising for longer than an hour.

- Have your child take 5-minute water breaks in the shade every 25 minutes. Teens should drink 8 ounces (240 ml) every 30 minutes. Encourage him to drink water even if he's not thirsty. Thirst is often delayed until a person is almost dehydrated.

- Avoid salt tablets, because they slow down stomach emptying and delay the absorption of fluids.

- Have your child wear a single layer of lightweight clothing. Change it if it becomes wet with perspiration.

- Athletic coaches recommend that exercise sessions be shortened and less vigorous if the temperature exceeds 82°F, especially if the humidity is high.

- When using a hot tub, limit exposure to 15 minutes and have a buddy system in case a heat reaction suddenly occurs. Hot tubs and saunas should be avoided by people with a fever, or following vigorous exercise when the body needs to release heat.

- Protect infants with fevers from heatstroke by not bundling them in blankets or excessive clothing.

POISONING

First, sweep any pills or solid poisons out of your child's mouth, using your finger. If your child swallowed a chemical, immediately give him 1 glass of water or milk to rinse the esophagus (not necessary for swallowed medicines). Then call the nearest Poison Center immediately for *all* ingestions. The National Poison Center hotline number is 1-800-222-1222. This number will automatically connect you with your local Poison Center. Do not induce vomiting. Syrup of ipecac is no longer used for poisonings. If you have any ipecac in your home, dispose of it by flushing it down the toilet. More than 50 percent of ingestions are of poisonous substances taken in a nontoxic amount or of nonpoisonous substances. In these cases, no treatment is necessary. Always suspect poisoning if your child is 1 to 4 years old and has the abrupt onset of unexplained symptoms (without fever). Be prepared to answer the following questions:

• What was swallowed?

• How much was swallowed? (Estimate the maximal amount.)

• When was it swallowed?

• Does your child have any symptoms? (For COMA or CONVULSIONS, go directly to those guidelines, pages 40–45.)

In the meantime, select from the following three guidelines the one that applies to your child's ingestion.

ACIDS, ALKALIS, OR PETROLEUM PRODUCTS (see below)
OTHER POISONOUS SUBSTANCES (see page 57)
PROBABLY HARMLESS SUBSTANCES (see page 57)

Some products have first aid for their ingestion listed on the label.

ACIDS, ALKALIS, OR PETROLEUM PRODUCTS

These include toilet bowl cleaners, drain cleaners, oven cleaners, lye, Clinitest tablets, ammonia, bleaches, kerosene, gasoline, benzene, furniture polish, and lighter fluid. If these agents are vomited, additional damage can occur to the esophagus or lungs.

First Aid

Don't induce vomiting! Have your child drink 2 or 3 ounces of water (or milk) to wash out the esophagus. Avoid excessive fluids, which could trigger vomiting. Keep your child sitting or standing to protect the esophagus. Don't let your child lie down. Bring with you the container the poison was in.

OTHER POISONOUS SUBSTANCES

Poisonous substances include most drugs, chemicals, and plants. The most dangerous prescription drugs of all (in overdosage) are barbiturates, clonidine, digitalis products, narcotics, Lomotil, Darvon, Tofranil, and other trycyclic antidepressants. Very dangerous over-the-counter medicines are iron and aspirin.

First Aid

Do not induce vomiting. Do sweep any pills or solid poisons out of your child's mouth by using a finger. If a chemical was swallowed, give 2 or 3 ounces of water (or milk) to rinse out the esophagus. Avoid excessive fluids which could trigger vomiting.

Drive to the nearest emergency department or call your child's physician immediately.

PROBABLY HARMLESS SUBSTANCES

Fortunately, many children ingest nonedible substances that do not produce any symptoms. Some examples of harmless substances are candles, chalk, crayons, ballpoint pens, felt-tip pens, lead pencils (which are actually graphite), dog or cat food, cat litter, dirt, hand soaps, hand lotions, lipstick, petroleum jelly, rouge, shampoos, shaving cream, silica granules, suntan lotions, and toothpaste. Some children like to chew on newspaper but don't swallow it. In general, the inks used in newspapers are harmless. The exception is that some of the colored inks are harmful, but one serving of the comics requires no intervention. Call your physician to be sure.

Prevention of Poisoning

You were lucky this time, but it's time to poison-proof the house.

- Remember to keep drugs and chemicals locked up or out of reach. Review where you keep drain cleaners, furniture polish, drugs, and insecticides, since these are the most common dangerous poisons.
- Also, remember that alcoholic beverages have caused serious poisonings. As little as 3 ounces of hard liquor has been fatal to a 2-year-old child. Remember that most mouthwashes contain 15 to 25 percent alcohol.

- Whenever you or your child is prescribed a new drug, remember to keep the safety cap on and carefully check the dosage before giving it.
- Don't leave drugs on countertops, especially when you are called to the door or telephone.
- Don't leave drugs in a purse, because children often search them for candy or gum. When you have guests, keep purses out of reach of children.
- Always read the label before giving any medicine. Be sure it's the right drug and that you are giving the correct dosage. Don't give medicines in the dark.
- Learn the names of all your house plants and remove any (e.g., dieffenbachia) that would cause more than vomiting or diarrhea. Teach your child never to put leaves, stems, seeds, or berries from any plant into the mouth.
- Don't store chemicals in soft-drink bottles or put gasoline into any type of food or beverage container.
- Keep the telephone number of the Poison Control Center handy: 1-800-222-1222.
- Remember that kids often get into poisons simply to satisfy their curiosity. Telling a young child not to put something in her mouth is not enough to prevent poisoning. To prevent poisonings, parents have to supervise consistently where young children are and what they are doing.

SUFFOCATION

Most infant suffocations occur when babies are placed facedown on a soft surface that they sink into. Infants from birth to 4 months old have the greatest risk of suffocating. These young infants don't have enough strength to lift their heads and turn their faces so that they can breathe. Many of these deaths occur when a baby naps at the home of a friend who doesn't have a crib or doesn't know the importance of having the baby sleep on his back.

Another cause of suffocation in young infants should be mentioned. Small babies have been smothered by mothers who inadvertently fell asleep on top of them. If you nurse your baby in your bed at night, be careful. It's best to keep your baby in a crib next to your bed.

Another reason not to let your baby sleep in your bed during the first 6 months is that the mattresses in most adult beds are too soft for babies. Blankets and pllows also increase the risk of suffocation.

Prevention of Suffocation in Infants

To be safe, always place your young baby to sleep on his back in a crib with a firm mattress. Also do this for naps. This is the sleep position recommended by the American Academy of Pediatrics for healthy infants during the first 6 months of life. Sleeping on the side is not an acceptable alternative because it is an unstable position and has twice the risk of sudden infant death syndrome (SIDS) than sleeping on the back. Sleeping on the tummy (facedown) carries 5 times greater risk.

Soft surfaces are unsafe for babies even if they are placed on their backs. Someone, such as another child or baby-sitter, might turn them over.

You can prevent these tragic deaths by suffocation by never putting young infants down to sleep on the following soft surfaces:

• Waterbeds or featherbeds

• Sheepskin rugs or mattress covers

• Any weak, spongy surfaces, including soft mattresses and comforters

• Mattresses covered with plastic bags

• Soft pillows or bean-bag chairs

Also, avoid stuffed toys, comforters, quilts, blankets, or soft objects that could bunch up around your child's face. Dress your infant warmly enough so blankets are not needed.

Prevention of Suffocation in Toddlers

Older infants and toddlers can be suffocated by plastic bags or sheets of plastic. These accidents usually occur when they pull the plastic over their heads or crawl into plastic bags. Carefully dispose of any plastic bags or keep them away from children less than 3 years old. Examples of such products are:

• Plastic dry-cleaning bags

• Plastic shopping bags

• Plastic trash bags

II. Trauma (Injuries)

BONE, JOINT, AND MUSCLE TRAUMA

This guideline covers injuries to bones, joints, and muscles. The legs are more commonly injured than the arms. *Fractures* (broken bones) and *dislocations* (bones out of joint) obviously need treatment by a physician. Stretches and tears of ligaments *(sprains)* are due to sudden twisting injuries and require medical attention unless they are very mild. By contrast, most stretches and tears of muscles *(strains)* are due to overexertion and can be treated at home. Excessive jumping gives muscle pain in the front of the upper leg. Excessive running (especially uphill) gives muscle pain in the front of the lower leg (called shin splints). *A muscle bruise* (called a charley horse) is the most common injury in contact sports and can also be treated at home. *Bone bruises* usually follow direct blows to the bone in exposed areas, like the elbow, hip, or knee, and are usually minor injuries.

Similar Condition—If appropriate, turn directly to the guideline for FINGER AND TOE TRAUMA, page 68.

First Aid for Suspected Fracture or Severe Sprain

Suspected Fracture—If you suspect a broken bone, take your child in for a medical exam and an X-ray. Don't let your child put pressure or weight on it. Splint the fracture before moving your child so the fracture edges won't damage blood vessels. Note: If your child sustains repeated fractures, be sure he is consuming a normal amount of calcium (800 to 1,200 mg) each day.

- *Shoulder or arm:* Use a sling made of a triangular piece of cloth to support the forearm at an 80- to 90-degree angle. At a minimum, support the injured part with the other hand.
- *Leg:* After placing a towel between the legs, use the uninjured leg as a splint by binding the thighs and legs together. At a minimum, carry

your child and don't permit any weight bearing on the injured leg. Transportation can be by car.

- *Neck:* Protect the neck from any turning or bending. Do not move your child until a neck brace or spine board has been applied. Call a rescue squad (911) for transportation.

Suspected Sprained Ankle or Knee—Treat most ankle and knee injuries with R.I.C.E. (rest, ice, compression, and elevation). Apply continuous compression with a snug elastic bandage for 48 hours. Numbness, tingling, or increased pain means the bandage is too tight. Apply crushed ice in a plastic bag or a cold pack wrapped in a wet cloth for 20 minutes out of every hour for 4 consecutive hours. Ice and compression reduce bleeding, swelling, and pain (all of which slow healing). Keep the injured ankle or knee elevated and at rest for 24 hours. While mild sprains could be cared for at home, most injuries to ligaments need to be evaluated by your physician. Transportation can be by car. (Note: While sprains are common in adults, under age 12 or 14, suspect a fracture.)

Call Your Child's Physician

Immediately If
- Your child is under 6 months old.
- The bone is deformed or crooked.
- Your child won't move an arm normally (especially if the injury followed someone's pulling on the arm; young children who won't straighten the elbow or turn the palm up usually have a subluxed radius, a partial dislocation of the elbow).
- Your child won't stand (bear weight) on the legs.
- A severe limp is present.
- The joint nearest the injury can't be moved fully.
- The pain is severe.
- A "snap" or "pop" was felt at the time of an injury to the knee.
- You think it's a serious injury.

During Office Hours If
- Your child can't walk without a limp.
- There is a large area of swelling (especially if it appeared within 30 minutes).

- The pain interferes with sleep.
- You think your child needs to be seen.

Home Care for Bone and Joint Trauma

Treatment of a Bruised Muscle or Bone

- Apply an ice bag or a cold pack wrapped in a wet cloth for 20 minutes. Repeat this 3 to 4 times the first day.
- Give your child acetaminophen or ibuprofen for pain. Ibuprofen is especially helpful for injuries and is available without a prescription. (Avoid aspirin in anyone with soft-tissue bleeding. Since aspirin is an anticoagulant, one aspirin can increase the tendency to bleed easily for up to a week.)
- Have your child rest the injured part as much as possible.
- The pain usually starts to ease after 48 hours, but there may be some discomfort for 2 weeks.

Treatment of Strained Muscles—These guidelines apply if several muscles hurt after a strenuous practice, athletic game, or long hike. Most muscle injuries can safely be cared for at home. Apply an ice bag or cold pack wrapped in a wet cloth to the sore muscles for 20 minutes. Repeat this 3 to 4 times the first day. Also give your child acetaminophen or ibuprofen for at least 48 hours. If stiffness persists after 48 hours, have your child soak in a hot bath for 20 minutes and gently massage the sore muscles. If the pain is localized, use a heating pad or hot compresses. Repeat this several times a day until improvement occurs. Have your youngster learn about stretching exercises and return to exercise gradually. Next time, he or she should be in better condition before going full throttle. Getting back in condition takes at least 7 days.

Call Your Child's Physician Later If

- The pain is not improving by 72 hours.
- The pain is not gone by 2 weeks.
- You feel like your child is getting worse.

Related Topic

For the home care of cuts and scrapes, and guidelines on tetanus boosters, see SKIN TRAUMA, page 78.

EAR TRAUMA

This guideline covers injuries to the outer ear (pinna) or ear canal (the channel that carries sound down to the eardrum). Most external injuries are bruises and scratches. If the ear is severely swollen, a blood clot is present that could permanently damage the ear's shape if it is not treated by a physician. Most bleeding from within the ear canal is from a scratch on the lining caused by a fingernail, cotton swab, or physician's otoscope. These scratches just bleed a few drops and then heal nicely. Long, pointed objects, such as pencils, sticks, straws, or wires, carry the risk of puncturing the eardrum or doing even greater damage to the hearing.

Call Your Child's Physician

Immediately If

- The skin is split open and probably needs sutures.
- The ear is very swollen.
- The pain is severe.
- A pointed object was inserted into the ear canal (e.g., a pencil, stick, straw, or wire) and caused pain.
- More than 4 drops of blood have come from the ear canal.
- Any clear fluid is draining from the ear canal.
- Walking is unsteady.
- The hearing is decreased on that side.
- You think your child needs to be seen.

Home Care for Superficial Cuts and Scrapes to the Ear

Wash the wound vigorously with soap and water. Then apply pressure for 10 minutes with a sterile gauze to stop bleeding. (See SKIN TRAUMA, page 78, for more details.)

EYE TRAUMA

This guideline covers injuries to the eye, eyelid, and area around the eye. Brushing against a small twig often causes more damage than collision with a large object like a door. The main concern is if the vision has been damaged. Older children can tell us if their vision is blurred or out of focus. Test them at home by covering each eye in turn and having them look at a distant object. Children under 3 years old usually need to be examined to answer this question.

Call Your Child's Physician

Immediately If

- The skin is split open and probably needs sutures.
- Any cut is present on the eyelid or eyeball.
- The pain is severe.
- The eyes are constantly tearing or blinking.
- Your child keeps the eye covered and won't open it.
- Vision is blurred or lost in either eye.
- Your child has double vision or can't look upward.
- The pupils are unequal in size.
- Blood or clouding is present behind the cornea (clear part).
- An object hit the eye at high speed (such as from a lawn mower).
- A sharp object hit the eye (such as a metallic chip).
- Your child is less than 3 years old *and* there are any findings of injury (like a black eye or bleeding in the white of the eyeball).
- You think your child needs to be seen.

Home Care for Eye Trauma

Superficial Cuts or Scrapes—Protect the eye with a clean cloth, then wash the wound vigorously with soap and water. Then apply pressure for 10 minutes with a sterile gauze to stop bleeding. (See SKIN TRAUMA, page 78, for more details.)

Swelling or Bruises with Intact Skin—Swelling usually follows injury to the soft tissues or bone around the eye. Apply ice for 20 minutes. Give your child acetaminophen or ibuprofen if necessary for pain. Don't be surprised if a black eye develops over the next 2 days. A black eye is harmless and needs no special treatment. A subconjunctival hemorrhage (flame-shaped bruise of the sclera or white of the eyeball) also shouldn't cause undue concern. These unsightly bruises do not spread to inside the eye. They generally last for 2 weeks and their disappearance cannot be hurried by any medicine or home remedy.

Call Your Child's Physician Later If

- There are any complaints about vision.

Prevention of Eye Trauma

- Objects that penetrate the eyeball often result in loss of vision. Don't buy your child an air-powered gun (BB gun).
- Don't allow your child to play nearby when someone is using a lawn mower.

FINGER AND TOE TRAUMA

This guideline covers injuries to the fingers or toes. Usually the impact simply causes a bruise or swelling of the soft tissues and underlying bone (as when a heavy object falls on a toe or when a hand is bumped against a wall). However, if the end of a straightened finger or thumb receives the blow (usually from a ball), the energy is absorbed by the joints' surfaces and the injury occurs there (a jammed finger). For jammed fingers, always check carefully that the end of the finger can be fully straightened. In crush injuries (as from slammed car or screen doors), usually the last digit receives a few cuts. Occasionally the nail is damaged. Rarely is there any fracture of the small underlying bone.

Call Your Child's Physician

Immediately If

- The skin is split open and probably needs sutures.
- Any bleeding won't stop after 10 minutes of direct pressure.
- The pain is severe.
- Blood collects under a nail *and* becomes quite painful.
- The fingernail is damaged following a crush injury.
- There is any dirt or grime in the wound that you can't get out.
- A finger joint can't be opened (straightened) and closed (bent) completely.
- You think it's a serious injury.

During Office Hours If

- The finger or toe is quite swollen.
- You think your child needs to be seen.

Home Care for Finger and Toe Trauma

The following topics are covered. Go directly to the part that pertains to your child:

BRUISED FINGER OR TOE
JAMMED FINGER
SMASHED OR CRUSHED FINGERTIP
TORN NAIL
SUPERFICIAL CUTS
SKINNED KNUCKLES
RING CAUGHT ON SWOLLEN FINGER

For puncture wounds, go to the guideline on SKIN TRAUMA, page 78.

Bruised Finger or Toe: Treatment—Soak it in cold water for 20 minutes. Give your child acetaminophen or ibuprofen as necessary for the pain. Call your physician later if the pain is not improving by 3 days or if your child is not using the finger or toe normally after a week.

Jammed Finger: Treatment—Soak the hand in cold water for 20 minutes. Give acetaminophen or ibuprofen as necessary for the pain. The finger will be sensitive for the next week, so protect it by "buddy-taping" it to the next finger. A splint could be used but often makes it more prone to getting bumped. Call your physician later if the pain is not improving by 3 days or if your child isn't using the finger normally within 2 weeks. If this problem is recurrent, tape the involved fingers (so the painful joints can't bend excessively) before sports for 3 or 4 weeks. To prevent future jammed fingers, have your child build up the small muscles of the fingers by daily squeezing exercises with a hand grip.

Smashed or Crushed Fingertip: Treatment—Before taking care of this yourself, recheck the guidelines for when to consult a physician. Soak the hand in cold water for 20 minutes. Give your child acetaminophen or ibuprofen as necessary for the pain. Wash the finger well with a liquid soap while soaking it. Trim any small pieces of torn skin with a sterile scissors. If there's a chance of a cut getting dirty, cover it with a Band-Aid. Change the dressing every 24 hours. The injured area will be sensitive for the next week, so protect it from re-injury. Call your physician later if the pain isn't improving by 3 days, any signs of infection develop, or your child isn't using the finger normally in 1 week.

Torn Nail: Treatment—These recommendations apply to a nail that has been torn by catching on something. If the nail was torn by a crush injury, your child needs to see a physician. If the nail is cracked but there are no rough edges, leave it alone. If the nail is almost torn through or there is a large flap of nail, use sterile scissors or nail clippers to cut along the line of the tear. Pieces of nail taped in place will catch on objects. Soak the finger for 20 minutes in cold water. Apply an antibiotic ointment and cover it with a Band-Aid. Each day, remove the dressing and soak the finger in a warm salt solution (1 teaspoon of salt to a pint of water) for 20 minutes once a day. By the seventh day, the nailbed should be covered with new skin, and both the soaking and the bandaging can be stopped. A new nail will grow in over the next 1 to 2 months. Call your physician later for any signs of infection.

Superficial Cuts: Treatment—Wash the wound vigorously with soap and water. Then apply pressure for 10 minutes with a sterile gauze to stop bleeding. (See SKIN TRAUMA, page 78, for details.)

Skinned Knuckles: Treatment—These wounds are deep scrapes of the upper surfaces of fingers or toes. Wash the wound vigorously with soap and water. Scrubbing with a sterile gauze may be necessary to get all the dirt out. Flaps of skin (especially if they are dirty) should be cut off with sterile scissors or nail clippers. When clean, apply pressure for 10 minutes with a sterile gauze to stop any bleeding. Apply an antibiotic ointment and cover with a Band-Aid. Remove the dressing and clean the wound each day. Call your physician for any signs of infection.

Ring Caught on Swollen Finger: Treatment—Call your physician immediately if the finger has turned blue or numb. In most cases, a high priority is to save the ring. The key to removing the ring is reducing the swelling of the finger. This approach requires patience. At 5-minute intervals, alternate soaking the hand in ice water and holding it (with all the fingers straightened) high in the air. At 30 minutes (after the hand has been elevated for the third time), mineral oil or cooking oil can be applied to the finger. While the hand remains elevated, steady upward pressure can be applied until the ring slides off. If it won't slide off, call your physician before the swelling becomes worse.

Swollen Toe or Finger in Infant—An unexplained swelling of a toe or finger requires medical attention. Fine human hair or a thin strand of thread can inadvertently become wrapped around a toe (occasionally a finger or penis). As your infant grows and the tourniquet of hair doesn't stretch, the blood supply from the toe is gradually cut off. A sharply demarcated groove with a swollen toe beyond it are the main findings. You will need medical help in removing this ring of hair.

GENITAL TRAUMA

This guideline covers injuries to the female or male genital area. Most are bruises (with swelling) or minor cuts that heal rapidly in 3 or 4 days.

Call Your Child's Physician Immediately If

- The skin is split open and probably needs sutures.
- Any external bleeding won't stop after 10 minutes of direct pressure.
- The pain is severe.
- Passing the urine is difficult.
- Blood is in the urine.
- Your child is a male *and* the scrotum is swollen.
- Your child is a female *and* there is any bleeding from inside the vagina.
- Your child is a female *and* the injury was from an object that could have penetrated the vagina.
- Your child feels dizzy or faints with standing up.
- Sexual abuse could be the cause.
- You think your child needs to be seen.

Home Care for Genital Trauma

For minor cuts, wash the area vigorously with soap and water. Then apply pressure for 10 minutes with a sterile gauze to stop bleeding. For swelling, apply a cold wet cloth for the next 20 minutes (if tolerated). (See SKIN TRAUMA, page 78, for additional information.) Call your physician later if passing the urine becomes difficult.

HEAD TRAUMA

Symptoms and Characteristics
- History of a blow to the head
- Scalp trauma (cut, scrape, bruise, or swelling)
- Crying and holding the head

Cause—Every child sooner or later strikes his head. Falls are especially common when your child is learning to walk.

Expected Course—Most head trauma simply results in a scalp injury. Big lumps can occur with minor injuries because the blood supply to the scalp is so plentiful. For the same reason, small cuts here can bleed profusely. Most bruises occur on the forehead. Sometimes a black eye appears after 3 days because the bruising spreads downward by gravity. Only 1 to 2 percent get a skull fracture. Since the presence of a simple skull fracture neither increases the chances of a complication nor changes the treatment, skull X-rays are rarely helpful and not routinely ordered. Usually there are no associated symptoms except for a headache at the site of impact. Children with concussions need to be examined by a physician, but concussions are uncommon following head trauma. Unless there is temporary unconsciousness, confusion, or amnesia, your child has not had a concussion.

Call 911 Immediately If
- Your child had a seizure (convulsion).
- Your child was unconscious or confused after the injury.
- Your child is unusually sleepy and difficult to awaken.
- Speech is slurred.
- Walking or crawling is unsteady.
- The arms are weak.
- There is any neck pain.

Call Your Child's Physician Immediately If
- The skin is split open and probably needs sutures.
- The accident was a severe one involving great force.
- Your child is under 1 year old.
- The crying lasted more than 10 minutes after the injury.

- Your child can't remember the accident (amnesia).
- A severe headache is present. (Young children with severe headaches either cry or are extremely restless.)
- Vomiting has occurred 2 or more times.
- Vision is blurred or double.
- Blood or watery fluid is coming from the nose or ears.
- The eyes are crossed.
- You think your child needs to be seen.

Home Care for Head Trauma

Wound Care—If there is a scrape, wash it off with soap and water. Then apply pressure with sterile gauze or a clean cloth for 10 minutes to stop any bleeding. For swelling, apply ice for 20 minutes. Although the swelling will go down in 3 to 4 days, the bruise may last for 2 to 4 weeks.

Rest—Encourage your child to lie down and rest until all symptoms are gone (or at least 2 hours). Your child can be allowed to sleep; you don't have to try to keep her awake. Just have her sleep nearby so you can periodically check on her. Don't give any pain medicine.

Diet—Give only clear fluids (ones you can see through) until your child has gone 2 hours without vomiting. Vomiting is common after head injuries and there is no need to have him vomit up his dinner.

Avoid Pain Medicines—Don't give acetaminophen or ibuprofen, because you need to follow closely your child's reaction to the injury. If the headache is bad enough to need a pain medicine, your child should be checked by a physician.

Special Precautions and Awakening—Although your child is probably fine, watching your child for 48 hours will insure that no serious complication is missed. Close observation is especially important during the first 8 hours after the injury. After 48 hours, however, your child should return to a normal routine and full activity.

Awakening at Night—Awaken your child twice during the night: once at your bedtime and once four hours later. (Awakening him every hour is unnecessary and next to impossible.) Arouse him until he is walking and talking normally. Do this for two nights and also sleep in the same room with your child. If his breathing becomes abnormal or his sleep is otherwise unusual, awaken him to be sure a coma is not developing. If you can't awaken your child, call your physician immediately. After two nights, return to a normal routine.

Checking Pupils—This is unnecessary. Some physicians may ask you to check your child's pupils (the black centers of the eyes) to make sure they are equal in size and become smaller when you shine a flashlight on them. Unequal pupils are never seen before other symptoms like confusion and difficulty walking. In addition, this test is difficult to perform with uncooperative children or dark-colored irises. In general, pupil checks are only necessary on children with severe head injuries, who are hospitalized.

Call Your Child's Physician Later If
- The headache becomes severe.
- Vomiting occurs 2 or more times.
- You feel your child is getting worse.

Prevention of Head Trauma
- When driving, place your child in a car safety seat. (See page 216 for details.)
- To prevent pedestrian accidents, teach your child to look both ways before crossing and while crossing. Teach him to use crosswalks and not to run across the street. Most children cannot safely cross the street alone until age 7 or 8.
- Never leave an infant of any age alone on a high place like a bed, sofa, changing table, or an exam table in the doctor's office. Your baby may unexpectedly roll over for the first time or wiggle off and fall on his head.
- Always keep the side rails up on the crib. Once your child can pull to standing in the crib, lower the mattress.
- Don't buy a bunk bed. If you already have one, keep children under age 6 out of the top bunk and use a side rail. Be sure the bed frame is strong enough to keep the mattress from falling through. And don't let your children jump on beds.
- Don't buy a baby walker (see page 124). They do not accelerate devel-

opment and 35 percent of infants using them have an accident requiring emergency care.

- Don't leave your child unattended in a shopping cart.
- Place a sturdy gate at the top of stairways. Keep the stairway cleared of clutter. When your child starts to climb stairs, teach him to hold on to the banister when descending.
- For doors leading to the basement or outdoors, keep them closed and secure with an extra latch above the child's reach.
- If you live on an upper floor of a building, install window locks or guards.
- Don't leave younger children under the supervision of an aggressive sibling.
- Always supervise your child's outside play until he or she can be trusted to stay in the yard (age 4 or 5). Three-year-olds can't be expected to keep promises not to go near the street.
- Don't allow your child to ride a bicycle in the street until your child is old enough (age 7 or 8) to understand such safety issues as emergency stops and rules about right of way.
- Never allow your child to ride a bike unless she is wearing a bicycle helmet. ATVs and motorcycles are too unsafe to ride, even with a helmet.
- Forbid trampolines. Serious accidents such as spinal cord injuries have occurred even with close supervision.

MOUTH TRAUMA

Small cuts and scrapes inside the mouth heal up beautifully in 3 or 4 days—twice as fast as skin injuries. Infections of mouth injuries are rare. You'll have difficulty finding where the injury was in a few weeks. Cuts of the tongue and insides of the cheeks due to accidentally biting oneself during eating are the most common mouth injury. Cuts and bruises of the lips are usually due to falls. A tear of the piece of tissue connecting the upper lip to the gum is very common. It can look terrible and bleed profusely until pressure is applied, but it is harmless. The potentially serious mouth injuries are those to the tonsils, soft palate, or back of the throat (as from falling with a pencil in the mouth). Prevent these by teaching your child not to run or play with any long object in the mouth. Cuts in the mouth usually don't require suturing except for loose flaps of tissue or gaping wounds of the tongue.

Similar Condition—If appropriate, turn directly to the guideline for TEETH TRAUMA, page 84.

Call Your Child's Physician Immediately If

- Any bleeding won't stop after 10 minutes of direct pressure.
- A deep or gaping cut is present and probably needs sutures.
- The injury is to the back of the throat.
- It resulted from falling down with a stick or other long object in the mouth.
- The pain is severe.
- You think your child needs to be seen.

Home Care for Mouth Trauma

Stop Any Bleeding—Stop any bleeding by pressing the bleeding site against the teeth or jaw for 10 minutes. For bleeding from the tongue, squeeze the bleeding site with a sterile gauze or piece of clean cloth. Don't release the pressure until 10 minutes are up. Once bleeding from inside the upper lip stops, don't pull the lip out again to look at it. Every time you do, the bleeding will start again.

Pain Relief—The area will probably hurt for 1 or 2 days. Apply a piece of ice or a Popsicle as often as necessary. If there is pain at bedtime, give acetaminophen or ibuprofen. For a day or so, offer your child a soft diet. Avoid any salty or citrus foods that might sting. Keep food out of the wound by rinsing the area well with water immediately after meals.

Call Your Child's Physician Later If

- You feel the area is becoming infected, especially increasing pain or swelling after 48 hours. (Keep in mind that any healing wound in the mouth is normally white for several days.)
- A fever occurs.
- You feel your child is getting worse.

NOSE TRAUMA

Most blows to the nose result in a bloody nose or swelling and bruising of the nose but no fracture. Even when a fracture is present, nasal X-rays often show nothing conclusive. The best course of action is to wait until day 4, when the swelling is gone. If the nose then appears to be crooked or different than it used to, you will probably be referred to an ear, nose, and throat surgeon. For mild fractures of the nose, this delayed correction leads to the best cosmetic results because the surgeon can see what he is correcting. Severe fractures of the nose are often reset immediately.

Call Your Child's Physician Immediately If

- The nose is definitely broken or crooked.
- The skin is split open and probably needs sutures.
- A nosebleed won't stop after 10 minutes of pinching the nostrils closed.
- Clear fluid is draining continuously from the nose.
- Pain is severe.
- Breathing is blocked on one side (when you close the other nostril with your finger) or both sides.
- A swelling of the septum (central dividing wall) is visible inside one nostril.
- You think your child needs to be seen.

Home Care for Nose Trauma

Bruises or Swelling—Apply ice to the area for the next hour. Give acetaminophen as necessary for pain. (Aspirin should be avoided, since it can increase the body's tendency to bleed easily and make nosebleeds worse.)

Superficial Cuts or Abrasions—Wash the area vigorously with soap and water for 5 minutes. Then apply pressure for 10 minutes with a sterile gauze to stop bleeding. To stop bleeding from the nostrils, see the guideline on NOSEBLEED, page 559.

Call Your Child's Physician Later If

- The shape of the nose has not returned to normal in 4 days.
- A yellow discharge, increasing tenderness, fever, or other signs of infection occur.
- You feel your child is getting worse.

SKIN TRAUMA

The following four skin injuries are covered. Go directly to the type of injury that pertains to your child.

BRUISES (see below)
CUTS AND SCRATCHES (see page 79)
PUNCTURE WOUNDS (see page 80)
SCRAPES (ABRASIONS) (see page 82)

BRUISES

Bleeding into or under the skin from damaged blood vessels gives a black-and-blue mark. Since the skin is not broken, there is no risk of infection. Bruises usually follow trauma with blunt objects. Unexplained bruises can indicate a bleeding tendency. (Exception: Bruises overlying the shins don't count, since children so commonly bump this area and then forget about it.)

Call Your Child's Physician Immediately If

• Bruises are unexplained *and* several in number.

Home Care for Bruises

Bruises—Apply ice for 20 minutes. No other treatment should be necessary. Give acetaminophen or ibuprofen for pain. Avoid massage. After 48 hours apply a warm washcloth for 10 minutes 3 times a day to help the skin reabsorb the blood. Bruises clear in 2 to 4 weeks after undergoing yellow, green, and brown color changes.

Blood Blisters—Do not open blisters; it will only increase the possibility of infection. They will dry up and peel off in 1 to 2 weeks.

Related Topic

BONE, JOINT, AND MUSCLE TRAUMA (see page 63)

CUTS AND SCRATCHES

Most cuts are superficial and extend only partially through the skin. They are caused by sharp objects.

What to Suture—Any cut that is split open or gaping probably needs sutures. Cuts longer than ½ inch (1 cm) usually need sutures. On the face, cuts longer than ¼ inch need sutures. The sooner a wound is closed, the lower the infection rate. If you think your child may need stitches, try to get her seen within 4 hours. Any open wound that may need sutures should be evaluated by a physician regardless of the time that has passed since the initial injury.

Call Your Child's Physician

Immediately If

- Bleeding won't stop after 10 minutes of direct pressure.
- The skin is split open or gaping and probably needs sutures.
- The cut is deep (e.g., you can see bone or tendons).
- There is any dirt in the wound that you can't get out.

During Office Hours If

- Your child hasn't had a tetanus booster in more than 10 years (5 years for dirty cuts).

Home Care for Cuts and Scratches

Treatment

- Apply direct pressure for 10 minutes to stop any bleeding.
- Wash the wound with soap and water for 5 minutes.
- Cut off any pieces of loose skin using a small scissors (for torn skin with scrapes).
- Apply an antibiotic ointment and cover it with a Band-Aid or gauze. Wash the wound, apply the ointment, and change the Band-Aid or gauze daily.
- Give acetaminophen or ibuprofen as needed for pain relief.

Liquid Skin Dressings—Liquid skin bandages that seal over cuts and scrapes are a major improvement over Band-Aids and antibiotic ointment. They only need to be applied once. They give faster healing and lower infection rates. After the wound is washed and dried, the liquid is applied by spray or with a swab. It dries in less than a minute and usually lasts a week. It's resistant to bathing. Check it out at your local pharmacy.

Common Mistakes in Treating Cuts and Scratches

- Don't use alcohol or Merthiolate on open wounds. They sting and damage the normal tissue. Hydrogen peroxide also is not used, because it can break down normal clots and is a feeble germ-killer.
- Don't kiss an open wound because the wound will become contaminated by the many germs in a normal person's mouth.
- Let the scab fall off by itself; picking it off may cause a scar.

Call Your Child's Physician Later If

- The cut looks infected (pus is visible, for instance).
- Pain, redness, or swelling increases after 48 hours.
- The wound doesn't heal within 10 days.

Related Topics

BITES: ANIMAL OR HUMAN (see page 15)
WOUND INFECTIONS (see page 87)
SUTURED WOUND CARE (see page 86)

PUNCTURE WOUNDS

The skin has been completely punctured by an object that is narrow and sharp. The most common puncture wound follows stepping on a nail. The wound is not wide enough to need sutures. Since puncture wounds usually seal over quickly and are not cleansed by any active bleeding, wound infections of all kinds are more common with this type of skin injury. Puncture wounds of the upper eyelid (as from a sharp pencil) are especially dangerous and can result in a brain abscess. A deep infection of the foot can begin with swelling of the top of the foot 1 to 2 weeks after the puncture. Tetanus (lockjaw) can occur if your child is not immunized.

Call Your Child's Physician

Immediately If

- A dirty object caused the puncture.
- The skin was quite dirty at the time.
- You can see some dirt or debris in the wound after soaking.
- The tip of the object could have broken off in the wound.
- The puncture is on the head, chest, abdomen, or overlying a joint.
- Your child has never received a tetanus shot.

During Office Hours If

- Your child hasn't had a tetanus booster in more than 5 years.

Home Care for Puncture Wounds

Cleansing—Soak the wound in warm water and soap for 15 minutes. Scrub the wound with a washcloth to remove any debris. If the wound rebleeds a little, that may help remove germs.

Trimming—Cut off any flaps of loose skin that cover the wound and interfere with drainage or removing debris. Use a fine scissors after cleaning them with rubbing alcohol.

Antibiotic Ointment—Apply an antibiotic ointment and a Band-Aid to reduce the risk of infection. Resoak the area and reapply antibiotic ointment every 12 hours for 2 hours.

Pain Relief—Give acetaminophen or ibuprofen for any pain.

Call Your Child's Physician Later If

- The wound looks infected.
- Pain, redness, or swelling increases after 48 hours.

Related Topic

WOUND INFECTIONS (see page 87)

SCRAPES (Abrasions)

An abrasion is an area of superficial skin that has been scraped off during a fall—a "skinned" knee from skidding on gravel, for instance. The mild ones are often called friction burns (such as a rope burn or floor burn).

Call Your Child's Physician

Immediately If

- There is any dirt or grime in the wound that you can't get out.
- It was a bicycle-spoke injury.
- It was a washing machine wringer injury.
- It is quite deep. (Note: If the complete layer of skin is removed, a skin graft may be necessary.)
- It involves a very large area.
- The pain is severe.

During Office Hours If

- Your child hasn't had a tetanus booster in more than 10 years.

Home Care for Scrapes

Cleaning the Scrape—First, wash your hands. Then wash the wound vigorously with soap and warm water. The area will probably need to be scrubbed several times with a wet gauze to get all the dirt out. You may have to remove some dirty particles (e.g., gravel) with a tweezers. If there is tar in the wound, it can often be removed by rubbing it with petroleum jelly, followed by soap and water again. Pieces of loose skin (especially if they are dirty) should be cut off with a sterile scissors. Rinse the wound well.

Antibiotic Ointments and Dressing—Apply an antibiotic ointment and cover the scrape with a Band-Aid or gauze dressing. This is especially important for scrapes over joints (such as the elbow, knee, or hand) that are always being stretched. Cracking and reopening at these sites can be prevented with an antibiotic ointment, which keeps the crust soft (no prescription needed). Cleanse the area once a day with warm water and then reapply the ointment and dressing until the scrape is healed.

Pain Relief—Since abrasions can hurt badly, give acetaminophen or ibuprofen for the first day. (For dosage, see tables on page 238–40.)

Call Your Child's Physician Later If

- The scrape looks infected.
- The scrape increases in size or spreads to good skin.
- The scrape doesn't heal within 2 weeks.

Related Topic

WOUND INFECTIONS (see page 87)

TAILBONE TRAUMA

The tailbone (or coccyx) is the small bone at the lower end of the spine. The tailbone is usually injured during a fall onto a hard surface, such as ice or stairs. The pain usually is due to bruising of the bone or stretching of the ligaments. Fractures of the tailbone are rare and they heal fine, so an X-ray is unnecessary for this injury. Dislocations of a fractured tailbone are extremely rare, but they need to be put back in place by a physician. Tailbone injuries can be diagnosed by finding tenderness of the bone located in the upper part of the groove between the buttocks.

Home Care for Tailbone Trauma

A bruised tailbone will usually hurt for 3 to 4 weeks. Give your youngster acetaminophen or ibuprofen for 2 or 3 days. Sitting on a large rubber ring or a cushion placed forward on the chair will take pressure off the tailbone. A heating pad may also help. Occasionally bowel movements will cause enough discomfort that 1 or 2 tablespoons of mineral oil will temporarily be needed twice a day. (See also CONSTIPATION, page 599, regarding a nonconstipating diet.) Call your physician if the pain is severe.

TEETH TRAUMA

This guideline covers injuries to the teeth (usually the front ones). Often, the only noticeable injury is bleeding from the gums. The tooth has been jarred and perhaps slightly loosened. These minor injuries heal in 3 days. The next most common injury is tooth displacement (usually pushed inward). It usually returns to its normal position within a few weeks without any treatment. Chipped (or fractured) teeth need to be seen by a dentist. Permanent teeth that are knocked out (avulsed) constitute an emergency.

First Aid for Replacing a Permanent Tooth

Although primary teeth can't successfully be reimplanted, permanent (second) teeth need to be returned to their sockets and the gumline as soon as possible. Best results occur if the tooth is reimplanted within 15 minutes. After 2 hours, replacement is worthless. Ideally, the tooth should be returned to the socket at the scene of the accident.

- Rinse off the tooth with saliva or water.
- Replace it in the socket facing the correct way.
- Press down on the tooth with your thumb until the crown is level with the adjacent tooth.
- Have your child bite down on a wad of cloth to stabilize the tooth until you can reach your dentist.

Call Your Child's Dentist

(Call your physician only if your dentist can't be reached and you are dealing with an emergency.)

Immediately If

- A permanent tooth has been knocked out. (If you haven't been able to replace it, bring it with you in a cup in some of your child's saliva or some milk.)
- A large piece of tooth has been chipped off.
- A red dot is visible inside a fractured tooth.
- The pain is severe.
- Any bleeding won't stop after 10 minutes of direct pressure. (For bleeding with missing teeth, have your child chomp down on a piece of gauze.)

• The tooth has been pushed out of its usual position.

During Office Hours If
• A baby tooth has been knocked out by trauma.
• A small piece of tooth has been chipped off.
• You can see a fracture line in the tooth.
• The tooth is sensitive to cold fluids.
• The tooth is more than slightly loose.
• You think your child needs to be seen.

Home Care for Teeth Trauma

Treatment—Apply a piece of ice or a Popsicle to the injured gum area, unless it increases the pain. If it still hurts, give your child some acetaminophen or ibuprofen. If any teeth are loose, put your child on a soft diet for 3 days. If a tooth is out of its normal position, try to reposition it with a little finger pressure. If a tooth is broken and dental care must be delayed, temporarily seal the sensitive area with melted candle wax. A delay of several days, however, may lead to a root-canal infection.

Prevention—Prevent tooth trauma in children who play contact sports by having them wear a mouth guard.

Call Your Child's Dentist Later If
• Any new symptoms develop.
• The tooth becomes sensitive to hot or cold fluids during the next week.
• The tooth becomes a darker color.

TETANUS BOOSTER FOLLOWING SKIN TRAUMA

Tetanus is a serious bacterial wound infection that progresses from local muscle spasms to total body rigidity and seizures. Tetanus is preventable if DTaP immunizations and tetanus boosters are kept up to date.

The need for a tetanus booster depends on the type of wound (whether or not it is tetanus-prone) and your child's immunization status. All puncture wounds and all cuts (breaks in the skin) caused by an unclean object pose a risk of tetanus. Cuts from a clean knife, piece of glass, etc., are not tetanus-prone wounds unless they become contaminated afterward. Neither are minor burns or scrapes, because these injuries are so superficial that they have adequate exposure to air. The tetanus bacteria can multiply only if buried in a wound where no air is present. Most children have scrapes from time to time; tetanus boosters for all of these wounds would be impractical.

Call Your Child's Physician

Within 24 Hours If

* *Tetanus-prone wounds:* Any puncture wound or dirty cut in children who have had no tetanus booter in more than 5 years.

During Office Hours If

* *Non-tetanus-prone wounds:* Any wound in patients who have had no tetanus booster in more than 10 years. (All immunized children and adults need a tetanus booster every 10 years.)

The administration of a tetanus booster is not an emergency. It can wait 24 hours without increasing the risk of tetanus. Most physicians give a Td booster at these times to help maintain adequate protection against diphtheria as well.

Cautions: If your child has not been immunized against tetanus and sustains a wound, he needs to be seen immediately. Also, if a wound needs suturing, it should be treated as soon as possible.

SUTURED WOUND CARE

Home Care of Sutured Wounds—Keep the wound completely dry for the first 24 hours. Then begin washing it gently with warm water and liquid soap 1 or 2 times a day. Apply an antibiotic ointment after you wash the wound to keep a thick scab from forming over the sutures (stitches). The wound should not be soaked. After 24 hours, your child can take brief showers. Avoid swimming, baths, or soaking the wound until the sutures are removed. Water in the wound can interfere with healing.

Suture Removal—The following guidelines can serve as a reminder that sutures (stitches) are ready for removal at different times, depending on the site of the wound.

AREA	NUMBER OF DAYS
Face	3–4
Neck	5
Scalp	6
Chest or abdomen	7
Arms and back of hands	7
Legs and top of feet	10
Back	10
Palms and soles	14

Have your child's stitches removed on the correct day. Stitches removed too late can leave unnecessary skin marks or even scarring. If any sutures come out too early, call your child's physician. In the meantime, reinforce the wound with tape or butterfly Band-Aids. Continue the tape until the date when the sutures would have been removed.

Protection—After removal of sutures, protect the wound from injury during the following month. Avoid sports that could reinjure the wound. If a sport is essential, apply tape before playing.

Scars—If your child needed sutures, he will develop a scar. All wounds heal by scarring. The scar can be kept to a minimum by taking the sutures out at the right time, preventing wound infections, and protecting the wound from being reinjured during the following month. The healing process goes on for 6 to 12 months; only then will the scar assume its final appearance. During this time, protect the area with sunscreen.

WOUND INFECTIONS

When your child has a break in the skin, watch for signs of infection. Wound infections need to be started on antibiotics.

Most contaminated wounds that are going to become infected do so 24 to 72 hours after the initial injury. An infected wound develops redness, swelling, tenderness, and pus. Keep in mind that a 2 to 3 mm rim of pinkness or redness, confined to the edge of a wound, can be normal, especially if the wound is sutured. However, the area of redness should not be spreading. Pain and tenderness also occur normally, but the pain and swelling are at a peak during the second day and thereafter diminish. If the infection spreads beyond the wound, it will follow the lymph channels and cause a red streak. If the infection reaches the bloodstream (blood poisoning), a fever will be present. The healing process can normally cause mild swelling and tenderness of the lymph nodes that drain the injured area.

Call Your Child's Physician

Immediately If

- The wound is extremely tender.
- An unexplained fever (over 100°F) occurs.
- A red streak runs from the wound.
- The wound infection is on the face.
- Your child looks or acts very sick.

Within 24 Hours If

- You can see pus in the wound, or there is pus draining from it.
- A pimple starts to form where a stitch comes through the skin.
- The wound is becoming more tender than it was on the second day.
- You think your child needs to be seen.

Home Care

Treatment of Mild Normal Redness—Use warm saltwater soaks or compresses (2 teaspoons of table salt per quart of water) to the wound for 15 minutes, 3 times a day. Dry the area thoroughly afterward. Never soak a sutured wound (reason: increases the risk of infection).

Prevention of Wound Infections—Wash all new wounds vigorously with soap and water for 5 to 10 minutes to remove dirt and bacteria. Soak puncture wounds in warm, soapy water for 15 minutes. Do this as soon as possible after the injury occurs, because the longer you wait, the smaller the benefit. Applying an antibiotic ointment after cleaning may be helpful. Encourage your child not to pick at insect bites, scabs, or other areas of irritated skin. Teach your children that kissing an open wound is dangerous because the wound will become contaminated by the many germs in the mouth.

Call Your Child's Physician Later If

- The redness starts to spread.
- You feel your child is getting worse.
- Your child develops any of the "Call Your Child's Physician" symptoms.

III. New Baby Care

NORMAL NEWBORNS

FIRST DAYS IN THE HOSPITAL: GETTING ACQUAINTED

Prenatal Tasks

Childbirth-preparation classes are especially important during the first pregnancy. These classes reduce the amount of fear that normal parents harbor about labor. They also teach mothers various techniques to control the pain of labor and delivery. In addition, they introduce the parents to the world of hospital obstetrics. If at all possible, both parents-to-be should attend these classes. During the prenatal period you will have carefully considered the following five questions:

• Will the father be present at labor and delivery? Most fathers find this a memorable experience, and most mothers are grateful to have their partners present for emotional support. In general, siblings should not be present at the delivery because some of them become frightened by the birth process.

• What baby equipment will you buy? (See NEWBORN EQUIPMENT AND SUPPLIES, page 118.)

• What will you name your baby? Try to narrow your list down to two male and two female names by the time of delivery.

• Will you breast-feed or bottle-feed? (See BREAST-FEEDING, page 150, and FORMULA-FEEDING, page 156.) In most communities, breast-feeding preparation classes are available.

• If your newborn is a boy, will you have him circumcised? (See CIRCUMCISION DECISION: PROS AND CONS, page 113.)

• If you have other children, who will baby-sit while you are in the hospital?

Who will help you during the first weeks after you come home from the hospital? (See page 97.)

Delivery- or Birthing-Room Contact with Your Baby

Parent bonding to an infant is one of the strongest human ties. This bonding gets off to a good start if the mother and father have close contact with their newborn during the first day of life. After your baby has been dried off and placed in a warm blanket, both parents can have some private time with the infant until he or she falls asleep. The period of wakefulness usually lasts from 30 to 60 minutes. Many studies over the past decade have found that early contact (preferably 6 hours during the first day) increases the parents' ability to soothe the baby, increases the likelihood of successful breast-feeding, enhances language development, and maximizes the sense that the baby belongs to the parents. This information underscores the importance of the father's being involved with his baby on the day of birth.

Rooming-In with Your Baby

Most hospitals now have units on the maternity ward where the mother and baby can constantly be together, with backup by the nursing staff. Increasing numbers of hospitals have gone over to this arrangement entirely. Others allow modified rooming-in, in which the baby is with the mother whenever the mother is awake. Rooming-in promotes bonding and a better feeding schedule. In this manner, the mother is quite familiar with her newborn by the time she is discharged. When you need some deep, restorative sleep, however, send your baby off to the newborn nursery. The nursing staff is available to help rather than replace the mother.

Feeding: Getting Started

Getting breast-feeding off to a good start will help guarantee success. During the first 30 minutes of quiet alert behavior after delivery, many babies will be interested in nursing at the breast. For others, the first real attempt at breast-feeding will occur when the baby awakens from his or her initial sleep, at 3 to 6 hours after delivery. Early sucking on the breast stimulates it to begin producing milk. Your baby should nurse for 10 minutes on the first breast and as long as he wants on the second breast.

Ask your nurse for help with correct breast-feeding positioning. Your baby's face and abdomen should be against your body so he doesn't have to turn his head to nurse. This position is 90 degrees different from the bottle-feeding position. Also keep his nose clear of the breast for breathing. Breast-feeding should be repeated on demand, approximately every 2 hours, including night feedings. Have your infant brought to your room at night to nurse if he or she is not rooming in with you around the clock. Supplementary formula should not be offered during the first 4 weeks, because it interferes with sucking and milk production. (An exception is a baby who is extremely hungry and the milk supply is delayed in coming in—see page 152.) Supplementation during the first week of life (especially in the newborn nursery) is the most common cause of inadequate breast milk production. Any mother who needs to be supplementing also needs to be working with a lactation specialist.

Don't expect a full milk supply until your milk comes in on the second to fourth day after delivery. A common error during this period of engorgement is failing to compress the areola so that the infant can grasp the nipple correctly. Take advantage of the brief hospital stay to get as much help with breast-feeding as possible before going home.

Healthy formula-fed babies should be offered formula as soon as they display an interest in feeding, which is usually 3 to 6 hours after delivery when they awaken from their first sleep. Bottle-fed babies typically take ½ ounce (15 ml) at the first feeding. By 3 days of age, full-term infants will usually take 2 ounces every 3 hours.

Learning Parenting Skills

During the hospital stay, both parents should take a crash course in caring for their newborn. Many of the skills will be demonstrated by the nursing staff. Some will be reviewed using video tapes or audio tapes. Your child's physician may give you written instruction sheets on some of these topics. Be certain that someone has taught you how to carry out each of the following tasks before you are discharged:

Feeding your baby (see BREAST-FEEDING, page 150, or FORMULA-FEEDING, page 156)

Soothing your baby with touching or holding when he or she is crying (see CRYING BABY [COLIC], page 253)

Normal skin care and bathing (see page 111)

Umbilical cord care (see page 112)

Circumcision care (see page 115)

Foreskin care, if not circumcised (see page 116)

Diapering (see DIAPER RASH, page 133)

Taking a temperature (rectal and armpit) and reading a thermometer (see FEVER, page 427)

Using a suction bulb (see under COLDS, page 550)

Using an approved car safety seat (see CAR SAFETY SEATS, page 216)

Helping siblings accept the new arrival (see SIBLING RIVALRY TOWARD A NEWBORN, page 126)

Helping your baby sleep on the back to avoid suffocation (see page 59)

You should also be aware there is nothing out of the ordinary about spitting up, loose bowel movements, straining with bowel movements, and unexplained crying.

Newborn Tests and Treatments

During your hospital stay, your child's physician will examine your new baby and answer any questions you might have about your baby's appearance (see NORMAL NEWBORN'S APPEARANCE, page 103). She will also review normal newborn behavior (see page 102), and symptoms to look for in the sick newborn (see page 130). During the hospital stay your baby will receive a vitamin K injection, which prevents hemorrhagic disease of the newborn, a condition that otherwise could cause severe bleeding in the first 7 days of life. Antibiotic eyedrops will be placed in each eye within one hour of birth to prevent eye infections with gonorrhea or chlamydia, two germs that can be present in the birth canal without any symptoms. A blood test to screen for metabolic diseases that could cause mental retardation and other serious medical conditions will be performed from a heel stick on the day of discharge. These genetic disorders (such as phenylketonuria or hypothyroidism) cannot be detected on a regular physical exam. A second metabolic screening test will be performed between 8 and 14 days after birth. Your baby's blood type will be determined only if the mother is blood group O or Rh negative.

Caution: All of these conditions may go untreated or undetected with a home delivery. If your baby is born at home and is well, arrange a medical checkup for the baby within 24 hours of birth.

Visitors—Friends, Relatives, and Children

The father is the most important visitor. He should come as often and stay as long as possible. He should hold his baby each day. Many hospitals now allow visits by siblings. Studies show that children who visit their mothers after the birth of a newborn are more responsive to their mother and the new baby than nonvisiting children are. Children should be supervised by parents or a responsible adult during the entire hospital visit. Siblings should not visit if they have an acute illness, a fever, or recent exposure to a contagious disease. Hospital visitors, however, can wear the mother out. People should telephone before they come by. If you are tired, consider temporarily canceling all visits (except from your partner).

Discharge from the Hospital

In our country most normal full-term newborns are discharged from the hospital with their mothers between 24 and 48 hours after birth. Early discharge is defined as discharge before 24 hours. Some parents desire early discharge because of limited insurance coverage, a need for the mother to be home with siblings, or personal preference. A baby should not be discharged before the temperature, pulse, and respirations have stabilized, the baby has urinated, and two successful feedings have occurred. (In a successful feeding, the baby demonstrates normal sucking, swallowing, and stomach-emptying mechanisms—all necessary for weight gain.) Babies who are discharged early should be seen on the third day of life to check them for weight, jaundice, and general health. Close medical follow-up is essential for infants who are discharged early. And finally, be sure to make your baby's first ride a safe ride. Leave the hospital with your infant in a car safety seat. It's illegal not to.

Recommended Reading

Laura Jana and Jennifer Shu, *Heading Home with Your Newborn: From Birth to Reality* (Elk Grove Village, IL: American Academy of Pediatrics, 2005).

FIRST WEEKS AT HOME: GETTING HELP

Preventing Fatigue and Exhaustion

For many mothers the first weeks at home with a new baby are often the hardest in their lives. You will probably feel overworked, even overwhelmed. Inadequate sleep will leave you with the feeling of fatigue. Caring for babies can be a lonely and stressful responsibility. You may wonder if you will ever catch up on your rest or work. The solution is asking for help. No one should be expected to care for a young baby

alone. Every baby awakens one or more times a night. The way to avoid
sleep deprivation is to know the total amount of sleep you need per day
and to get that sleep in bits and pieces. Go to bed earlier in the evening,
after your baby's final feeding of the day. When your baby naps, you must
also nap. Your baby doesn't need you hovering over him while he's asleep.
If he is sick he will have symptoms. While you are napping, take the telephone off the hook and put up a sign on the door stating MOTHER AND
BABY SLEEPING. If your total sleep remains inadequate, hire a baby-sitter
or bring in a relative to allow yourself a good nap. (See the role of helpers
and the father, page 99.) If you don't take care of yourself, you won't be
able to take care of your baby.

Postpartum Blues

More than 50 percent of women experience postpartum blues on the
third or fourth day after delivery. The symptoms include irrepressible
crying, tiredness, sadness, and sometimes difficulty in thinking clearly.
The main cause of this temporary reaction is probably the sudden decrease of maternal hormones. The full impact of being totally responsible
for a dependent newborn may also be a contributing factor. If caring for
your baby leads to a state of exhaustion, you may find yourself in a downward spiral. Many mothers feel guilty about these symptoms, because
they have been led to believe they should be overjoyed about caring
for their newborn. In any event, these symptoms usually clear in 1 to
3 weeks as the hormone levels return to normal and as the mother develops routines and a sense of control over her life.

There are several ways to cope with the postpartum blues. First, acknowledge your feelings. Discuss them with your partner or a close
friend, as well as your sense of being trapped and the feeling that these
new responsibilities are insurmountable. Don't feel you need to suppress
crying or put on a "Supermom show" for everyone. Second, get adequate
rest. Third, get help with all your work. Fourth, renew contact with
other people; don't become isolated. Get out of the house at least once a
week—going to the hairdresser, shopping, or visiting friends. By the
fourth week, setting aside an evening a week for a "date" at home with
your husband is also helpful. Take-out food and a rental movie can help
you tap back into your marriage. If you don't feel better by the time your
baby is 1 month old, see your physician about the possibility of needing
counseling for depression. If the blues are making it impossible for you to
care for yourself and your baby, seek help sooner.

Helpers: Relatives, Friends, Sitters

As already emphasized, everyone needs extra help during the first few weeks alone with a new baby. Ideally, you were able to make arrangements for help before your baby was born. The best person to help is usually your mother or mother-in-law. If not, teenagers or adults can be hired to come in several times a week to help with housework or look after your baby while you get a nap. If you have other young children, you will need daily help. Clarify that your role is looking after your baby. Your helper's role is to shop, cook, clean house, and wash clothes and dishes. If your newborn has a medical problem that requires special care, ask for home visits by a public health nurse.

Father's Role

The father needs to take time off from work to be with his partner during labor and delivery, as well as on the day she and the child come home from the hospital. If the couple has a relative who will temporarily live in and help, the father can continue to work. However, when the relative leaves, the father can take some saved-up vacation time as paternity leave. At a minimum he needs to work shorter hours until his wife and baby have settled in. The age of noninvolvement of the father is a thing of the past. Not only does the mother need the father to help her with household chores, but the baby also needs contact with the father to develop a close relationship with him. Today's fathers get involved with feeding, changing diapers, bathing, putting to bed, reading stories, dressing, disciplining, helping with homework, playing games, and calling the physician when the child is sick. The father needs to be his wife's support system. He needs to spell her in the evenings so she can nap or get a brief change of scenery. The father's work needs to stay at the office during these tough months. Some fathers avoid interacting with the baby during the first year of life because they are afraid they will hurt their baby or, if the baby cries, that they won't be able to calm the baby. The longer they go without learning these skills, the harder it becomes to master them. At a minimum, fathers should hold and comfort their babies at least once a day (something commonly overlooked in our culture).

Visitors

During the first month at home, only close friends and relatives should be allowed to visit. They should call before they visit to be sure that it is a convenient day and time. They should not visit if they are sick. To prevent unannounced visitors, the parents can put up a sign stating MOTHER AND BABY SLEEPING. NO VISITORS. PLEASE CALL FIRST. Friends without children may not understand your needs. During visits, the visitor should also give special attention to older siblings (see SIBLING RIVALRY TOWARD A NEWBORN, page 126).

Feeding: Achieving Weight Gain

Your main assignments during the early months of life are loving and feeding your baby. All babies lose a few ounces during the first few days after birth. However, they should rarely lose more than 7 percent of the birth weight (about 8 ounces for a 7 pound birth weight). Most bottle-fed babies are back to birth weight by 7 days of age, and breast-fed babies by 10 days of age. Then, infants gain approximately an ounce per day during the early months. If milk is provided liberally, the normal newborn's hunger drive sees to it that enough weight is gained.

Breast-feeding mothers often wonder if their baby is getting enough calories, since they can't see how many ounces the baby takes. Your baby is doing fine if he or she demands to nurse every 1½ to 2½ hours, appears satisfied after feedings, takes both breasts at each nursing, wets 6 or more diapers each day, and passes 3 or more soft stools per day. Whenever you are worried about your baby's weight gain, take your baby to your physician's office for a weight check. Feeding problems detected early are much easier to remedy than those of long standing. A special weight check 1 week after birth is a good idea for infants of first-time breast-feeding mothers or those concerned about their milk supply. (See BREAST-FEEDING, page 150, or FORMULA-FEEDING, page 156.)

Dealing with Crying

Crying babies need to be held. They need someone with a soothing voice and a soothing touch. You can't spoil your baby during the early months of life. Overly sensitive babies may need a more gentle kind of touch. For additional help on this subject, see CRYING BABY (COLIC), page 253, or PREVENTION OF SLEEP PROBLEMS: BIRTH TO 6 MONTHS, page 257.

Sleep Position

Remember to place your baby in his crib on his back. As of 1992, this is the sleep position recommended by the American Academy of Pediatrics for healthy babies. The back (supine) position reduces the risk of sudden infant death syndrome (SIDS).

Taking Your Baby Outdoors

Your baby can be taken outdoors at any age; just dress for the weather. You already took him outdoors when you left the hospital, and you will be going outside again when you take him for the two-week checkup. Dress him with as many layers of clothing as an adult would wear for the outdoor temperature. The most common mistake is overdressing babies in the summertime. (See also SUNBURN, page 503.) In the wintertime, babies need a hat because they often don't have much hair to protect against heat loss. The idea that cold air or winds can cause ear infections or pneumonia is a myth. Camping and crowds should probably be avoided during the first month of life. Also try to avoid close contact with sick people during the first year of life.

Medical Checkup on the Third or Fourth Day of Life

Early discharge from the newborn nursery has become commonplace for full-term babies. Early discharge means going home before 24 hours after giving birth. In general this is a safe practice if the baby's hospital stay has been uncomplicated. These newborns need to be re-checked 2 days after discharge to see how well they are feeding, urinating, producing stools, maintaining weight, and breathing. They will also be checked for jaundice and overall health. In some cases, this special re-check will be provided in your home.

The Two-Week Medical Checkup

This checkup is probably the most important medical visit during the first year of life. Any physical condition that was not detectable during the hospital stay will usually have developed symptoms by 2 weeks of age. From your baby's height, weight, and head circumference, your child's physician will be able to judge how well your child is growing. This is also the time during which your family is under the most stress of adapting to a new baby. Try to develop a habit of jotting down questions about your child's health or behavior at home. Bring this list with you to office visits for discussion with your child's physician. Most physicians welcome the opportunity to address your agenda, especially if your questions are ones not easily answered by reading or talking with other mothers. If at all possible, have your husband join you on these visits to the physician's office. Most physicians prefer to get to know the father during a checkup rather than during the crisis time of an acute illness. If you think your newborn starts to look or act sick between health supervision visits, be sure to call your physician for help (see SICK NEWBORN: SUBTLE SYMPTOMS, page 130).

NORMAL NEWBORN'S REFLEXES AND BEHAVIOR

Some findings in newborns that concern parents are not signs of illness. The best evidence that these behaviors are harmless is that the infant does not seem to mind them. Most of these reflexes are due to an immature nervous system and will disappear in 3 or 4 months:

- Chin trembling
- Lower lip quivering
- Hiccups
- Irregular breathing (it's normal if your baby is content, the rate is less than 60 breaths per minute, a pause is less than 10 seconds, and your baby doesn't turn blue). Occasionally infants take rapid, progressively deeper, stepwise breaths to expand their lungs completely.
- A seesaw motion of the chest and abdomen with breathing due to the diaphragm moving up and down.
- Passing gas (not a temporary behavior). (See GAS, EXCESSIVE, page 610.)
- Sleep noise from breathing and moving. Also during light sleep, babies can normally whimper, cry, groan, or make other strange noises. If you use a nursery monitor don't overreact to these normal variations in sleep sounds.
- Sneezing
- Spitting up or belching. (See SPITTING UP, page 138, for details.)
- Startle reflex or brief stiffening of the body (also called the Moro or embrace reflex) following noise or abrupt movement
- Straining with bowel movements
- Throat clearing (or gurgling sounds of secretions in the throat)
- Trembling or jitteriness of arms and legs during crying is normal. Convulsions are rare. During convulsions, babies also have jerking or blinking of the eyes, rhythmic sucking of the mouth, and they don't cry. If your baby is trembling and not crying, it could be abnormal. Give her something to suck on. If the trembling doesn't stop during sucking, call your child's physician immediately.
- Yawning

NORMAL NEWBORN'S APPEARANCE

Even after your child's physician assures you that your baby is normal and has all his parts, you may find that he looks a bit odd. He does not have the perfect body you have seen in baby books. Be patient. Most newborns have some peculiar characteristics due to the birth process. Fortunately they are temporary. Your baby will begin to look normal by 1 to 2 weeks of age.

The discussion of these temporary newborn characteristics is arranged by parts of the body. A few minor congenital defects that are harmless but permanent will also be included. Talk with your child's physician if you are not sure that what you see on your baby matches what is described on this list. Better yet, find out when he is coming to the hospital so he can examine your baby in your presence.

Head

Molding—Molding refers to the long, narrow, cone-shaped head that results from passage through a tight birth canal. This compression of the head can temporarily hide the fontanel. The head returns to a normal shape in a few days.

Caput—This refers to swelling on top of the head or throughout the scalp due to fluid squeezed into the scalp during the birth process. Caput is present at birth and clears in a few days.

Cephalohematoma—This is a collection of blood on the outer surface of the skull. It is due to friction between the skull and the pelvic bones during the birth process. The lump is usually confined to one side of the head. It first appears on the second day of life and may increase in size for up to 5 days. It doesn't resolve completely until 2 or 3 months of age.

Anterior Fontanel—The "soft spot" is found in the top front part of the skull. It is diamond-shaped and covered by a thick fibrous layer. Touching this area is quite safe. The purpose of the soft spot is to allow rapid growth of the brain. The soft spot will normally pulsate with each beat of the heart. It normally closes over with bone between 12 and 18 months of age.

Eyes

Swollen Eyelids—The eyes may be puffy due to pressure on the face during delivery. They may be puffy and reddened if silver nitrate eyedrops were used at birth. This irritation should clear in 3 days.

Subconjunctival Hemorrhage—A flame-shaped hemorrhage on the white of the eye (sclera) is not uncommon. It's harmless and due to birth trauma. The blood is reabsorbed in 2 to 3 weeks.

Iris Color—The iris generally comes in variations of four colors: blue, green, gray, or brown. The permanent color of the iris is often uncertain until your baby reaches 6 months of age. White babies are usually born with blue-gray eyes. Black babies are usually born with brown-gray eyes. Children who are going to have dark irises often change color early (by 2 months of age). Children who are going to have light-colored irises usually change closer to 5 or 6 months of age.

Tear Duct, Blocked—See page 140.

Ears

Folded Over—The ears of newborns are commonly soft and floppy. Sometimes one of the edges is folded over. The outer ear will assume normal shape as the cartilage hardens over the first few weeks.

Earpits—About 1 percent of normal children have a small pit or dimple in front of the outer ear. This minor congenital defect is of no importance unless it becomes infected.

Nose

Flattened—The nose can become misshapen during the birth process. It may be flattened or pushed to one side. It will look normal by 1 week of age.

Mouth

Sucking Callus (or Blister)—Sucking callus occurs in the center of the upper lip and is due to constant friction at this point during bottle- or breast-feeding. It will disappear when your child begins cup feedings. Babies can also be born with a sucking callus on the thumb or wrist.

Tongue-Tie—The normal tongue in newborns has a short, tight band that connects it to the floor of the mouth. This band normally stretches with time, movement, and growth. Tongue-tie rarely causes any symptoms (see page 575).

Epithelial Pearls—Little white-colored cysts can occur along the gumline or on the hard palate. These are due to blockage of normal mucous glands from friction associated with sucking. They disappear by 1 to 2 months of age.

Teeth—The presence of a tooth at birth is a rare event. Approximately 10 percent of them are extra teeth without a root structure. The other 90 percent are prematurely erupted normal teeth. The distinction can be made with an X-ray. The extra teeth should be removed, usually by a dentist. The normal teeth need to be removed only if they become loose (with a danger of choking) or if they cause sores on your baby's tongue.

Breasts

Breast Engorgement—Swollen breasts are present during the first week of life in many girl and boy babies. They are caused by the passage of female hormones across the mother's placenta. Sometimes the breast will actually leak a few drops of milk, which is normal. Swollen breasts generally last for 2 to 4 weeks, but longer in breast-fed babies. One breast may become less swollen before the other one by a month or more. Never squeeze the breast because this can cause infection. Be sure to call your child's physician if the swollen breast develops any redness, streaking, or tenderness.

Genitals, Girls

Swollen Labia—The labia minora can be quite swollen in newborns due to the passage of female hormones across the placenta. The swelling will resolve in 2 to 4 weeks.

Hymenal Tags—The hymen can also be swollen due to maternal estrogen and have smooth ½-inch projections of pink tissue. These normal tags occur in 10 percent of newborn girls and slowly shrink over 2 to 4 weeks.

Vaginal Discharge—As the maternal hormones decline in the baby's blood, a clear or white discharge can flow from the vagina during the latter part of the first week of life. Occasionally the discharge will become pink or blood-tinged (false menstruation). This normal discharge should not last more than 2 or 3 days.

Genitals, Boys

Hydrocele—The newborn scrotum can be filled with clear fluid. This fluid usually is squeezed into the scrotum during the birth process. (See SWELLING, GROIN OR SCROTUM, page 632, for details.)

Undescended Testicle—The testicle is not in the scrotum in about 4 percent of full-term newborns. Many of these testicles gradually descend into the normal position during the following months. By 1 year of age only 0.7 percent of all testicles are undescended. These need to be brought down surgically.

Tight Foreskin—Most uncircumcised babies have a tight foreskin that doesn't allow one to see the head of the penis. This is normal and should not be retracted. (See FORESKIN CARE AND PROBLEMS, page 116, for details.)

Erections—Erections occur commonly in the newborn male, as they do at all ages. They are usually triggered by a full bladder. Erections demonstrate that the nerves to the penis are normal.

Urine Stream—The normal urine stream is forceful and may travel 2 feet at what seems like the speed of light. If your son's stream is weak or dribbly or he has to strain to urinate, he needs to see his physician to be sure he doesn't have an obstruction (posterior urethral valves or meatal stenosis).

Bones and Joints

Tight Hips—Your child's physician will test how far your child's legs can be spread apart to be certain the hips are not too tight. Bending the upper legs outward until they are horizontal is called 90 degrees of spread. (Less than 50 percent of normal newborn hips permit this much spreading.) As long as the upper legs can be bent outward to 60 degrees and are the same on each side, they are fine. The most common cause of a tight hip is a dislocation.

Tibial Torsion—The lower legs (tibia) normally curve in because of the cross-legged posture that your baby was confined to while in the womb. If you stand your baby up, you will also notice that the legs are bowed.

Both of these curves are normal and will straighten out after your child has been walking for 6 to 12 months.

Feet Turned Up, In, or Out—Feet can turn any which way because of the cramped quarters inside the womb. As long as the feet are flexible and can be easily moved to a normal position, they are normal. The direction of the feet will become more normal between 6 and 12 months of age.

Long Second Toe—The second toe is longer than the great toe by heredity in some ethnic groups who originated along the Mediterranean.

"Ingrown" Toenails—Many newborns have soft nails that easily bend and curve. However, they are not truly ingrown because they don't curve into the flesh.

Hair

Scalp Hair—Most hair at birth is dark-colored. This hair is temporary and begins to shed by 1 month of age. Some babies lose it gradually while the permanent hair is coming in; others lose it rapidly, and temporarily become bald. The permanent hair will begin to appear by 6 months. It may be an entirely different color from the newborn hair.

Body Hair (Lanugo)—Lanugo is the fine, downy hair that is sometimes present on the back and shoulders. It is more common in premature infants. It is rubbed off with normal friction by 2 to 4 weeks of age.

Skin

See NEWBORN RASHES AND BIRTHMARKS, page 108.
Some bruises on the head or face from the birth process are not unusual. They don't require any treatment.

Minor Birth Defects

Minor defects of the body surface are found at birth in over 13 percent of newborns. Most of them have no other medical significance (e.g., an extra toe). A few are markers for major internal abnormalities. Examples are an ear tag, which can be accompanied by deafness, or a birthmark overlying the midline of the lower back, which can be accompanied by spinal cord defects. Such children need a hearing test and spinal X-rays, respectively.

NEWBORN RASHES AND BIRTHMARKS

After the first bath, your newborn will normally have a ruddy complexion due to the extra-high count of red blood cells. He can quickly change to a pale or mottled blue color if he becomes cold, so keep him warm. During the second week of life, the skin will normally become dry and flaky. In this guideline, the following seven rashes and birthmarks are covered. Save time by going directly to the one that pertains to your baby.

ACNE (see below)
DROOLING RASH (see below)
ERYTHEMA TOXICUM (see page 109)
FORCEPS OR BIRTH CANAL INJURY (see page 109)
MILIA (see page 110)
MONGOLIAN SPOTS (see page 110)
STORK BITES (PINK BIRTHMARKS) (see page 110)

ACNE

More than 30 percent of newborns develop acne of the face—mainly small red bumps. This neonatal acne begins at 3 to 4 weeks of age and lasts until 4 to 6 months of age. The cause appears to be the transfer of maternal hormones just prior to birth. Since it is temporary, no treatment is necessary. Baby oil or ointments make it worse.

DROOLING RASH

Many babies have a rash on the chin or cheeks that comes and goes. This is often due to contact with food and acid that has been spit up from the stomach. Rinsing the face with water after feedings or spitting up can help. Having babies sleep on the back has also reduced the frequency of face rashes.

Other temporary rashes on the face are heat rashes in areas held against the mother's skin during nursing (especially in the summertime).

Change your baby's position more frequently and put a cool washcloth on the area. No baby has perfect skin. The babies in advertisements wear makeup.

ERYTHEMA TOXICUM

More than 50 percent of babies get a rash called erythema toxicum on the second or third day of life. The rash is composed of ½-inch to 1-inch red blotches with one little white or yellow "pimple" in the center. They look like insect bites but are not. They are numerous, keep reoccurring for a week, can be present anywhere on the body surface (except the palms and soles), and look terrible. Their cause is unknown, they are harmless, and they resolve by 2 weeks of age (rarely, 4 weeks).

FORCEPS OR BIRTH CANAL INJURY

If your baby's delivery was difficult, a forceps may have been used to help him through the birth canal. The pressure of the forceps on the skin can leave bruises, scrapes, or damaged fat tissue anywhere on the head or face. Skin overlying bony prominences (such as the sides of the skull bone) can become damaged even without a forceps delivery by pressure from the birth canal. Fetal monitors can also cause scrapes and scabs on the scalp. The bruises and scrapes will be noted on day 1 or day 2 and disappear by 1 to 2 weeks. The fat tissue injury (subcutaneous fat necrosis) won't be apparent until day 5 to day 10. A firm coin-shaped lump, attached to the skin and sometimes with an overlying scab, is the usual finding. This lump may take 3 or 4 weeks to resolve. For any breaks in the skin, apply an antibiotic ointment (no prescription needed) 4 times a day until healed. If it becomes tender to the touch, soft in the center, or shows other signs of infection, call your child's physician.

MILIA

Milia are tiny white bumps that occur on the faces of 40 percent of newborn babies. The nose and cheeks are most often involved, but milia are also seen on the forehead and chin. Although they look like pimples, they are smaller and not infected. They are blocked-off skin pores and will open up and disappear by 1 to 2 months of age. No ointments or creams should be applied to them.

Any true blisters (tiny bumps containing clear fluid) or pimples that occur on the skin (especially in the scalp) during the first month of life must be examined and diagnosed quickly. If they are caused by the herpes virus, treatment is urgent to prevent complications.

MONGOLIAN SPOTS

A Mongolian spot is a bluish-green or bluish-gray flat birthmark that is found in over 90 percent of Native American, Asian, Hispanic, and black babies. They are also seen in 10 percent of white babies, especially those of Mediterranean descent. They occur most commonly over the back and buttocks, although they can be present on any part of the body. They vary greatly in size and shape. They have no relationship to any disease. Most fade away by 2 or 3 years of age, although a trace may persist into adult life.

STORK BITES (Pink Birthmarks)

Flat pink birthmarks (also called capillary hemangiomas or salmon patches) occur over the bridge of the nose, the eyelids, or the back of the neck (stork bites) in more than 50 percent of newborns. The ones in front are often referred to as "angel's kisses." All the birthmarks on the bridge of the nose and eyelids clear completely. Those on the eyelids clear by 1 year of age; those on the bridge of the nose may persist for a few additional years. Most birthmarks on the nape of the neck also clear, but 25 percent can persist into adult life. Those on the forehead that run from the bridge of the nose up to the hairline usually persist into adult life. Laser treatment during infancy should be considered. Talk with your child's physician during regular visits about blood-vessel birthmarks that are raised or increasing in size (strawberry hemangiomas). These run a small risk of bleeding with trauma. They persist until 6 to 8 years of age but go away without any treatment.

NEWBORN SKIN CARE AND BATHING

Bathing

Bathe your baby daily in hot weather, once or twice a week in cool weather. Keep the water level below the navel or give sponge baths until 2 days after the cord has fallen off. (Reasons: Sitting in germy bath water can cause a cord infection. Also, submerging the cord may interfere with its drying out and falling off. Getting it a little wet doesn't matter.) Use tap water without soap or use a nondrying baby soap sparingly. Don't forget to clean the face and neck; otherwise, chemicals from dribbled milk or other foods can build up and cause an irritated rash. Also rinse off the eyelids with clean water. The ear canals don't need cleaning. Putting cotton swabs in them just pushes the earwax back in and leads to blockage and possible hearing problems. The earwax moves outward naturally; just pick off flakes of earwax as they come to the surface. Don't forget to wash the genital area. The male genitals can be washed with either plain water or a mild soap. However, when you wash the inside of the female genital area (the vulva), never use soap, as this tissue is very sensitive. Rinse the area with plain water, wiping from front to back. This practice and the avoidance of any bubble baths before puberty may prevent many urinary tract infections and vaginal irritations. At the end of the bath, rinse your baby well; soap residue can be irritating.

Related Topics

CIRCUMCISION CARE AND PROBLEMS (see page 115)
FORESKIN CARE AND PROBLEMS (see page 116)

Changing Diapers

After wet diapers are removed, just rinse your baby's bottom off with a wet washcloth or diaper wipe. After soiled diapers, you must rinse the bottom under running warm water. You can't clean BMs off the skin with diaper wipes alone. Millions of bacteria will remain and cause diaper rashes. After you finish the rear, cleanse the genital area by wiping front to back with a wet cloth. In boys, stool can hide under the scrotum so rinse more carefully there.

Related Topic

DIAPERS: REUSABLE VERSUS DISPOSABLE (see page 119)

Shampoo

Wash your baby's hair once or twice a week with a special baby shampoo that doesn't sting the eyes. You can use an adult shampoo if you are careful about the eyes. Don't be concerned about hurting the anterior fontanel (soft spot). It is well protected.

Related Topic

CRADLE CAP (see page 132)

Lotions, Creams, and Ointments

Newborn skin normally does not require any ointments or creams. Especially avoid the application of any oil, ointment, or greasy substance, since this will almost always block the small sweat glands and lead to pimples and/or a heat rash. If the skin starts to become dry and cracked, use a baby lotion or moisturizing cream twice a day, just as you would for yourself. For deep cracks (as around the ankles), petroleum jelly is better. Cornstarch powder can be used to prevent rashes in areas of friction (as under the diaper). But avoid talcum powder because of the risk of a serious chemical pneumonia if your baby inhales some of the powder into the lungs.

Umbilical Cord

Try to keep the cord dry. Apply rubbing alcohol to the base of the cord (where it attaches to the skin) twice a day (including after the bath) until 1 week after it falls off. Clean underneath the cord with rubbing alcohol and a cotton swab by lifting and bending the cord to each side. Although using alcohol can delay the separation of the cord by 1 to 2 days, it does prevent cord infections, and that's what's really important. Air exposure also helps with drying and separation, so keep the diaper folded down below the cord area or use a scissors to cut away a wedge of the diaper in front.

Related Topics

UMBILICAL CORD, DELAYED SEPARATION (see page 144)
UMBILICAL CORD, OOZING (see page 144)

Fingernails

Cut the toenails straight across to prevent ingrown toenails, but round off the corners of the fingernails to prevent scratches. Trim the nails once a week after a bath when the nails are softened. Long fingernails or those with sharp corners can cause unintentional scratches to your baby or others. Occasionally a baby scratches the clear part of the eye (causing a corneal abrasion), screams bloody murder, and needs the eye checked and patched by your physician for 1 or 2 days. Use a special baby nail clipper, special baby scissors, or a fine emery board. This job usually takes two people unless you do it while your child is asleep. Having someone cut your baby's nails during breast- or bottle-feeding sometimes works. If you don't hold the finger still, you can cause a cut of the fingertip.

CIRCUMCISION DECISION: PROS AND CONS

Circumcision means cutting off the foreskin or ring of tissue that covers the head (glans) of the penis. If you decide to have your newborn son circumcised, it is usually done the day he goes home from the hospital. Fewer children in the United States are being circumcised now than several years ago. In 1980, 90 percent of American males were circumcised, compared to 60 percent now. The following information should help you decide what is best for your son.

Cultural Aspects

Followers of the Jewish and Islamic faiths perform circumcision for religious reasons. Nonreligious circumcision became popular in English-speaking countries between 1920 and 1950, in hopes it would prevent sexually transmitted diseases. It never caught on in Asia, South America, Central America, or most of Europe. Over 80 percent of the world's male population is not circumcised. Circumcision rates have fallen to 1 percent in Britain, 10 percent in New Zealand, and 30 percent in Canada.

Purpose of the Foreskin

The presence of the foreskin is not some cosmic error. The foreskin protects the glans against urine, feces, and other types of irritation. Although rare events, infections of the urinary opening (meatitis) and scarring of the opening (meatal stenosis) almost exclusively occur in the circumcised penis. The foreskin may also serve a sexual function, namely protecting the sensitivity of the glans. (See FORESKIN CARE AND PROBLEMS, page 116, for information on hygiene.)

Benefits of Circumcision

Some of the reasons you may want to circumcise are:

- Protects against urinary tract infections (UTIs) during the first year of life. However, UTIs are rare and treatable.

- Prevents infections under the foreskin. It also prevents persistent tight foreskin. Both of these problems are rare and are usually due to pulling back the foreskin too often or too hard.

- Decreases the risk of getting some sexually transmitted diseases (STDs) later in life. This includes HIV. However, it does not completely prevent any STD.

- Lowers the risk of cancer of the penis. However, good hygiene offers equal protection against this very rare cancer.

- Keeps your son's appearance "like other boys" or "like his dad." Boys may not mind looking different from other men in their family. However, they do mind being harassed in the locker room or shower about their foreskin. This could happen if most of their buddies are circumcised.

Risks of Circumcision

Some of the reasons not to circumcise include:

- Problems with surgery. Problems that may occur are skin or bloodstream infections, bleeding, gangrene, scarring, and various surgical accidents. One study showed that 1 of every 500 circumcised newborns suffered a serious side effect.

- Pain. The procedure causes pain. However, the doctor can use a local anesthetic around the area to block much of the pain.

- Cost. You may have to pay for the surgery yourself because many insurance companies do not cover the cost.
- You must decide quickly. If you initally decide not to have your son circumcised and then change your mind after your son is 2 months old, the procedure will require a general anesthesia. So try to make your final decision during the first month of life.

Recommendations

Circumcision for religious purposes will continue. Routine circumcision for other boys is open to question. Just because a father was circumcised doesn't mean that this elective procedure must be performed on the son. Since the foreskin comes as standard equipment, I lean toward leaving it intact, unless your son will be attending a school where everyone else is likely to be circumcised. But I don't feel strongly about it. The risks and benefits are both too small to swing the vote either way. This is a parental decision, not a medical decision.

CIRCUMCISION CARE AND PROBLEMS

A circumcision is the surgical removal of most of the normal male foreskin. The incision is initially red and tender; the tenderness should be minimal by the third day. The scab at the incision line comes off in 7 to 10 days. If a Plastibel ring was used, it should fall off by 14 days (10 days on the average). While it cannot fall off too early, don't pull it off, because you may cause bleeding. Any cuts, scrapes, or scabs on the head of the penis may normally heal with yellowish-colored skin if your baby has been jaundiced. This bilirubin in healing tissue is commonly mistaken for an infection or pus.

Call Your Child's Physician

(The following statements apply to recent circumcisions in newborns.)

Immediately If

- The urine comes out in dribbles.
- The urine stream is weak.
- The head of the penis is blue or black.
- The incision line bleeds more than a few drops.

- The circumcision looks infected (yellow pus, spreading redness, red streaks).
- Your baby develops a fever over 100.4°F (38.0°C) rectally.
- Your baby is acting sick.

During Office Hours If

- The circumcision looks abnormal to you.
- You think your child needs to be seen.

Home Care for Circumcision Problems

Treatment

- Plastibel ring type. Gently cleanse the area with water 2 times a day or whenever it becomes soiled. Soap is usually unnecessary. A small amount of petroleum jelly or an antibiotic ointment can be applied to the incision line once a day to keep it soft during healing.
- Incision type (i.e., no plastic ring is present). Remove the dressing (which is usually gauze with petroleum jelly) with warm compresses 24 hours after the circumcision was done. Then care for the area as described for the Plastibel.

Call Your Child's Physician Later If

- It looks infected.
- The Plastibel ring does not fall off by day 14.
- The Plastibel ring starts moving in the wrong direction.
- Your child develops any of the "Call Your Child's Physician" symptoms.

FORESKIN CARE AND PROBLEMS

At birth the foreskin is normally attached to the head of the penis (glans) by a layer of cells. Over the next 5 or 10 years the foreskin will naturally separate from the head of the penis without any help from us. It gradually loosens up (retracts) a little at a time. Normal erections during childhood probably cause most of the change by stretching the foreskin.

The foreskin generally causes no problems. However, overzealous retraction can cause it to get stuck behind the head of the penis (the glans) and cause severe pain and swelling (an emergency). If retraction causes bleeding, scar tissue may form and interfere with natural retraction.

Occasionally the space under the foreskin becomes infected from forced retraction. Most of these problems can be prevented.

Call Your Child's Physician

Immediately If

- The foreskin is pulled back and stuck behind the head of the penis.
- Your child can't pass any urine.
- A fever is present.
- It looks infected (yellow pus, spreading redness, red streaks).
- Your child starts to look or act very sick.

During Office Hours If

- The urine stream is weak or dribbly.
- You think your child needs to be seen.

Normal Foreskin Retraction

Some physicians feel that parents should not engage in any attempts at retraction, but this runs the risk of smegma collection and infection. In general, the foreskin requires minimal care. The following suggestions are a modest attempt to assist the natural process and maintain good hygiene.

- During the first year of life, clean only the outside of the foreskin. Don't engage in any attempts at retraction. Don't put any cotton swabs in the opening.
- Begin gentle partial retraction at 1 or 2 years of age. It can be done once a week during bathing. Perform retraction by gently pulling the skin on the shaft of the penis downward toward the abdomen. This will make the foreskin open up, revealing the end of the glans.
- During retraction, the exposed part of the glans should be cleansed gently with water. Wipe away any whitish material (smegma) that you find there. Smegma is simply the accumulation of dead skin cells that are normally shed from the glans and lining of the foreskin throughout life. Do not use soap or leave soapy water under the foreskin, because this can cause irritation and swelling. (Note: A collection of smegma that is seen or felt through the foreskin, but which lies beyond the level to which the foreskin is retractable, should be left alone until normal separation exposes it.)

- After cleansing, always pull the foreskin forward to its normal position.

- Avoid vigorous retraction, because this can cause pain or bleeding or the foreskin to become stuck behind the head of the penis (paraphimosis). Retraction is excessive if it causes any discomfort or crying.

- By age 5 or 6, teach your son to retract his own foreskin and clean beneath it once a week during bathing to prevent poor hygiene and infection. Gentle reminders are necessary in the early years.

- In summary, foreskin retraction is overdone in our country.

  Keep in mind that any degree of foreskin movement is normal as long as your boy has a normal urine stream. There should be no rush to achieve full retraction. Full retraction always occurs naturally during early puberty. As the foreskin becomes retractable on its own, cleanse beneath it to prevent infections.

NEWBORN EQUIPMENT AND SUPPLIES

Before the baby is born, most parents prepare a special room. They buy a layette including clothing, a place to sleep, feeding equipment, bathing equipment, and changing supplies. This preparation is called nesting behavior. The most common mistake parents on a limited budget can make during this time is buying something they don't need at all or buying an expensive (often fancy) version of an essential piece of equipment. Sometimes parents can borrow some of the equipment from friends or relatives. The first list describes essential equipment. It may also come in handy next time you need a shower gift. The second list includes helpful but nonessential items. The final list reviews items that are unnecessary for most families.

Essential Equipment

Car Safety Seat—Child restraint seats are essential for transporting your baby in a car. They are required by law in all 50 states. Consider buying one that is convertible and usable until your child reaches 40 pounds and 40 inches. Until your child is 1 year old and weighs more than 20 pounds, the car seat faces backward; after that time it is moved to a forward-facing position. While car seats must conform to federal safety standards, they are also ranked by consumer product magazines. Many hospitals have a rental program for car safety seats, which can save you money unless you are going to have several children. (See CAR SAFETY SEATS, page 216, on how to select and use a car seat.)

Crib—Since your baby will spend so much unattended time in the crib, make certain it is a safe one. Federal safety standards require that all new cribs have spaces between the crib bars of 2⅜ inches or less. This restriction is to prevent a child from getting the head or body stuck between the bars. If you have an older crib, be sure to check this distance, which is approximately the width of 3 fingers. Also check for any defective crib bars. The mattress should be the same size as the crib so that your baby's head can't get caught in the gap. It should also be firm and waterproof. Bumper pads are unnecessary because infants rarely strike their head on the railings. The pads have the disadvantage of keeping your baby from seeing out of the crib; they are also something to climb on at a later stage. During the first 2 or 3 months of life it may be more convenient for feeding during the night to have your baby sleep next to your bed in a bassinet, a cradle, or even a drawer or sturdy cardboard box with a firm pad on the bottom.

Bathtub—Small plastic bathtubs with sponge linings are available. A large plastic dishpan will also suffice for the purpose. A molded sponge lining can be purchased separately. As a compromise, a kitchen sink works well if you are careful about preventing your child from falling against hard edges or turning on the hot water, thereby causing a burn. Until the umbilical cord falls off, keep the water level below the navel. Most children can be bathed in a standard bathtub by 1 year of age.

Bottles and Nipples—If you are feeding your baby formula, you will need about ten 8-ounce bottles. While clear plastic bottles cost twice as much as glass ones, you will be glad you bought the unbreakable type the first time you or your baby drops one. If you use disposable bottle liners, you probably will only need 5 bottles. You will also need a corresponding number of nipples. If you prepare more than one bottle at a time, you will need a 1-quart measuring cup and a funnel for mixing a batch of formula.

Diapers: Reusable Versus Disposable—Whether to use disposable or cloth diapers is a controversial issue. Disposable diapers have become almost universal in our country. However, disposable diapers are thrown away after just one use into already overflowing landfills. Let's compare disposable diapers with cloth diapers.

- *Rashes.* Disposable diapers are better for preventing diaper rashes.
- *Pins.* Disposable diapers don't require diaper pins. But you don't need diaper pins for cloth diapers either if you buy diaper covers with Velcro straps.
- *Convenience.* Disposable diapers are very convenient. They make it easier to travel. They are also useful at child care centers. Also, super-absorbent disposable diapers do not leak.
- *Cost.* The average cost of disposable diapers is about 20 cents a diaper. Cloth diapers from a diaper service cost about 12 cents a diaper. If you wash your own diapers the cost is about 3 cents a diaper after the initial purchase. A diaper service will save you over $500 per child. Washing your own diapers will save you over $1,200 per child.
- *Wetness.* If you are breast-feeding you may want to know how often your baby wets so you can check if your baby is getting enough breast milk. It is easy to know when a cloth diaper is wet. It is more difficult to know when a disposable diaper is wet, but you can insert a cotton ball or piece of tissue.

If you choose cloth diapers and plan to wash them yourself, you will need 3 dozen to 6 dozen cloth diapers as well as several pairs of plastic pants. You will also need a diaper pail for storing dirty diapers until washtime. Regardless of the type of diaper you use, bowel movements should be scraped into the toilet for sanitary reasons.

Which type of diaper to use is a controversial issue. My advice is to take advantage of both options. Use cotton diapers when you are at home. Use disposable diapers when you are traveling or as a backup if you are out of the home. Use disposables when your child has diarrhea because they prevent leakage of watery stools. (Some parents prefer disposables at night because they are leakproof.) During the first 2 or 3 months of life, when most mothers are exhausted by new-baby care, consider a diaper service rather than washing the diapers yourself. You will find that modern diaper services are very efficient, provide excellent sterilized diapers, and pick them up once a week.

Pacifier—A pacifier is useful in soothing many babies. To prevent choking, the pacifier's shield should be at least 1½ inches in diameter and the pacifier should be one single piece. Some of the newer ones are made of silicone (instead of rubber), which lasts longer because it doesn't dry out. The orthodontic-shaped pacifiers are accepted by some babies but not by others. (See PACIFIERS, page 367, for additional information.)

Nasal Suction Bulb—A suction bulb is essential for helping young babies with breathing difficulties due to sticky or dried nasal secretions. A suction bulb with a blunt tip is more effective and less likely to irritate the nasal lining than the ones with long tapered tips (which are used for irrigating ears). The best ones on the market have a small clear plastic tip (mucus trap), which can be removed from the rubber suction bulb for cleaning. (See under COLDS, page 550, for proper use.)

Thermometer—A rectal thermometer is most helpful if your baby becomes sick. Digital thermometers display the temperature in 30 seconds and are the most accurate and easiest to read. (See TYPES OF THERMOMETERS, page 436.)

Diaper and Bottle Bag—For traveling outside the home with your baby, you will need an all-purpose backpack to carry the items that allow you to feed your baby and change diapers. They often fit on the back of strollers. Backpacks are more comfortable and convenient than shoulder bags.

High Chair—During the first 6 months of life your baby can be held when he or she is being fed. Once your child can sit unsupported and take solid foods, a high chair is needed. The most important feature is a wide base that prevents tipping. The tray needs to have a good safety latch. The tray should also have adjustable positions to adapt to your infant's growth. A safety strap is critical. Plastic or metal chairs are easier to clean than wooden chairs. Small, portable, hook-on high chairs that attach directly to the tabletop are gaining in popularity. They are convenient and reasonably priced. The ones with a special clamp that keeps your child from pushing the chair off the tabletop with his feet have a good safety record. By 2 years of age, most toddlers can sit in a youth chair.

Training Cup—By the time your child is 1 year old, he will want to hold his own cup. Buy a spillproof one with a weighted base, a lid, and a spout. By 2 years of age, most children can use a regular cup.

Bib—To keep food off your baby's clothes, find a molded plastic bib with an open scoop on the bottom to catch the mess.

Safety Gadgets—Once your child is crawling, you will need electric-outlet safety plugs, cabinet door safety locks, bathtub spout protectors, toilet clamps, plastic corner guards for sharp table edges, and so forth.

Helpful Equipment

The following items mainly provide your child with forms of transportation or special places to play. While they all have some advantages, if none of them is available, your child could also be carried and permitted to play on a blanket on the floor.

Changing Table—Diapers need to be changed 10 to 15 times a day. While a bed can be used for changing, performing this task without bending over prevents back strain. A regular table or buffet covered with a changing pad can work as well as a special changing table.

Automatic Swing—While swings are entertaining to most babies, they are especially helpful for crying babies. They come in windup-spring, pendulum-driven, or battery-powered models. The latter two have quieter mechanisms. Again, a sturdy base and crossbars are important for safety.

Front Carrier or Sling—Front packs or slings are great for new babies. They give your child a sense of physical contact and warmth. The slings are helpful during breast-feeding. They allow you freedom to use your hands. Buy one with head support. Carrying a baby in front after 5 or 6 months of age can cause a backache for the parent.

Backpack—Backpacks are useful in carrying babies who are 5 or 6 months old and have good head support. They are an inexpensive way to carry your baby outside when you go shopping, hiking, or walking anywhere. The inner seat can usually be adjusted to different levels.

Stroller—Another way to transport a baby who has outgrown the front pack is in a baby stroller. The most convenient ones are the umbrella type, which fold up and have at least 1 reclining position. A safety belt is important to keep your baby from standing up and falling. A sun shade is also great for inspiring an afternoon snooze.

Infant Seat or Bouncer Seat—An infant seat is a good place to keep a young baby when he or she is not eating or sleeping. A bouncer seat has the added advantage that your baby can self-initiate movement. Infants prefer this inclined position so they can see what is going on around them. Buy one with a safety strap, but don't substitute it for a car seat. Once children reach 3 to 4 months of age, they can usually tip the infant seat over, so discontinue using it.

Playpen—A playpen is a handy and safe place to leave your baby when you need uninterrupted time to cook a meal or do the wash. Babies like playpens because the slatted or mesh sides afford a good view of the environment. Most playpens are portable and can be used both indoors and outdoors. As with cribs, the slats should be less than 2⅜ inches apart. Bottomless playpens or fencing off areas with plastic walls are gaining in popularity. Your baby should be introduced to the playpen by 4 months of age so that he or she builds up positive associations with it. It is very difficult to introduce a playpen after a baby has learned to crawl. Avoid stringing any objects on a cord across the playpen, because your baby could become entangled in them and strangle.

Gates—A gate is essential if your house has stairways that your baby must be protected from. A gate also helps to keep a child in a specific room with you and out of the rest of the house, as when you are working in the kitchen. Many rooms can be closed off with doors. All gates should be climb-resistant. The strongest gates are spring-loaded.

Humidifier—A humidifier will be helpful in dry climates or areas with cold winters.

Food Grinder—The time comes when your baby must make the transition from baby foods to table foods. A baby-food grinder takes the work out of mashing up table foods. It's as effective as a blender, easier to clean, and less expensive. Food processors have the advantage of allowing you to make larger quantities faster than in a grinder. If you buy all baby food in jars, this item is not necessary.

Teethers—During teething, many infants like to chew on something. Teethers are available in many shapes, sizes, and colors to help comfort and distract your baby.

Unnecessary Equipment

Some baby equipment is usually not worth the investment, but your judgment may be different. You can bathe your baby without a special bathinette. Nursery monitors or intercoms will not prevent crib deaths, may interfere with the learning of self-comforting behavior, and lead to sleep deprivation in the parent. Baby carriages or buggies generally have been replaced by baby strollers, front packs, or backpacks.

You can determine if your baby is being fed enough without a baby scale (see BREAST-FEEDING, page 150, and FORMULA-FEEDING, page 156). An infant feeder is a bottle with a nipple on one end and a piston on the other, used to feed young babies strained foods. They are advertised as a "natural" step between bottle- and spoon-feeding. Since babies don't need any food except formula or breast milk until at least 4 months of age (at which time spoon-feeding works quite nicely), this item is unnecessary and can lead to forced feedings. You can prepare warm formula without a bottle warmer.

Finally, shoes are not needed until your child has to walk outdoors (see SHOES, page 220).

Harmful Equipment: Baby Walkers

Over 40 percent of children who use walkers have an accident requiring medical attention. They get skull fractures, concussions, broken legs and arms, dental injuries, and lacerations. Each year over 8,000 children are treated in emergency rooms for walker-related injuries. There have even been some deaths from major brain injuries. Most of the serious walker injuries occur from falling down a stairway. When a crawling child falls down some unprotected steps, he tumbles and breaks his fall. When a child goes down a stairway in a walker, he accelerates and crash-lands at the bottom. Gates **do not** prevent babies from tumbling down stairs in walkers. Children in walkers have crashed right through them.

Why, then, do parents use walkers? Mainly because children like to be upright, especially after they have learned to sit with support but can't sit alone. Once they learn to crawl, however, they usually prefer to be out of the walker. Some parents believe walkers help children learn to walk. On the contrary, walkers can delay both crawling and walking.

In summary, don't buy a walker. If you already own one, throw it in the trash (don't pass it on to some unwary family). Stationary activity centers are a safe substitute for baby walkers. In fact, in 2001 the

American Academy of Pediatrics recommended a ban on the manufacture and sale of infant walkers, and some countries have already done so.

SLEEP POSITION FOR YOUNG INFANTS: PREVENTING SIDS

The Safest Sleep Position: On the Back

The American Academy of Pediatrics (AAP) recommends that all healthy infants sleep on their backs the first 6 months of life. Studies have shown sleeping on the back reduces the risk of sudden infant death syndrome (SIDS). SIDS is the sudden, unexplained death of a healthy infant. Thousands of babies die each year from SIDS. Typically, a baby dies from SIDS while sleeping. The AAP started recommending that babies sleep on their backs in 1992. Eighty percent of parents now follow this advice and there has been a 40 percent drop in the rate of SIDS.

Reasons Sleeping on the Stomach Increases the Risk of SIDS

Laying a baby on his stomach puts pressure on his jawbone. This causes the airway in the back of the mouth to become narrower. Also, if the baby sleeps on a soft surface, the nose and mouth may sink in, so the child breathes from a small pocket of stale air.

If your baby sleeps on his stomach, the risk of SIDS is 3 to 9 times greater. Sleeping on the side is safer than the stomach but still has twice the risk of SIDS as the back position. If you use a child-care center or baby-sitter, be sure they know how important it is to put your baby on his back to sleep.

Other Ways to Reduce the Risk of SIDS

You can also reduce the risk of SIDS by:

• Using a firm mattress (avoid soft bedding). Young infants should never be placed on waterbeds, sheepskin, soft pillows, bean-bag chairs, or other soft, spongy surfaces. Also makes sure that none of these surfaces is placed in the crib. Even if you place your child to sleep on her back, it is possible that she will roll over during the night.

• Not letting your baby sleep in your bed during the first 12 months. The mattresses in most adult beds are too soft for babies. Blankets and pillows in your bed also increase the risk. The SIDS rate is 20 times higher for babies sleeping in an adult bed compared to sleeping in a crib.

• Breast-feeding your baby, if possible.

• Protecting your infant from exposure to cigarette, cigar, or pipe smoke.

Disadvantages to Sleeping on the Back

There are 2 minor disadvantages. When lying on the back, young infants are more likely to have a startle reflex (Moro reflex) that awakens them. Swaddling your baby in a snug blanket can prevent this. To swaddle your baby use the 3-step "burrito-wrap" technique. Start with your baby lying on the blanket and the arms at the sides. Then (1) pull the left side of the blanket over the body and tuck, (2) pull the bottom up, and (3) pull the right side over and tuck.

The other disadvantage is that some babies get a flattening of the back of the head. Prevent this cosmetic problem by changing the baby's head position slightly during sleep. Also provide some "tummy time," as described next.

Tummy Time During Playtime

It is good for your baby to spend some time on his stomach when he is awake during the day. The back position is only recommended for bedtime and naps. Letting your baby play on his stomach helps strengthen his shoulder muscles. Changing positions also keeps your baby's head from becoming flattened from lying in the same position all of the time.

SIBLING RIVALRY TOWARD A NEWBORN

Sibling rivalry refers here to the natural jealousy of older siblings toward the arrival of a new baby. The peak age for sibling rivalry is 1 to 3 years, but it also can be seen in 4- and 5-year-olds. Not surprisingly, most children prefer to be the only child during these years. Basically, they don't want to share your time and affection. The arrival of a new baby is especially stressful for the firstborn. The jealousy stems from the sibling's viewpoint that the newcomer receives all the attention, visitors, gifts, and special handling. The most common symptom is lots of demands for attention. The sibling wants to be held and carried about, especially when the mother is busy with the newborn. Other symptoms include regressive behavior, such as thumbsucking, wetting, or soiling. Aggressive behavior, such as handling the baby roughly, can also occur. All of these symptoms are normal. While some can be prevented, the remainder can be improved within a few months.

Prevention of Sibling Rivalry

During Pregnancy

- Prepare the older sibling for the newcomer. Talk about the pregnancy. Have him or her feel your baby's movements.
- Try to find a hospital that provides sibling classes where children can learn about babies and sharing parents.
- Try to give your older child a chance to be around a new baby so that he has a better idea of what to expect.
- Encourage your older child to help you prepare the baby's room.
- Move your older child to a different room or big bed several months before the baby's birth so she won't feel pushed out by the new baby. If he or she will be enrolling in a play group or nursery school, start it well in advance of the delivery.
- Praise your older child for mature behavior, like talking, using the toilet, feeding or dressing himself, and playing games.
- Don't make any demands for new skills (such as toilet training) during the 2 months just preceding the delivery. Even if your child appears ready, postpone these changes until your child has made a good adjustment to the new baby.
- Tell your child where she'll go and who will care for her when you go to the hospital if she won't be home with her father.
- Read books together about what happens during pregnancy as well as after the baby is born.
- Look through family photographs and talk about your older child's first year of life.

In the Hospital

- Call your older child daily from the hospital.
- Try to have your older child visit you and the baby in the hospital. Many hospitals are accepting this practice.

- If your older child can't visit you, send him a picture of the new baby.
- Encourage Dad to take your youngster on some special outings at this time (e.g., to the park, zoo, museum, or fire station).

Coming Home

- When you enter your home, spend your initial moments with the older sibling. Have someone else carry the new baby into the house.
- Give the sibling a gift "from the new baby."
- Ask visitors to give extra notice to the older child. Have your older child unwrap the baby's gifts.
- From the beginning, refer to your newborn as "our baby."

The First Months at Home

- Give your child the extra attention he needs. Help him feel more important. Try to provide at least 30 minutes a day of exclusive, uninterrupted time. Hire a baby-sitter and take your older child outside or look through his baby album with him. Make sure that the father and relatives spend extra time with him during the first month. Give him lots of physical affection throughout the day. If your older child wants more outings than you can provide, ask a relative or hire a sitter to take him places.
- Encourage your older child to touch and play with the new baby in your presence. Allow him to hold the baby while sitting in a chair with side arms. Avoid such warnings as "Don't touch the baby." Newborns are not fragile and it is important to show your trust. However, you can't allow your older child to carry the baby until he reaches school age.
- Enlist your older child as a helper. Encourage him to help with baths, dry the baby, get a clean diaper, find a pacifier, or fetch toys. At other times encourage him to feed or bathe a doll as you do the same for the baby. Emphasize how much the baby "likes" the older sibling. Make comments such as: "Look how happy she gets when you play with her," or "You can always make her laugh."
- When you are busy attending to the baby, try to include your older child by talking with him. When you are nursing or bottle-feeding, read a story, play a game, or do a puzzle with your older child.
- Accept regressive behaviors (such as thumbsucking or clinging) as things your child needs to do temporarily. Do not criticize them.

- Intervene promptly for any aggressive behavior. Tell him, "We never hurt babies." Send your child to time-out for a few minutes. Don't spank your child or slap her hand at these times, because if you hit her, she will eventually get back at the baby. For the next few weeks don't leave the two of them alone.
- If your child is old enough, encourage her to talk about her mixed feelings about the new arrival. Give her an alternative behavior: "When you're upset with the baby, come to me for a big hug."

Spacing Children—The ideal spacing between children is 2 or more years. Children less than 2 years apart tend to have a greater number of negative interactions. Another reason for spacing children is that a separate, special early childhood enhances development. More importantly, spacing children increases the ability of the parents to cope successfully with child-rearing. The care of three or more preschoolers can be overwhelming, with all their needs to be fed, toileted, dressed, and entertained.

Call Your Child's Physician During Office Hours If

- Your older child tries to hurt the baby.
- Regressive behavior doesn't improve by 1 month.

NEWBORN PROBLEMS

SICK NEWBORN: SUBTLE SYMPTOMS

A newborn is a baby less than 1 month old. Newborns mainly eat, sleep, cry a little, and need lots of love and their diapers changed frequently. If a newborn is ill, the symptoms can be subtle. Also, a newborn can deteriorate quickly. If a newborn is sick at all, the illness can be serious.

Call Your Child's Physician Immediately If

- Your baby is less than 1 month old and sick in any way (e.g., vomiting, cough, poor color, or diarrhea).
- Your newborn's appetite or suck becomes poor.
- Your newborn sleeps excessively—for instance, past feeding times.
- Your newborn cries excessively. (See also CRYING BABY [COLIC], page 253.)
- Your newborn develops a fever over 100.4°F (38.0°C) rectally or over 99.0°F (37.2°C) axillary.
- Your newborn's temperature drops below 96.8°F (36°C) rectally, or below 95.4°F (35.5°C) axillary. (Note: In general, do not take an infant's temperature unless he feels hot or looks sick.)
- You have other urgent questions.

Related Topic

NORMAL NEWBORN'S REFLEXES AND BEHAVIOR (see page 102)

SICK INFANT: JUDGING THE SEVERITY OF ILLNESS

During the first 2 years of a child's life, most parents feel inexperienced and inadequate in determining how sick their child is during a cold or other infection. Since these children can't talk, they can't help much with diagnosis. How sick your child looks or acts is much more relevant than the level of fever. Also, some children look much better 30 to 40 minutes after the fever is lowered with medicine.

Guidelines to Severe Illness

Call Your Child's Physician Immediately If

- Your child is a newborn (less than 1 month old) with any sign of illness (exception: mild nasal congestion).
- Your child looks or acts very sick.
- Your child cannot be made to smile, or hardly responds.
- Your child refuses to play.
- Your child is too weak to sit up or stand.
- Your child cries constantly for more than 3 hours.
- Your child cries more when you touch him or hold him.
- The cry becomes high-pitched or strange-sounding.
- The cry becomes a weak whimper or moan.
- Your child cannot sleep for more than 30 minutes at a time.
- Your child cannot be comforted for more than 30 minutes at a time.
- Your child cannot be fully awakened.
- The breathing becomes labored.
- The mouth and lips become bluish.
- The skin becomes grayish.

Related Topics

CRYING BABY (COLIC) (see page 253)
FEVER (see page 427)
SICK NEWBORN: SUBTLE SYMPTOMS (see page 130)

CRADLE CAP

Symptoms and Characteristics

Cradle cap is a commmon scalp condition in babies. Cradle cap appears as pink patches with oily, yellow scales or crusts on the scalp. It often begins in the first weeks of life.

Cause—Cradle cap is probably caused by hormones from the mother that crossed the placenta before birth. The hormones cause the oil glands in the skin to become overactive and release more oil than normal. This causes the dead skin cells that normally fall off to "stick" to the skin and form yellow crusts and scales. It's not caused by poor hygiene.

Expected Course—With treatment it will clear up in a few weeks. Without treatment it will go away on its own after several months. Cradle cap is not contagious and does not recur.

Call Your Child's Physician During Office Hours If

- The rash has spread beyond the scalp.
- A weepy, raw rash is present behind the ears.
- You have other questions.

Home Care for Cradle Cap

Antidandruff Shampoo—Buy an antidandruff shampoo (no prescription needed) at the drugstore. Wash your baby's hair with it twice a week. While the hair is lathered, massage your baby's scalp with a soft brush or a rough washcloth for 5 minutes. Don't worry about hurting the soft spot; it's well protected. Once the cradle cap has cleared up, use a regular shampoo twice a week.

Softening Thick Crusts—If the scalp is very crusty, put some baby oil or olive oil on the scalp 1 hour before washing to soften the crust. Wash all the oil off, however, or it may worsen the cradle cap.

Resistant Cases—If the rash is red and irritated, apply 1 percent hydrocortisone cream (no prescription needed) once a day. Rub in a small amount. After 1 hour wash the area with soap and water. Do this for no longer than 7 days.

Call Your Child's Physician Later If

- The cradle cap lasts more than 2 weeks with treatment.

DIAPER RASH

Symptoms and Characteristics

- Any rash in the skin area covered by a diaper

Causes—Almost all children get diaper rashes. Diaper rashes are more common in children with fair, sensitive skin, especially in redheads. Most diaper rashes are due to the prolonged contact with wetness, bacteria, digestive enzymes, and ammonia that comes with wearing diapers. The skin irritants (such as ammonia) are made by the action of bacteria from bowel movements on certain chemicals in the urine. Bouts of diarrhea cause rashes in almost all children. Diaper rashes occur less frequently with disposable diapers. You don't have to switch diapers, however, to clear up a diaper rash. Diaper rashes are worse with airtight plastic pants, so avoid them until your baby makes enough urine to soak through the diaper. In societies where diapers aren't worn, babies don't acquire diaper rashes.

Allergies to soaps, detergents, whiteners, and bleaches are very rare, and you needn't worry about these.

Expected Course—With proper treatment these rashes are usually better in 3 days. If they do not respond, a yeast infection (candida) has probably occurred. Suspect this if the rash becomes bright red and raw, covers a large area, and is surrounded by red dots. You will need a special cream for yeast infections.

Call Your Child's Physician

Immediately If

- The diaper rash has any big (larger than 1 inch across) blisters or open sores.
- Your child's face is bright red and tender to the touch.
- Your child looks or acts very sick.

Within 24 Hours If

- The diaper rash is a solid bright red.
- Open, weeping sores are present.
- The rash is raw or bleeding.
- Pimples, blisters, boils, or crusts are present.

- An unexplained fever is present.
- The rash causes enough pain to interfere with sleeping.
- The rash has spread beyond the diaper area.
- Your child is male and circumcised *and* the end of the penis has a sore or scab (meatal ulcer).
- You think your child needs to be seen.

Home Care for Diaper Rash

Change Diapers Frequently—The key to successful treatment is keeping the area dry and clean so it can heal itself. Check the diaper about every hour, and if it is wet or soiled, change it immediately. Exposure to stools causes most of the skin damage.

Increase Air Exposure—Leave your baby's bottom exposed to the air as much as possible each day. Practical times are during naps or after bowel movements. Put a towel or diaper under your baby. When the diaper is on, fasten it loosely so that air can circulate between it and the skin. Avoid airtight plastic pants until the rash is gone. Put a towel between you and your baby's bottom instead. Warm air from a hair dryer for 3 minutes on the low setting can encourage healing.

Rinse the Skin with Warm Water—All you need is warm tap water. Washing with soap following every diaper change will dry out and irritate the skin. A mild soap is needed only after bowel movements to help remove the film of bacteria left on the skin. After using a soap, rinse thoroughly and pat dry. If the diaper rash is quite raw, use lukewarm water soaks in a tub for 15 minutes 3 times a day. Adding 1 or 2 tablespoons of baking soda to the water may help healing. (Note: Running water is far superior to disposable diaper wipes. Disposable wipes should be used only for traveling, but avoid those containing alcohol.) You can't clean BMs off the skin with diaper wipes alone. Millions of bacteria will remain and cause diaper rashes.

Nighttime Care of Diaper Rashes—Awaken once during the night to change your baby's diaper until the rash is better. Avoid plastic pants at night.

Creams and Ointments—Creams are optional. Most babies don't need any cream unless the diaper rash becomes infected with yeast. In addition, unless the hygiene measures outlined above are carried through, creams can't help the rash. If your baby's skin is dry and cracked, apply an ointment after a diaper change to protect the skin. A barrier protection ointment is also needed when your child has diarrhea. If your child develops a heat rash, change to a cream.

After the diaper rash is healed, cornstarch powder can be used to prevent the shiny pink diaper rash that comes from friction against the diaper. Recent studies show that cornstarch does not encourage yeast infections. Avoid talcum powders because of the risk of serious pneumonia if your baby breathes some in.

Yeast Infections—If the rash is bright red or does not respond to 3 days of warm-water cleansing and air exposure, suspect a yeast infection. Apply Lotrimin cream (no prescription necessary) 4 times a day or after each bottom rinse for BMs.

Washing Cloth Diapers—If you wash cloth diapers yourself, you will need to use a laundry bleach (such as Clorox) to sterilize them. During the first wash cycle, use the hot temperature setting and any detergent. During the second cycle, use warm water and 1 cup of bleach. Unlike bleach, vinegar is not effective in killing germs.

Call Your Child's Physician Later If
• The rash isn't much better in 3 days.
• Your child develops any of the "Call Your Child's Physician" symptoms.

Prevention of Diaper Rashes
• Change the diapers frequently, especially after bowel movements (BMs).
• Rinse the skin with plenty of warm water after BMs.
• Fasten the diaper loosely, so air can circulate under the diapers.
• Give your child some genes for industrial-strength skin.

JAUNDICE OF THE NEWBORN

Jaundice is a yellow (or orange) color of the skin and the whites of the eyes (the sclera). The yellow color is due to increased amounts of a yellow pigment in the body called bilirubin. Bilirubin is produced by the normal breakdown of red blood cells. Bilirubin accumulates in the body if the liver doesn't excrete it into the intestines at a normal rate.

Types of Jaundice

Physiological Jaundice—Physiological (normal) jaundice occurs in more than 50 percent of babies. An immaturity of the liver leads to a slowdown in the processing of bilirubin. The jaundice first appears at 2 to 3 days of age. By 5 or 6 days, the liver kicks in. The jaundice usually disappears by 1 to 2 weeks of age and the levels reached are harmless. In prematures, jaundice occurs more commonly and lasts longer.

Breast-Feeding Jaundice—Breast-feeding jaundice occurs in 5 to 10 percent of newborns. It's caused by an insufficient intake of breast milk (calories and fluid). It follows the same pattern as physiological jaundice.

Breast-Milk Jaundice—Breast-milk jaundice occurs in 1 to 2 percent of breast-fed babies. It is caused by a special substance (inhibitor) that some mothers produce in their breast milk. This substance increases the resorption of bilirubin from the intestines. This type of jaundice starts at 4 to 7 days of age, and may last from 3 to 10 weeks normally.

Blood-Group Incompatibility (Rh or ABO Problems)—If a baby and mother have different blood types, sometimes the mother produces antibodies that destroy the newborn's red blood cells. This causes a sudden buildup in bilirubin in the baby's blood. This type of jaundice usually begins during the first 24 hours of life. High levels of bilirubin may be reached. Rh problems formerly caused the most severe form of jaundice but now are preventable with an injection of RhoGAM to the mother within 72 hours after delivery, which prevents her from forming antibodies that might endanger her subsequent babies.

Treatment of Jaundice

Treatment of Severe Jaundice—High levels of bilirubin can cause deafness, cerebral palsy, or brain damage in some babies. High levels usually occur with blood-type differences. These complications can be prevented by lowering the bilirubin using phototherapy (blue light that breaks down bilirubin in the skin). In many communities, phototherapy can be used in the home. In rare cases where the bilirubin reaches dangerous levels, an exchange transfusion may be used. This technique replaces the baby's blood with fresh blood. Physiological jaundice does not rise to levels requiring this type of treatment.

Treatment of Breast-Feeding Jaundice—Try to increase breast milk production. Read about breast-feeding or talk with a lactation specialist. Increase the frequency of feedings. Nurse your baby every 1½ to 2½ hours during the day. Don't let your baby sleep more than 4 hours at night without a feeding. If you must supplement, supplement with formula, not glucose water.

Treatment of Breast-Milk Jaundice—The bilirubin level can rise above 20 in less than 1 percent of children with breast-milk jaundice. Usually elevations to this level can be prevented by more frequent feedings. Nurse your baby every 1½ to 2½ hours. Since the bilirubin is carried out of the body in the stools, passing frequent BMs is helpful. If your baby sleeps more than 4 hours at night, awaken him for a feeding. If your baby goes more than 24 hours without a BM, insert a lubricated thermometer carefully ½ inch (1 cm) into the anus and gently move it from side to side a few times to stimulate a BM.

Occasionally the bilirubin will not come down with frequent feedings. In this situation the bilirubin level can be reduced by alternating each breast-feeding with formula-feeding for two or three days. (Supplementing with glucose water is not helpful for moving the bilirubin out of the body.) Talk to your baby's physician for the latest instructions on lowering bilirubin in these babies. Whenever you miss a nursing, be sure to use a breast pump to keep your milk production flowing. Breast-feeding should not be permanently discontinued because of breast-milk jaundice. Once the jaundice clears, you can return to full breast-feeding and you needn't worry about the jaundice coming back.

Treatment of Physiological Jaundice—No treatment is necessary other than normal feedings.

Call Your Baby's Physician

Immediately If
- Jaundice is noticed during the first 48 hours of life.
- The jaundice involves the arms or legs.
- Your baby looks deep yellow or orange.
- Your baby hasn't passed urine in more than 8 hours.
- Your baby develops a fever over 100.4°F (38.0°C) rectally.
- Your child also starts to look or act sick (see page 130).

- Your baby passes less than 3 good-sized BMs per day.
- Your baby has less than 6 wet diapers per day.

During Office Hours If
- The color gets deeper after day 7.
- The jaundice is not gone by day 14.
- Your baby is not feeding well or gaining weight well.

Since newborns are going home earlier than they used to, the parent must be more involved with observations about the degree of jaundice. The amount of yellowness is best judged by viewing your baby unclothed in natural light by a window. Most babies look more yellow under house lighting. The best way to check for yellow skin is to press on it with your finger, then assess the underlying color before the pink color returns.

SPITTING UP (Reflux)

Symptoms and Characteristics
Spitting up (also called regurgitation or reflux) is the effortless spitting up of one or two mouthfuls of stomach contents. Formula or breast milk just rolls out of the mouth, often with a burp. It usually happens during or shortly after feedings. It begins in the first 2 weeks of life.

Spitting up is harmless as long as your infant doesn't spit up large amounts that interfere with normal weight gain. This condition is also called gastroesophageal reflux.

Similiar Condition—If appropriate, turn directly to the guideline for VOMITING, page 619. Vomiting is more forceful, causes discomfort, and involves larger amounts.

Cause—Spitting up results from poor closure of the valve (ring of muscle) at the upper end of the stomach. Spitting up is normal and harmless for over half of all babies. It becomes a problem if it causes poor weight gain (from spitting up large amounts), choking with aspiration, or acid damage to the lower esophagus (esophagitis).

Expected Course—Spitting up improves with age. By 7 months of age, most reflux has decreased or is gone. The reasons for this are probably because the baby is old enough to sit up or is eating solid foods. By the time your baby has been walking for 3 months, even severe reflux should be totally cleared up.

Call Your Child's Physician

Immediately If

- You see blood in the spit-up material.
- The spitting up causes your child to choke or stop breathing for more than 10 seconds.

During Office Hours If

- Your baby does not gain weight normally.
- You have other concerns or questions.

Home Care for Spitting Up

Feed Smaller Amounts—Overfeeding always makes spitting up worse. If the stomach is filled to capacity, spitting up is more likely. Give your baby smaller amounts (at least 1 ounce less than you have been giving). Your baby doesn't have to finish a bottle. Wait at least 2½ hours between feedings because it takes that long for the stomach to empty itself.

Avoid Pressure on Your Child's Abdomen—Avoid tight diapers. They put added pressure on the stomach. Don't put pressure on the stomach or play vigorously with him right after meals.

Burp Your Child to Reduce Spitting Up—Burp your baby two or three times during each feeding. Do it when he pauses and looks around. Don't interrupt his feeding rhythm in order to burp him. Keep in mind that burping is less important than giving smaller feedings and avoiding tight diapers. Also cut back on pacifier time. Constant sucking can pump the stomach up with air.

Keep Your Child in a Vertical Position After Meals—After meals, try to keep your baby in an upright position using a front pack, backpack, or swing for 30 minutes. When your infant is in an infant seat, keep him from getting scrunched up by putting a pad under his buttocks so he's more stretched out. After your child is over 6 months old, a jumpy seat or infant activity station can be helpful for maintaining an upright posture after meals.

Use a Proper Sleep Position—Most infants with spitting-up problems can sleep on their backs, the position recommended by the American Academy of Pediatrics to reduce the risk of SIDS. Try to elevate the head of the bed a bit. Sleeping in a car seat with also reduce reflux. Again, put a pad under his bottom so your baby isn't too scrunched up. If your child is having breathing problems (choking or sleep apnea), talk to your doctor.

Add Rice Cereal to Formula—If your infant still spits up large amounts after all the previous treatments have been tried, you can try thickening the formula with rice cereal. Add 1 level teaspoon of rice cereal to each ounce of formula. You will need to make the nipple opening bigger.

Call Your Child's Physician Later If
- Your baby doesn't seem to improve with these approaches.

TEAR DUCT, BLOCKED

Symptoms and Characteristics
- A continuously watery eye.
- Tears run down the face even without crying.
- During crying, the nostril on the blocked side remains dry.
- Onset in the first 2 months of life.
- The eye is not red and the eyelid is not swollen.

If your child's symptoms are different, call your child's physician for help.

Cause—Your child probably has a blocked tear duct (dacryostenosis). This means that the channel that normally carries tears from the eye to the nose is blocked. Although the obstruction of the tear duct is present at birth, the occasional delay in onset of symptoms can be explained by the delay in tear production until the age of 3 or 4 weeks in a few babies.

Expected Course—This is a common condition that affects 6 percent of newborns. Both sides are blocked 30 percent of the time. Over 90 percent of tear ducts open up spontaneously by the time the child is 12 months of age. If the obstruction persists beyond 12 months of age, an ophthalmologist can open it using a special probe.

Call Your Child's Physician

Immediately If
- The eyelids are red or swollen.
- A red lump appears at the inner lower corner of the eyelid.

Within 24 Hours If

- The eyelids are stuck together with pus after naps.
- Lots of yellow discharge is present.
- The cornea (clear part) becomes cloudy.
- You think your child needs to be seen.

Home Care for Blocked Tear Duct

Preventing Infections—Because of poor drainage, eyes with blocked tear ducts easily become infected. The infected eye produces a yellow discharge. To keep the eye free of infection, massage the lacrimal sac (where tears collect) twice a day to empty it of old fluids. Always wash your hands carefully before doing this. The lacrimal sac is in the inner lower corner of the eye. Start at the inner corner of the eye and press upward using a cotton swab. The massage technique is somewhat controversial. Some physicians recommend massaging downward in hopes of washing out the plug that blocks the lower duct. Some physicians recommend not massaging the sac at all. Massage in either direction must be done gently, since it may irritate the eyelid tissue and contribute to infection. If the eye becomes infected, it is very important to begin antibiotic eyedrops.

Call Your Child's Physician Later If

- Your child reaches 12 months of age and the eye is still watering.
- Your child develops any of the "Call Your Child's Physician" symptoms.

Related Topic

RED OR PINKEYE WITH PUS (see page 527)

THRUSH

Symptoms and Characteristics

- White, irregularly shaped patches
- Coats the insides of the lips and cheeks and sometimes the tongue (if the only symptom is a uniformly white tongue, it's due to a milk diet, not thrush)

- Adherent to the mouth (cannot be washed away or wiped off easily like milk curds)
- Your child is bottle-fed or breast-fed.
- Thrush causes mild discomfort.

If your child's symptoms are different, call your physician for help.

Cause—Thrush is caused by a yeast (called candida) that grows rapidly on the lining of the mouth in areas abraded by prolonged sucking (as when a baby sleeps with a bottle or pacifier). A large pacifier or nipple can more easily injure the lining of the mouth. Antibiotics also make a child more susceptible by eliminating the normal bacteria in the mouth. Note: Thrush is not contagious, since yeast do not invade normal tissue.

Call Your Child's Physician During Office Hours If

- An unexplained fever is present.
- You think your child needs to be seen.

Home Care for Thrush

Nystatin Oral Medicine—The drug for clearing up thrush is nystatin oral suspension. It requires a prescription. Call your physician during office hours with the name and telephone number of your pharmacy. Some physicians will want to examine the child before prescribing. Give 1 ml of nystatin 4 times a day. Place it in the front of the mouth on each side; it doesn't do any good once it's swallowed. If the thrush isn't responding, rub the nystatin directly on the affected areas with a cotton swab or gauze wrapped on your finger. Apply it after meals, or at least don't feed your baby anything for 30 minutes after application. Keep this up for at least 7 days, or until all thrush has been gone for 3 days. If you are breast-feeding, apply nystatin to any irritated areas on your nipples. Thrush is not a reason to stop nursing.

Decrease Sucking Time to 20 Minutes per Feeding—Prolonged sucking (as when a baby sleeps with a bottle or pacifier) can abrade the lining of the mouth and make it more prone to a yeast infection. If sucking on a nipple is painful for your child, temporarily use a cup. If the thrush recurs and your child is bottle-fed, switch to a nipple that has a different shape and is made from silicone.

Restrict Pacifier Use—Eliminate the pacifier temporarily, except when it's really needed to calm your baby. If your infant is using an orthodontic pacifier, switch to a smaller, regular one. Special washing of bottle nipples or pacifiers is not helpful or necessary.

Diaper Rash Associated with Thrush—If your child has an associated diaper rash, assume it is due to yeast. Buy some Lotrimin cream (no prescription necessary) and apply it 4 times a day. (Also see the guidelines on DIAPER RASH, page 133.)

Call Your Child's Physician Later If
- Your child refuses to drink.
- The thrush becomes worse on treatment.
- The thrush lasts more than 10 days with treatment.
- Your child develops any of the "Call Your Child's Physician" symptoms.

UMBILICAL CORD, BLEEDING

A few drops of blood at the point of separation of the cord is common. The area may bleed a few times from the friction of the diaper or your baby's normal movements against clothing.

Call Your Child's Physician Immediately If
- The clamp has come undone and the cord is bleeding.
- Any spot of dried blood is the size of a quarter or greater.
- Bleeding doesn't stop after 10 minutes of direct pressure.

Home Care

Apply Direct Pressure—The bleeding usually stops by itself or can easily be stopped by direct pressure with a sterile gauze.

Call Your Child's Physician Later If
- Re-bleeding continues for more than 3 days.
- Your child develops any of the "Call Your Child's Physician" symptoms.

UMBILICAL CORD, DELAYED SEPARATION

Although most cords fall off between 10 and 14 days of age, an occasional cord may stay for 6 weeks. Cords can also hang by a strand of tissue for 2 or 3 days. Eventually they all fall off by themselves, so just be patient about it. In the meantime:

Home Care

Clean the base of the cord (where it attaches to the skin) with rubbing alcohol twice a day. To do this properly, you must lift the cord stump away from the body surface. Recent studies showed that cords fall off 2 days earlier if allowed to heal naturally without any alcohol. Therefore if the cord is still attached at 2 weeks of age, stop using alcohol. Prior to that, do use alcohol to prevent cord infections. Also help the cord dry faster by keeping the diaper folded below it. An easier approach if you're using disposables is to cut off a wedge of diaper with a scissors so the cord is uncovered. In addition, give sponge baths or keep the level of bath water below the cord until it falls off.

Call Your Child's Physician Later If

- The cord is still attached after 6 weeks. (Note: The cord can't fall off too early.)
- You have any other questions.

Related Topic

If the cord begins to look infected, see UMBILICAL CORD, OOZING, below.

UMBILICAL CORD, OOZING

The umbilicus (navel) is oozing, moist, or may even have some dried pus on the surface. Sometimes the cord has already fallen off; more often it is still attached and contributes to the problem. Your baby probably has a superficial infection of the navel from surface bacteria. It usually can be cleared up fairly quickly. Infection of the umbilicus must be treated with respect because of the risk of spreading to the liver or the abdominal cavity.

Call Your Child's Physician

Immediately If

• Red streaks develop on the normal skin surrounding the navel.

• Pimples or blisters appear around the navel.

• Lots of drainage is coming out of the navel.

• Your baby develops a fever over 100.4°F (38.0°C) rectally.

• Your baby acts sick.

During Office Hours If

• There is a nubbin of tissue inside the navel that looks abnormal to you.

• You think your child needs to be seen.

Home Care for Umbilical Cord Oozing

Cleansing the Umbilicus—Four times a day, clean the navel with rubbing alcohol for several minutes. Use a cotton swab and be vigorous about it. The umbilical area does not have any sensation, so the alcohol won't sting. If the cord is still present, you must clean underneath it by lifting it and bending it to each side. If the cord has fallen off, you can pour some alcohol into the depression and remove it after 2 or 3 minutes. It takes that long to kill all the bacteria. Although using alcohol can delay the separation of the cord by 1 to 2 days, it does prevent cord infections, and that's what's really important. Air exposure and dryness help healing, so be sure to keep the diaper folded down below the cord area or cut off a wedge of diaper (if you use disposables) with a scissors.

Common Mistakes—Do not put talcum powder on the umbilicus; it can cause irritation and tissue reaction (talc granulomas).

Call Your Child's Physician Later If

• The infection seems to spread.

• The umbilical area is not completely dry and clean by 48 hours on this treatment.

• Your child develops any of the "Call Your Child's Physician" symptoms.

Related Topics

UMBILICAL CORD, BLEEDING (see page 143)
UMBILICAL CORD, DELAYED SEPARATION (see page 144)

UMBILICAL HERNIA

An umbilical hernia is a navel that bulges (pops out) with crying or straining. The bulge may disappear when your baby is quiet. If you feel the area with your finger, you will find a small round opening in the muscles of the abdominal wall. During pregnancy, the umbilical cord's blood vessels pass through this ring, and normally it closes off after birth. Umbilical hernias are very common. They are not painful and they never break. Crying does not make them any bigger or last any longer. Most close spontaneously by school age. Half of the persistent ones close by adolescence.

Treatment

No treatment is needed unless the hernia persists beyond age 5 or 6. At that age, day (outpatient) surgery can be performed to close the defect if the hernia presents a cosmetic problem, the hernia always protrudes, or the defect is larger than 2 cm (about 1 inch) across. The smaller ones usually continue to close. Covering them with tape, a coin, or a belly band does not speed healing and can lead to a skin rash or infection. Your child's physician will be glad to check the hernia on regular office visits. The only complication (which occurs in far less than 1 per 1,000 cases) is getting a loop of intestine stuck in the opening. If you think this has happened (if, for instance, the hernia becomes hard, tender, and won't go back in), call your child's physician immediately for help.

Related Topic

SWELLING, GROIN OR SCROTUM (see page 632)

IV. Health Promotion: Keeping Your Child Healthy

FEEDING, EATING, AND GROWTH

NORMAL GROWTH

Normal growth is one of the best indicators of good health and nutrition. Normal heights and weights, however, are difficult to define. Short parents tend to have short children. Tall parents tend to have tall children. For any given height, an ideal weight can be determined from a growth chart. An infant with failure to thrive is one who is underweight for his height. A child with obesity is one who is overweight for his height.

Your child's physician weighs and measures your child on each health supervision visit. These numbers are plotted on a standard growth chart. If you wish, ask your child's doctor for a copy. Your child's growth rate over time tells us the most about his nutritional health. The following facts and figures may answer some of your questions about normal growth.

Average Newborns (Full-Term)
Weight: 7 pounds, 5 ounces (normal range: 6 to 10 pounds)
Length: 20 inches (50 cm) (normal range: 18½ to 21½ inches)
Head circumference: 13.8 inches (35 cm) (normal range: 33 to 37 cm)
A premature baby is born before 37 weeks gestation and usually weighs
  less than 5½ pounds (2.5 kilograms)

Average Weights at Different Ages
5 months: double birthweight
12 months: triple birthweight
2 years: quadruple birthweight
Remember: 1 pound = 16 ounces; 1 kilogram = 2.2 pounds

Average Heights at Different Ages
4 years: double birth length
13 years: triple birth length
Remember: 1 foot = 12 inches; 1 inch = 2.5 centimeters

Predicting Adult Heights
The adult height cannot be predicted, except with a growth chart. If a child has consistently followed one height line or trajectory (e.g., the 30th percentile), he or she probably will end up in the 30th percentile as an adult. The only formula that can give an approximate adult height is based upon the "mid-parent height." But again there is tremendous normal variation. The mid-parent height is the sum of the parents' heights divided by 2. Using this number:

Adult height (boys) = mid-parent height plus 2½ inches
Adult height (girls) = mid-parent height minus 2½ inches

BREAST-FEEDING

Babies who are breast-fed have fewer infections (especially diarrhea) and allergies during the first year of life than babies who are fed formula. Breast milk is also inexpensive, sterile, and served at the perfect temperature. Breast-feeding becomes especially convenient when a mother is traveling with her baby. Overall, breast milk is nature's best food for young babies. Even if you need to return to work early, breast-feeding for 1 month can be beneficial for your baby. After you return to work, breast-feeding can be continued or discontinued, depending on your situation.

How Often to Feed
The baby should nurse for the first time in the delivery room. The second feeding will usually be at 4 to 6 hours of age, after he awakens from a deep sleep. Until your milk supply is well established and your baby is gaining weight (usually 2 weeks), nurse your infant whenever he cries or seems hungry ("demand feeding"), usually 1½ hours or greater. After your baby is 1 month of age and your milk supply is in, babies can receive

adequate breast milk by nursing every 2 to 2½ hours. If your baby cries and less than 2 hours have passed, he can be rocked or carried in a front pack, but if you're convinced he's hungry, feed him. If the baby is sleeping and more than 3 hours have passed since the last feeding during the day, wake him up. During the night, allow one 5-hour interval if the baby is sleeping. Your baby will not gain adequately unless he nurses 8 or more times per day initially. The risks of continuing to nurse at short intervals (less than 1½ hours) is that "grazing" will become a habit, your baby won't be able to sleep through the night, and you won't have much free time. Although your baby's appetite will determine feeding intervals (called demand feeding), the guidelines for bottle feedings per day (see page 156) generally also apply to breast-feeding after the first 2 months of life.

How Long per Feeding

During the first week, bring in your full milk supply by offering both breasts with each feeding. Try 10 minutes on the first breast and as long as your baby wants on the second breast (at least 10 minutes). Alternate which breast you start on. Needing to stimulate your baby to take the second breast is normal.

After your milk supply has come in (by day 8 at the latest), encourage your baby to nurse as long as she wants to on the first breast (up to 20 minutes) (reason: to get the high-fat, calorie-rich hind milk). You can tell your baby has finished the first breast when the sucking slows down and your breast becomes soft. Then offer the second breast if she's interested. Alternate the breast you start with at each feeding.

How to Know Your Baby Is Getting Enough Breast Milk

In the first couple weeks, if your baby has 3 or more good-sized bowel movements per day and 6 or more wet diapers per day, he is receiving a good supply of breast milk. (Caution: Infrequent bowel movements are not normally seen before the second month of life.) In addition, most babies will act satisfied after completing a feeding. Your baby should be back to birth weight by 10 days of age if breast-feeding is going well. Therefore, the 2-week checkup by your baby's physician is very important. The presence of a letdown reflex is another indicator of good milk production.

The Letdown Reflex

The letdown reflex is the automatic release of breast milk into the milk ducts. A letdown reflex develops after 2 to 3 weeks of nursing and is indicated by tingling or milk ejection in the breast just before feeding (or when you are thinking about feeding). It also occurs in the opposite breast while your baby is nursing. Initally, milk letdown may require 60 to 90 seconds of sucking. Letdown is enhanced by adequate sleep, adequate fluids, a relaxed environment, and reduced stress (such as lower expectations about how much housework needs to be done). If your letdown reflex is not present yet, take extra naps and ask your husband and friends for more help. Also consider calling the local chapter of La Leche League (a support group for nursing mothers) or a lactation nurse at your hospital.

Supplemental Bottles

Try not to offer your baby any routine bottles during the first 4 weeks after birth because this is when you establish your milk supply. Good lactation depends on frequent emptying of the breasts. Supplemental bottles can take away from sucking time on the breast. If your baby is not gaining well, see your physician or a lactation specialist for a weight check and advice.

After your baby is 4 weeks old and nursing is well established, you should offer your baby a bottle of expressed milk or 1 ounce of formula once a day so he can become accustomed to the bottle and the artificial nipple. Once your baby accepts bottle feedings, you can occasionally leave your baby with a sitter and go out for the evening or return to work outside the home. You can use pumped breast milk that has been refrigerated or frozen. Keep 1 or 2 bottles of expressed breast milk (or ready-to-use formula) handy in case you are unexpectedly delayed and your baby is hungry. If practical, supplement with pumped breast milk rather than commercial formula, since taking formula will cancel some of the advantages that breast milk provides.

Extra Water

Babies do not routinely need extra water. Even when they have a fever or the weather is hot and dry, breast milk provides enough water.

Pumping the Breasts to Relieve Pain or Collect Milk

Severe engorgement (severe swelling) of the breasts decreases milk production. To prevent engorgement, nurse your baby more often.

Also, compress the area around the nipple (the areola) with your fingers at the start of each feeding to soften the areola. For milk release, your baby must be able to grip and suck on the areola as well as the nipple. Every time you miss a feeding (e.g., if you return to work outside the home), pump your breasts. Also, whenever your breasts hurt and you are unable to feed your baby, pump your breasts until they are soft. If you don't relieve engorgement, your milk supply can dry up in 2 to 3 days.

A breast pump is usually necessary. Sometimes pumping can be done by hand; ask someone to teach you the Marmet technique. If you use a breast pump, you will also need some initial assistance.

Pumped breast milk can be stored for 6 days in a refrigerator or up to 6 months in a freezer. To thaw frozen milk, put the container of breast milk in the refrigerator, where it will take a few hours to thaw, or place it in a pan of warm water until it has warmed up to the temperature your baby prefers. Never warm it up in a microwave or boiling water; this would destroy the protective antibodies.

Sore Nipples

Clean a sore nipple with water after each feeding. Do not use soap or alcohol, because they remove natural oils. At the end of each feeding, the nipple can be coated with some breast milk to keep it lubricated. For cracked nipples, apply 100 percent lanolin (no prescription needed) after feedings. Try to keep the nipples dry with loose clothing, air exposure, and nursing pads.

Sore nipples usually are due to poor latching on and a feeding position that causes undue friction on the nipple. Position your baby so he directly faces the nipple without turning his neck. At the start of the feeding, compress the nipple and areola between your thumb and index finger so your baby can latch on easily. Throughout the feeding, hold your breast from below so the nipple and areola aren't pulled out of your baby's mouth by the weight of the breast. Slightly rotate your baby's body so his mouth applies pressure to slightly different parts of the areola and nipple at each feeding.

Start your feedings on the side that is not sore. If one nipple is extremely sore, temporarily limit feedings to 10 minutes on that side. The pain won't improve, however, until the previous instructions on correct latching on and positioning are carried out.

Vitamin D

Breast milk contains all the necessary vitamins and minerals except vitamin D and flouride. Starting at 2 months of age, all breast-fed babies need to receive 200 IU per day of vitamin D, according to the 2003 policy of the American Academy of Pediatrics' Committee on Nutrition. Until separate vitamin D drops become available, use drops containing vitamins A, D, and C (available without a prescription) in a dosage of 0.5 ml.

Some parents prefer not to give vitamin D. They should consider the following facts: Most full-term light-skinned babies who are breast-fed do receive adequate vitamin D from its natural production in their skin during sun exposure. To prevent inadequate vitamin D and soft bones (rickets), all premature babies need vitamin D each day. Full-term dark-skinned babies regardless of the climate and light-skinned babies who have little sun exposure (less than 10 minutes of sun exposure twice a week) also need vitamin D supplements.

Fluoride

Breast milk doesn't contain fluoride. From 6 months to 16 years of age, children need fluoride to prevent tooth decay. Give 0.25 mg of fluoride drops each day. In the United States this is a prescription item that you can obtain from your child's physician. When you discontinue breast-feeding, also stop the fluoride supplements if your municipal water supply contains fluoride and your baby drinks 4 to 8 ounces of water per day.

Breast milk contains adequate iron during the first 6 months of life. To prevent iron deficiency anemia, add iron-containing solid foods (e.g., cereals) to your infant's diet after 4 months of age.

Vitamins for the Mother

A nursing mother can take a multivitamin tablet daily if she is not following a well-balanced diet. She especially needs 400 units of vitamin D and 1,200 mg each of calcium and phosphorus per day. A quart of milk (or its equivalent in cheese or yogurt) can also meet this requirement.

The Mother's Medications

Almost any drug a breast-feeding mother consumes will be transferred in small amounts into the breast milk. Therefore, try to avoid any drug that is not essential, just as you did during pregnancy. Fortunately, the dose your baby receives via breast milk is much less than he or she would receive if we were prescribing it for the baby. Therefore, side effects are uncommon.

Some commonly used drugs that are safe for you to take while nursing are acetaminophen, ibuprofen, penicillins, cephalosporins, erythromycin, stool softeners, antihistamines, cough drops, nose drops, eyedrops, and skin creams. Most nonprescription cold and cough medicines are fine, but avoid pseudoephedrine because it can reduce milk production in some mothers. Sulfa drugs can be taken once your baby is beyond 4 weeks of age *and* not jaundiced. Avoid aspirin because of a small risk of Reye's syndrome. Consult your physician about all other drugs. Acceptable drugs should nonetheless be taken immediately following breast-feedings so that their level in the breast milk at the time of the next feeding is low. A high intake of caffeine-containing beverages or herbal teas (or excessive smoking of cigarettes) can cause restlessness, crying, even diarrhea. Alcohol can cause drowsiness, so limit yourself to 1 beer or glass of wine per day. Diarrhea in the baby can also be caused by some laxatives (but not by chocolate). Used in moderation, these products shouldn't cause any symptoms. The effect on the baby of foods in the mother's diet is overrated.

Burping

Burping is optional. While it may decrease spitting up, air in the stomach does not cause pain. Burping twice during a feeding and for about 1 minute is plenty. Try burping your baby when switching from the first breast to the second and at the end of the feeding.

Cup-Feeding

Introduce your child to a cup at approximately 6 months of age. Total weaning to a cup will probably occur somewhere between 9 and 18 months of age, depending on your baby's individual preference (see WEANING, NORMAL, page 162). Regardless of when you start, weaning should proceed gradually. If you discontinue breast-feeding before 9 months of age, switch to bottle-feeding first. If you stop breast-feeding after 9 months of age, you may be able to go directly to cup-feeding.

Call Your Child's Physician During Office Hours If

- Your baby doesn't seem to be gaining adequately (a weight check at 1 week is a good idea for babies of mothers who are breast-feeding for the first time).
- Your baby has less than 6 wet diapers per day.

- During the first month, your baby has less than 3 bowel movements per day.
- You suspect your baby has a food allergy.
- You need to take a medication that was not discussed.
- Your breasts are not full (engorged) before feedings by day 5.
- You have painful engorgement or sore nipples that do not respond to the recommended treatment.

Call Your Obstetrician If

- You have a fever.
- You have a breast infection.

FORMULA-FEEDING

Breast milk is best for babies, but breast-feeding isn't always possible. Use an infant formula if:

- You decide not to breast-feed.
- You need to discontinue breast-feeding and your infant is less than one year of age.
- You need to supplement your infant's diet occasionally after breast-feeding is well established.
- Note: If you want to breast-feed but feel your milk supply is insufficient, don't discontinue breast-feeding. Instead seek help from your physician or a lactation nurse.

Infant Formulas

Infant formulas are a safe alternative to breast milk. Infant formulas have been designed to resemble breast milk and fulfill the nutritional needs of your infant by providing all known essential nutrients in their proper amounts. Most formulas are derived from cow's milk. A few are derived from soybeans and are for infants who may be allergic to the type of protein in cow's milk. Bottle-feeding can provide your child with all the emotional benefits and many of the health benefits of breast-feeding. Bottle-fed babies grow as rapidly and are as happy as breast-fed babies. A special advantage of bottle-feeding is that the father can participate.

Use an infant formula that is iron-fortified to prevent iron deficiency anemia, as recommended by the American Academy of Pediatrics. The amount of iron in iron-fortified formula is small and won't cause any symptoms. The formulas that are not iron-fortified (with the confusing name of low-iron formulas) are not appropriate for any infant and will eventually be removed from the market.

Most infant formulas are available in three forms: powder, concentrated liquid, and ready-to-serve liquid. Powder and ready-to-serve liquid are the most suitable forms when formula is used to supplement breast milk, because concentrated liquid forces you to prepare 26 ounces at a time. Powder and concentrated liquid formulas are less expensive per feeding than ready-to-serve formulas.

Preparing Infant Formulas

The concentrated formulas are mixed 1:1 with water. The powdered formulas are mixed 2 ounces of water per each level scoop of powder. Never make the formula more concentrated by adding extra powder or extra concentrated liquid. Never dilute the formula by adding more water than specified. Careful measuring and mixing ensure that your baby is receiving the proper formula.

If you use tap water for preparing formula, use only water from the cold water tap. If the water hasn't been used for several hours, let the water run for 2 minutes before you use it. (Old water pipes may contain lead-based solder, and lead dissolves more in warm water or standing water.) Fresh, cold tap water from city water supplies is considered safe for infants in this country. If you make one bottle at a time, you don't need to use boiled water. Just heat cold tap water to the preferred temperature. If you have well water, either boil it for 10 minutes (plus one minute for each 1,000 feet of elevation) or use distilled water until your child is 6 months of age.

If you prefer to prepare a batch of formula, you must use boiled or distilled water and closely follow the directions printed on the side of the formula can. This prepared formula should be stored in the refrigerator and must be used within 48 hours. Boiling water for a single bottle went out in the 1970s.

Whole Cow's Milk

Whole cow's milk should not be given to babies before 12 months of age for many reasons, including increased risks of iron deficiency anemia and allergies. The ability to drink from a cup doesn't mean you should switch to cow's milk. While it used to be acceptable to introduce whole cow's milk after 6 months of age, recent studies have shown that infant formula is the optimal food for non-breast-fed babies during the first year of life. (Note: Evaporated milk mixed with water becomes whole milk.)

Skim milk or 2 percent milk should not be given to babies before 2 years of age, because the fat content of regular milk (approximately 3.5 percent butterfat) may be needed for rapid brain growth. (Note: Powdered milk mixed with water becomes skim milk.) The American Academy of Pediatrics recommends that parents not use raw (even though certified) milk for children because of the risk of transmitting serious infectious diseases. Stay with the safety record of pasteurized milk products.

Traveling

When traveling, use powdered formula for convenience. Put the required number of scoops in a bottle, add cold tap water, and shake. A more expensive alternative is to use individual, throwaway bottles of ready-to-use formula sold by the formula companies for this purpose. This product can be stored at room temperature and avoids problems with contaminated water.

Formula Temperature

In the summertime, many children prefer cold formula. In the wintertime, most prefer warm formula. By trying various temperatures, you can find out which your child prefers. If you do warm the formula, be certain to check the temperature of a few drops on your skin before giving it to your baby. If it is too hot, it will burn your baby's mouth. Microwave heating deserves special caution, as high temperatures can be reached quickly.

Amounts and Schedules

Newborns usually start with 1 ounce per feeding, but by 7 days they may take 3 ounces. The amount of formula that most babies take per feeding (in ounces) can be calculated by dividing your baby's weight (in pounds) in half. Another way to calculate the ounces per feeding is to add 3 to your baby's age (in months) with a maximum of 8 ounces per feeding at 5 or 6 months of age. The average ounces of formula a baby needs in 24 hours is the baby's weight in pounds multipied by 2. The maximal amount recommended per day is 32 ounces. Overfeeding can cause vomiting, diarrhea, or excessive weight gain. If your baby needs more than this amount and is not overweight, consider starting solids.

If your baby is not hungry at some of the feedings, the feeding interval should be increased. Although the feeding schedule should be flexible, the following guidelines apply to most babies:

From Birth to 1 Month
- 6 to 8 milk feedings per day
- No more than every 2½ hours
- To reduce night feedings, awaken your baby if he naps for more than 3 consecutive hours during the day.

From 1 to 3 Months
- 5 or 6 milk feedings per day
- No more than every 3 hours

From 3 to 6 Months
- 4 or 5 milk feedings per day
- No more than every 3 hours

By 6 Months
- 4 milk feedings a day (solids with 3 of these)
- 2 snacks per day

By 9 Months
- 3 milk feedings a day (solids with all meals)
- 3 snacks per day (see SOLID [STRAINED] FOODS, page 167)

Length of Feeding

A feeding shouldn't take more than 20 minutes. If it does, you are overfeeding your baby or the nipple is clogged. A clean nipple should drip about 1 drop per second when the bottle of formula is inverted.

Formula Storage

Prepared formula should be stored in the refrigerator and must be used within 48 hours. Prepared formula left at room temperature for more than 1 hour should be discarded. At the end of each feeding, discard any formula left in the bottle, because it is no longer sterile.

Extra Water

Babies do not routinely need extra water. They can be offered a bottle of water twice a day, however, when they have a fever or the weather is hot and dry.

Feeding Position

Feeding should be a relaxing time—a time for you to provide both food and comfort for your baby. Make sure that both you and the baby are comfortable:

• Your arm is supported by a pillow.

• Your baby is in a semi-sitting position supported in the crook of your arm.

• The bottle is tilted so that the nipple and the neck of the bottle are always filled with formula. (This prevents your baby from taking in too much air.)

Burping

Burping is optional. It doesn't decrease crying. While it may decrease spitting up, air in the stomach does not cause pain. If you burp your baby, be sure to wait until he reaches a natural pause in the feeding process. Burping 2 times during a feeding and for about 1 minute is plenty. More burping may be needed if your baby is a "spitter" (see SPITTING UP [REFLUX], page 138). To reduce the amount of swallowed air, hold the bottle tipped at an angle that keeps the nipple full of formula.

Breast Discomfort in Bottle-Feeding Mothers

Your breasts will make milk for several days even though you chose not to breast-feed. Breast milk comes in on day 2 or 3 and swollen breasts can be painful for a few days. Here is what to do:

• *Ibuprofen.* Take 400 mg of ibuprofen 3 times per day to reduce pain and swelling.

• *Ice.* Apply a cold pack or ice bag wrapped in a wet cloth to your breasts for 20 minutes as often as needed. This will reduce milk production. Do not apply heat because it will increase milk production.

• *Pumping.* For moderate pain, hand express or pump off a little breast milk to reduce your pain. While pumping breast milk can increase milk production, doing this to take the edge off your discomfort is not detrimental.

• *Binding.* Binding the breasts by wearing a tight bra or elastic wrap is no longer recommended. It can increase the risk of breast infections (mastitis).

Vitamins and Iron

Infant formulas contain all of your baby's vitamin and mineral requirements except for fluoride. In our country, the most common cause of anemia in children under 2 years old is iron deficiency (largely because it's not present in cow's milk). Therefore, be sure to use iron-fortified formula (not the low-iron type). (Note: All soy-based formulas are iron-fortified.) Iron also can be provided at 4 months of age by adding iron-fortified cereals to the diet.

Fluoride

From 6 months to 16 years of age, children need fluoride to prevent dental caries. If the municipal water supply contains fluoride and your child drinks at least 1 pint each day, this should be adequate. Otherwise, fluoride drops or tablets should be given. Formula-fed infants should receive fluoride supplements without vitamins. This is a prescription item that can be obtained from your child's physician. Try to give fluoride on an empty stomach because mixing it with milk reduces its absorption to 70 percent.

Cup-Feeding

Introduce your child to a cup at approximately 4 to 6 months of age. Total weaning to a cup will probably occur somewhere between 9 and 18 months of age, depending on your baby's individual preference (see WEANING, NORMAL, page 162).

Baby Bottle Tooth Decay: Prevention

Sleeping with a bottle of formula, breast milk, cow's milk, juice, or any sweetened liquid in the mouth can cause severe decay of the newly erupting teeth. The sugar in these drinks is converted to acid by the normal bacteria of the mouth. Since liquids tend to pool in the mouth during sleep, the acid etches the enamel. Prevent this tragedy by not using the bottle as a daytime or nighttime pacifier. If you cannot discontinue the nighttime bottle or replace it with a pacifier, fill it with water. This approach will prevent tooth decay, although it may not improve sleep problems. Of note, dental decay has also resulted when a mother repeatedly falls asleep with her baby asleep on the breast.

NIGHTTIME FEEDINGS

The first weeks are crazy. Your baby will probably need to be fed every 1½ to 3 hours. His voracious appetite precludes any schedule. You'll be up for feedings at least twice each night. But by 1 month of age you can start to shape his feeding behaviors. Here are some tips:

- After the first month of life and your milk supply is in, keep daytime feeding intervals to at least 2 hours. More frequent daytime feedings (such as hourly) lead to frequent awakenings at night. For every time you nurse your baby, there should be 4 or 5 times that you snuggle him without nursing. Don't let him get into the bad habit of nursing every time you hold him (called grazing) or every time he fusses (called comfort nursing).

- Place your baby in the crib drowsy but partially awake. His last waking memory needs to be of the crib, not of the breast or bottle. If he learns how to put himself to sleep, then the only reason he will cry at night is if he's hungry.

- Make middle-of-the-night feedings brief and boring, compared to daytime feedings. Don't turn on the lights or talk to him. Feed your child quickly and quietly. Provide that extra rocking and playtime during the day.

- In the meantime, you need to learn to take naps during the day to survive these nighttime demands. Also lower your housekeeping standards.

- With this approach and a little luck, your bottle-fed baby will give up middle-of-the-night feedings between 2 and 4 months of age. Your breast-fed baby will do the same between 4 and 6 months of age.

WEANING, NORMAL

The definition of weaning is replacing the bottle or breast (i.e., nipple feedings) with cup-drinking and solid foods. Weaning occurs easily and smoothly unless the breast or bottle has become overly important to the child. Then we have to deal with weaning resistance (see page 164).

How to Prevent Weaning Problems

Children normally develop a reduced interest in breast and bottle feedings between 6 and 12 months of age if they are also taking cup and spoon feedings. Brazelton has found that the onset of crawling (at 7 or 8 months) and walking (at 11 or 12 months) are associated with a diminished interest in breast-feeding. Both of these bursts in motor development provide a natural time to start weaning. Between 12 and 18 months of age the parent often has to initiate weaning, but the child is still receptive. After 18 months of age, weaning is usually resisted because the child has become overly attached to the breast or bottle. If your child shows a lack of interest in nipple feedings at any time after 6 months of age, start to phase them out.

You can tell that your baby is ready to begin weaning when he or she throws the bottle down, takes only a few ounces of milk and then stops, chews on the nipple rather than sucking it, refuses the breast, or nurses for only a few minutes, then wants to play. The following steps make early natural weaning at 9 to 12 months most likely:

- Keep formula feedings to 4 times a day or less after your child reaches 6 months of age. (Some breast-fed babies may need 5 feedings per day until 9 months of age.) Even at birth, formula feedings should be kept to 8 times per day or less.

- Give older infants their daytime milk at mealtimes with solids. Once your child is on just 4 milk feedings a day, be sure 3 of them are given at mealtimes with solids (rather than as part of a pre-nap-time ritual). Your child can have the fourth feeding prior to going down for the night.

- After your baby is 4 weeks old and breast-feeding is well established, offer him a bottle of expressed breast milk or formula once a day. This experience will help your baby become accustomed to a bottle so that you can occasionally leave him with a sitter. This step is especially important if you will be returning to work or school. The longer after 2 months you wait to introduce the bottle, the more strongly your infant will initially reject it. If you wait until 4 months of age, the transition period may take up to 1 week. Once bottle feedings are accepted, you will need to continue them at least 3 times a week to maintain acceptance.

- Hold your child to soothe her discomfort and stress rather than nursing her. Try to separate simple holding from holding with nursing. You can comfort your child and foster a strong sense of security and trust without nursing every time she is upset and not hungry. If you don't follow this guideline, your child will learn to eat whenever she is upset and you may become an "indispensable mother."

- Don't let the bottle or breast substitute for a pacifier. Learn to recognize the need for nonnutritive sucking when your young baby is not hungry. At these times encourage him to suck on a pacifier or thumb rather than giving him food. Feeding your baby every time he needs to suck can lead to obesity.

- Don't let the bottle or breast become a substitute for a transitional (security) object at bedtime. Your child should be able to go to sleep at night without having a breast or bottle in his mouth. He needs to learn how to put himself to sleep. If he doesn't, he will develop sleep problems that require the parents' presence during the night.

- Don't let your child hold the bottle or take it to bed. Your child should think of the bottle as something that belongs to you; hence, she won't protest giving it up, since it never belonged to her in the first place.

- Don't let a bottle become a daytime toy. Don't let your child carry a bottle around as a companion during the day. This habit will keep him or her from engaging in more stimulating activities.

- Offer your child formula or breast milk in a cup by 6 months of age. For the first few months your child will probably accept the cup only after he or she has had some milk from bottle or breast. However, by 9 months of age your child should be offered some milk from a cup before bottle feedings.

- Help your baby become interested in foods other than milk by 4 months of age. Introduce solids by spoon by 4 months of age. Introduce finger foods by 8 months of age. As soon as your child is able to use finger foods, have him or her sit with the family during mealtime. This custom will stimulate your child to ask for other foods that he sees you eating. Consequently, his or her interest in exclusive milk feedings will diminish.

WEANING PROBLEMS

When Is Weaning Delayed or Abnormal?

Breast-feeding or bottle-feeding can be considered prolonged after about 18 months of age. The older toddler who only occasionally nurses or bottle-feeds doesn't necessarily need any pressure to give up the breast or bottle. Delayed weaning should be considered abnormal only if it is causing one or more of the following types of harm:

- Refusal to eat any solids after 6 months of age
- Anemia confirmed on a routine screening test at 1 year of age

- Tooth decay (baby-bottle caries)
- Obesity from overeating
- Daytime withdrawal and lack of interest in play because the child is always carrying a bottle around
- Frequent awakening at night for refills of a bottle
- Inability to stay with a baby-sitter because the child is exclusively breast-fed and refuses a bottle or cup

If any of these criteria apply to your baby, proceed to the following section. Otherwise, continue to nipple-feed your baby when he or she wants to (but 4 times or less a day) and don't worry about complete weaning at this time.

How to Eliminate Excessive Breast- or Bottle-Feeding

To decrease breast- or bottle-feedings to a level that won't cause any of the preceding side effects, take the following steps:

- Reduce milk-feedings to three or four a day. When your child comes to you for additional feedings, give him extra holding and attention instead. Get your child on a schedule of three main meals per day plus two or three nutritious snacks.
- Introduce cup-feedings if this was not done at 6 months of age. Cup-feedings are needed as substitutes for breast- or bottle-feedings regardless of the age at which weaning occurs. The longer the infant goes without using a cup, the less willing he will be to try it. Starting daily cup-feedings by 5 or 6 months of age is a natural way to keep breast- or bottle-feedings from becoming overly important.
- Immediately stop allowing your child to carry a bottle around during the day. The companion bottle can interfere with normal development that requires speech or two-handed play. It also can contribute to problems with tooth decay. You can tell your child, "It's not good for you" or "You're too old for that."
- Immediately stop allowing your child to take a bottle to bed. Besides causing sleep problems, taking a bottle to bed carries the risk of causing tooth decay. You can offer the same explanations as above.

Once you have made these changes, you need not proceed further unless you wish to eliminate breast- or bottle-feedings completely. Attempt total weaning only if your family is not under stress (such as might be caused by moving or some other major change) and your child is not in crisis (e.g., from illness or trying to achieve bladder control). Weaning from breast or bottle to cup should always be done gradually and with love. The "cold turkey" or abrupt withdrawal approach will only make your child angry, clingy, and miserable. While there is no consensus about the best time to wean, there is agreement about the appropriate technique.

How to Eliminate Breast-Feeding Completely

- Offer formula in a cup before each breast-feeding. If your child refuses formula, offer expressed breast milk. If that fails, add some flavoring he likes to the formula. If your child is older than 12 months, you can use whole milk. Some infants won't accept a cup until they've nursed for several minutes. (Note: If your child is less than 9 months of age and you wish to discontinue breast-feeding, follow this procedure but try switching to bottle-feedings rather than a cup.)
- Gradually eliminate breast-feeding. First, eliminate the feeding that is least important to your child (usually the midday one). Replace it with a complete cup-feeding. About once a week drop out one more breast-feeding. The bedtime nursing is usually the last to be given up, and there's no reason why you can't continue it for months if that's what you and your child want. Some mothers prefer to wean by decreasing the length of feedings. Shorten all feedings by 2 minutes each week until they are 5 minutes long. Then eliminate them one at a time.
- Relieve breast engorgement. Since the breast operates on the principle of supply and demand, reduced sucking time eventually reduces milk production. In the meantime, express just enough milk to relieve breast pain resulting from engorgement. (This is better than putting your baby to the breast for a minute, because she probably won't want to stop nursing.) Remember that complete emptying of the breast increases milk production. An acetaminophen or ibuprofen product also may help relieve discomfort.
- If your child asks to nurse after you have finished weaning, respond by holding her instead. You can explain that "the milk is all gone." If she has a strong sucking drive, more pacifier time may help.

How to Eliminate Bottle-Feeding Completely

- Offer formula in a cup before each bottle-feeding. Use whole milk if your child is 1 year of age or older.

- Make the weaning process gradual. Eliminate 1 bottle-feeding every 3 to 4 days, depending on your child's reaction. Replace each bottle-feeding with a cup-feeding and extra holding.

- Eliminate bottle-feedings in the following order: midday, late afternoon, morning, and bedtime. The last feeding of the day is usually the most important one to the child. When it is time to give up this feeding, gradually reduce the amount of milk each day over the course of a week.

- After you have completed the weaning process, respond to requests for a bottle by holding your child. You can explain that bottles are for little babies. You may even want to have your child help you carry the bottles to a neighbor's house. If your child has a strong need to suck, offer a pacifier.

Call Your Child's Physician During Office Hours If

- Your child is over 6 months of age, won't eat any food except milk, and won't drink from a cup.

- You think your child has anemia.

- This approach to weaning has not been successful after trying it for 1 month.

- Your child is over 3 years old.

- You have other questions or concerns.

SOLID (STRAINED) FOODS

Age for Starting Solid Foods

The best time to begin using a spoon is when your baby can sit with some support and voluntarily move his head to engage in the feeding process—i.e., when he or she is ready. This time is usually between 4 and 6 months of age. From a nutritional standpoint, breast milk and iron-fortified formulas meet all of your baby's needs until 4 to 6 months of age. He or she needs nothing else. Introducing strained foods earlier just makes feeding more complicated. Waiting also reduces the likelihood of food allergies in your baby. By all means, don't give strained foods in a bottle; wait until your child can accept spoon feedings. An exception to the above guideline is to start solids at 3 months of age if your baby is drinking more than 1 quart of formula per day and remains quite hungry.

A common myth is that solids at bedtime will help your baby sleep through the night. Three research studies have shown this is not true. The only exceptions are those few breast-fed babies who are not receiving enough calories or gaining adequately. If your baby is not sleeping through the night, see PREVENTION OF SLEEP PROBLEMS: BIRTH TO 6 MONTHS, page 257.

Types of Solid Foods

Cereals—Cereals are usually the first solid food added to your baby's diet. Generally these are introduced to infants between 4 and 6 months of age. Cereals should be fed with a small spoon and should not be given in the baby's bottle. This is because an infant should be taught to differentiate between what he eats and what he drinks. Start with rice cereal, which is less likely to cause allergies than other cereals. Barley and oatmeal may be tried 2 or 3 weeks later. A mixed cereal should be added to your baby's diet only after each kind of cereal in the mixed cereal has been separately introduced.

Vegetables and Fruit—Strained or pureed vegetables and fruits are the best solid foods introduced to your baby. The order in which you add vegetables and fruits to your baby's diet is not important. However, you should introduce only 1 new food at a time and no more than 3 new foods per week.

Meat and Protein Alternatives—By 7 to 8 months of age your baby should be ready for strained or pureed meats and protein alternatives (such as beans, peas, lentils, cottage cheese, and yogurt). Babies who are only getting breast milk and no other solids can develop a zinc and iron deficiency. This can be prevented by starting pureed red meats between 6 and 8 months.

Homemade Baby Foods—Between 8 and 12 months of age, introduce your baby to mashed table foods or junior foods, now also called stage 3 foods. If you make your own baby foods in a baby-food grinder or electric blender, be sure to add enough water to get a consistency that your baby can easily swallow. For convenient individual portions, these homemade baby foods can be poured into ice cube trays, frozen, removed, and stored in plastic freezer bags.

Foods to Avoid

Avoid sweet foods and desserts in the first year of life, since they may interfere with your baby's willingness to try other new, unsweet foods. Also avoid honey during the first year because of the risk of botulism.

Although there is controversy about them, egg whites, peanut butter, and seafood may be more likely to cause allergies than other solids and should be avoided until 1 year of age (especially in infants with allergies). Very allergic children should avoid all seafood, peanuts, and nuts until 2 years old. Orange juice is no longer restricted because the rash orange juice sometimes causes around the mouth is from an oil in the orange peel; it's not an allergy.

Amounts of Solids

Start with a few small spoonfuls. Initially your baby may just want a taste. Then gradually work up to larger portions. A good rule of thumb during the first year of life is 2 to 4 tablespoons (1 to 2 ounces) of each kind of food per meal. If your child is still hungry after finishing that amount, serve her more.

Spoon-Feeding

Spoon-feeding is begun at 4 months of age. By 9 to 12 months of age, most children want to try to feed themselves, and can do so with finger foods. By 15 to 18 months of age, most children can use a spoon independently for foods they can't pick up with their fingers, and the parent is no longer needed in the feeding process. Here's how to start:

• Be sure to place food on the middle of the tongue. If you place it in front, your child will probably push it back at you. Some infants get off to a better start if you place the spoon between their lips and let them suck off the food.

• Some children constantly bat at the spoon or try to get a grip on it during feedings. These children need to be distracted with finger foods (such as Cheerios) or by having a spoon of their own to play with.

• If your child previously liked spoon-feeding and now clamps his mouth shut when the spoon approaches, he's probably not hungry or someone has tried to force him to eat more than he wants. Spoon-feed your child only when he is hungry. If he turns his head away more than once, mealtime should be over.

• Spoon-feeding can be very messy in the beginning. Use a small baby spoon and a scooped-out bib to catch the dribble. Also, put some plastic under the high chair to reduce your cleanup time.

Finger Foods

Finger foods are small, bite-size pieces of soft foods. Most babies love to feed themselves and gain this added sense of independence. Finger foods can be introduced between 9 and 10 months of age or whenever a child develops a pincer grip (finger-thumb pickup). Since most babies will not be able to feed themselves with a spoon until 15 months of age, finger foods keep them actively involved in the feeding process. Start with dry cereals that easily dissolve in saliva (Cheerios are hard to beat). Other good finger foods are toast, cheese wedges, pieces of scrambled egg, cooked vegetable strips, slices of canned fruit (peaches, pears, or pineapple), slices of banana, crackers, cookies, and breads. With each passing month, try to increase the amount of finger foods and decrease the amount of mashed foods that require a spoon.

Snacks

Once your baby goes to 3 meals a day or 5-hour intervals, small snacks will often be necessary to tide him over to the next meal. Most babies go to this pattern between 6 and 9 months of age. The midmorning and midafternoon snack should be a nutritious, nonmilk food. Fruits and dry cereals are recommended. If your child is not hungry at mealtime, the snacks should be made smaller or eliminated.

Table Foods

Your child should be eating the same meals as you do by approximately 1 year of age. This assumes that your family consumes a well-balanced diet low in animal fats, and that you carefully dice any foods that would be difficult for your baby to chew. Avoid foods like raw carrots that could be aspirated into the lungs. (See CHOKING, page 10, for a list of dangerous foods.)

Heating Solid Foods

Overheated foods can cause mouth burns. Be careful. Test them before serving to an infant. Microwaves have the disadvantage of heating from the inside out, leaving some parts of the food hotter than others. The cooler temperature of the container can also be misleading. Stir microwave-heated food to distribute the heat evenly before testing it.

Iron

Throughout our lives we need iron in our diet to prevent anemia. Certain foods are especially good sources of iron. Red meats, fish, and poultry are best. Some young children will only eat lunch meats, and the low-fat ones are fine. Adequate iron is also found in iron-enriched cereals, beans of all types, egg yolks, peanut butter, raisins, prune juice, sweet potatoes, and spinach.

Vitamins

Before 1 year of age, infants receive all necessary vitamins in breast milk or formula. The only exception is that breast-fed babies need supplemental vitamin D starting at 2 months of age to prevent rickets (soft bones). Added vitamins are unnecessary after your child has reached 1 year of age and is on a regular balanced diet. If he's a picky eater, give him 1 chewable vitamin pill at least twice per week.

APPETITE SLUMP IN TODDLERS

Symptoms and Characteristics

• You think your child doesn't eat enough, is never hungry, won't eat unless you feed him, or eats slower than anyone else.
• Your child is between 1 and 5 years of age.
• Your child's energy level remains normal.
• Your child is growing normally.
• Your child is not losing weight.

Causes—Between 1 and 5 years of age, many children normally gain only 4 or 5 pounds per year, in contrast to the 15 pounds gained during the first year of life. Children in this age range can normally go 3 or 4 months without any weight gain. This normal slowdown in growth results in a reduced need for calories and a normal decline in appetite (called physiological anorexia). Food intake is governed by the appetite center in the brain. Kids eat as much as they need for growth and energy. Any hungry child will eat if food is available. No child will voluntarily starve himself at this age.

The appetite may decrease even further if parents try to force the child to eat more than he needs (even though he is of normal height and weight). They may apply pressure because they fear that decreased eating might cause poor health or a nutritional deficiency—neither of which is true. But forced feedings interfere with the normal pleasure of eating and actually decrease the appetite. If the child also is going through a normal phase of negativism, the struggle can accelerate.

Two other reasons that parents attempt to force their children to eat are short stature and normal shifting linear growth. The 3 percent of children under the third percentile in height are said to have short stature. The majority of them are well nourished. Feeding them more cannot increase their height—but it can make them fat. Children with shifting linear growth concern their parents, because their growth rate falls off before 1 year of age. Many children with short parents are born with average height. During the second half of the first year of life, however, they may shift to a lower height percentile (or line on the growth curve) because it corresponds to the height of their parents. Once they get to the new growth channel, they continue to grow along it at a normal rate. They never appear to be underweight during any of this gradual shifting to a lower height curve.

Expected Course—Once you allow your child to control his own food intake, the "problem" will disappear in a matter of 2 to 4 weeks. Rest assured, your child's appetite will reach gigantic proportions by adolescence.

Improving Poor Appetites

Put Your Child in Charge of How Much He Eats at Mealtime— Trust your child's appetite center. All children eat as much as they need. Your child's brain will make sure he eats enough calories for normal energy and growth. Your only job is to serve well-balanced meals. If your child is hungry, he will eat. If he's not, he will be by the next meal. Even reminding him to eat or to eat more will work against you.

Allow One Small Snack Between Meals—The most common reason for some children never appearing hungry is that they have so many snacks that they never become truly hungry. Be sure your child arrives at mealtime with an empty stomach. Offer your child no more than two small snacks of nutritious food each day, and provide them only if your child requests them. Keep the size of the snack to one-third of what you would expect him to eat at mealtime. If your child is thirsty between meals, offer water. Limit the amount of juice your child drinks to less than 6 ounces each day. Let your child miss snacks if she chooses. Even skipping an occasional meal is harmless.

Never Feed Your Child If He Is Capable of Feeding Himself—The greatest tendency for parents of a child with a poor appetite is to pick up the utensils, load up the spoon, smile, and try to trick or coerce the child into taking it. Once your child is old enough to use a spoon (usually age 12 to 15 months), never again pick it up for him. If your child is hungry, he will feed himself. Forced feeding is the main cause of power struggles around food.

Offer More Finger Foods—Finger foods can be started at 9 to 10 months of age. They allow your child a major role in self-feeding even if he is not yet able to use a spoon.

Limit Milk Intake to Less Than 16 Ounces Per Day—If your child eats cheese or yogurt, reduce milk by an equivalent amount. Most children in our society receive excessive milk, which fills kids up and dulls the appetite. Milk is a food and contains as many calories as most solid foods. Excessive milk or juice is a common cause of a poor appetite for solids.

Serve Small Portions of Food—A child's appetite is decreased by being served more food than he could possibly eat. Serving a small amount (less than you think he will eat) on a large plate leads to a sense of accomplishment. If your child seems to want more, wait for him to ask for seconds.

Consider Giving Your Child Vitamins Every Other Day If Food Intake Is Borderline—Although vitamins are probably unnecessary, they are not harmful in normal dosages and may allow you to relax about your child's eating patterns. However, they won't increase the appetite.

Make Mealtimes Pleasant—Draw your children into the conversation. Tell them what's happened to you today and ask about their day. Talk about fun subjects unrelated to food. Avoid making it a time for criticism or struggle over control.

Avoid Conversation About Eating at Any Time—Don't discuss food intake in your child's presence. Trust the appetite center to look after your child's food needs. Don't even provide praise for appropriate eating. Don't give bribes or rewards for meeting your eating expectations. Children should eat because it satisfies their hunger. Occasionally the child can be praised for trying new foods that he does not like the taste or texture of.

Don't Extend Mealtime—Don't keep your child sitting at the dinner table after the rest of the family is done. This only causes your child to develop unpleasant associations with mealtime.

Common Mistakes

Parents who are worried that their child isn't eating enough may initiate some irrational patterns of feeding. Some awaken the child at night to feed him or her. Some offer the child snacks at 15- or 20-minute intervals throughout the day. Others permit snacks that are larger than a regular meal. Some try to make the child feel guilty by talking about other children in the world who are starving. Others threaten: "If you don't eat what I cook, it means you don't love me." Some parents force the child to sit in the high chair or at the table for long periods of time after the meal has ended. The most common mistake, of course, is picking up a spoon or fork and trying various ways to get food into the child's mouth. Another mistake is cooking special foods for the child. Although the child may eat these, the total calories consumed per day will probably not increase (since it does not need to increase).

Prevention of Feeding Battles

The main way to prevent feeding struggles is by teaching your child how to feed himself or herself from as early an age as possible. You needn't wait until your child is old enough to use a spoon independently. For the young child, you can allow your child to initiate the feeding (by reaching or leaning forward) and to pace the feeding (by turning the head or gesturing). Food should not be placed in the mouth just because it is inadvertently open. The hands should be free and not pinned down during feedings. Do not insist that your child empty the bottle, finish a jar of baby food, or clean the plate. By time your child is 9 to 10 months old, start giving him or her finger foods. By 12 months of age your child should start to learn how to use a spoon and should be completely self-feeding by 15 months of age.

Call Your Child's Physician During Office Hours If

- Your child has not had a medical checkup in the last year.
- Your child is losing weight.
- Your child has not gained any weight in 6 months.
- Your child has associated symptoms of illness (such as diarrhea or fever).
- Your child gags on or vomits some foods.
- Someone is punishing your child for not eating.
- This approach has not improved mealtimes in your house within 1 month.
- You have other questions or concerns.

Related Topics

MEDICINES: HELPING CHILDREN SWALLOW THEM (see page 244)
OVEREATING: PREVENTION OF (see page 201)

PICKY EATERS

Symptoms and Characteristics

The peak time for picky eating is the toddler or preschool years. A picky eater:

- complains about or refuses specific foods, especially vegetables and meats
- pushes foods around the plate
- hides foods or gives them to a pet under the table
- eats enough total foods and calories per day, as evidenced by normal growth.

Causes—Children of all ages (and adults) commonly have a few food dislikes. A picky eater is a child with many food dislikes. At age 2 or 3, up to 20 percent of children are picky eaters. Most young children dislike foods with a bitter or spicy taste, and that should be considered normal. Sometimes children dislike foods because of their color, but more often it's because they are difficult to chew. Children accept tender meals better than tough ones, and well-cooked vegetables better than raw. Learning to accept these foods should not be expected before the teenage years. Occasionally a child who gags on large pieces of all foods has large tonsils that make it difficult to swallow.

Expected Outcome—Most children who are picky eaters grow out of it. They start trying new foods during the early school years. The voracious appetite during the adolescent years also increases the willingness to experiment. If you try to force your child to eat a food he doesn't like, he may gag or even vomit. Forced feedings always interfere with the normal pleasure of eating and eventually decrease the appetite.

Living with a Picky Eater

Try to Prepare a Main Dish That Everyone Likes—Try to avoid an unusual main dish that your child strongly dislikes. Some children don't like foods that are mixed together, such as casseroles. Try reintroducing such dishes when your child is older.

Allow Occasional Substitutes for the Main Dish—If your child refuses to eat the main dish and this is an unusual request, you may allow a substitute dish. An acceptable substitute would be breakfast cereal or a simple sandwich the child prepares for himself. Never become a short-order cook and prepare any extra foods for mealtime. The child should know that you expect him to learn to eat the main dish that has been prepared for the family.

Respect Any Strong Food Dislikes—If your child has a few strong food dislikes (especially any food that makes her gag), do not serve that food to her when it's prepared as part of the family meal.

Don't Worry About Vegetables, Just Encourage More Fruits—Because vegetables tend to be hard to chew and some of them are bitter, they are commonly rejected by children and even by many adults. Keep in mind that fruits and vegetables are from the same food group. There are no essential vegetables. Vegetables can be entirely replaced by fruits without any nutritional harm to your child. This is not a health issue. Don't make your child feel guilty about avoiding some vegetables.

Don't Allow Complaining About Food at Mealtimes—Have a rule that it's okay to decline a serving of a particular food or to push it to the side of the plate. But complaining about it is unacceptable.

Encourage Your Child to Taste New Foods—Many tastes are acquired. Your child many eventually learn that she likes a food she initially refused. Research shows it may take seeing other people eat a new food

10 times before a child is even willing to taste it, and another 10 times of tasting it before she develops a liking for it. Don't try to rush this normal process of adapting to new foods. Trying to force a child to eat one bite of a food per year of age is not helpful with most picky eaters. Instead, it's better to simply serve it repeatedly, ask the child to taste it, and then trust her when she says she has tasted it.

Avoid Pressure or Punishment at Mealtime—Never pressure your child to eat all foods. Never punish your child for refusing to take one bite of a new food. It will only lead to liking that food less over time, gagging, or even vomiting. If your child has a stubborn, strong-willed nature, pressure around eating can progress to a power struggle, which in turn prolongs the picky eating.

Don't Argue About Dessert—An unnecessary area of friction for picky eaters is a rule that if you don't clean your plate, you can't have any dessert. Since desserts are not necessarily harmful, a better approach is to allow your child 1 serving of dessert regardless of what she eats. However, there are no seconds on dessert for children who don't eat an adequate amount of the main course. Desserts don't have to be sweets; they can be nutritious desserts such as fruit.

Don't Extend Mealtime—Don't keep your child sitting at the dinner table after the rest of the family is done. This will only cause your child to develop unpleasant associations with mealtime.

Keep the Mealtime Atmosphere Pleasant—Make it an important family event. Draw your children into friendly conversation. Tell them what's happened to you today and ask about their day. Talk about fun subjects unrelated to food. Avoid making it a time for criticism or struggle over control.

Avoid Conversation About Eating at Any Time—Don't discuss what your child eats in your child's presence. Trust your child's appetite to look after your child's caloric needs. Also don't give praise for appropriate eating. Don't give bribes or rewards for meeting your eating expectations. Children should eat to satisfy their appetite, not to please the parent. Occasionally you might praise your child for trying a new food that he does not like the taste or texture of.

Consider Giving Your Child a Daily Vitamin-Mineral Supplement—If your child is not eating at least 1 serving of meat per day, give a multivitamin with iron to prevent iron deficiency anemia. Although supplemental vitamins are probably unnecessary for most of us, they are not harmful in normal amounts and may allow you to be less concerned about your child's eating patterns.

Call Your Child's Physician During Office Hours If

- Your child is losing weight.
- Your child gags on or vomits certain foods.
- Your child has heartburn.
- Your child has constipation.
- You have other questions or concerns.

A HEALTHY DIET

Health Problems Related to Diet

In the United States, at least 7 health conditions have been proven to relate to diet. The first 4 problems occur in children as well as in adults. The last 3 primarily occur in adults.

Iron Deficiency Anemia—This type of anemia usually occurs between 6 months and 2 years of age. Many children have no symptoms. The most common symptoms are pale skin, becoming tired easily, and delayed motor development. Iron deficiency anemia can also cause behavioral symptoms such as restlessness, irritability, and poor attention span.

Overweight—Obesity is one of the most common nutritional problems in our country (see OVEREATING: PREVENTION OF, page 201). Obesity is also one of the most important contributing factors in heart disease, hypertension, type 2 diabetes, and some cancers.

Tooth Decay—Tooth decay is accentuated by the intake of sugars in association with poor tooth-brushing habits (see TOOTH DECAY PREVENTION, page 194).

Intestinal Symptoms—Too little fiber intake can cause intestinal symptoms such as constipation, abdominal discomfort, appendicitis, gallstones, and some intestinal cancers.

Osteoporosis—Soft bones (osteoporosis) in later adulthood causes curvature of the spine and increased fractures (especially hip fractures). Most of the calcium that gives strong bone density is laid down between 9 and 18 years of age.

Coronary Artery Disease—An increased intake of animal fats (especially cholesterol) contributes to coronary artery disease. This disease hardly exists in poor countries where the population subsists on low-fat, high-carbohydrate diets. It is also less common among vegetarians.

High Blood Pressure—High blood pressure has been associated with an increased salt intake or a decreased calcium intake in some susceptible individuals. Most individuals, however, get rid of extra salt through their kidneys and don't develop hypertension.

Recommendations for a Healthy Diet

Learn the Four Food Groups—Food can be divided into four basic groups: milk products, meats/eggs, grains, and fruits/vegetables. The USDA revised the Dietary Guidelines for Americans in 2005. The recommended servings per day as listed are for teens and adults.

- Milk products include milk, cheese, yogurt, and ice cream. Eat 3 servings per day (a serving equals 1 cup).
- Meats include red meats, poultry, fish, and eggs. Eat 2 servings per day (6 ounces total).
- Grains include breads, cereals, rice, pasta, and so forth. Eat 6 or more servings per day (a serving equals ½ cup or 1 slice of bread). At least half the amount should be whole grains.
- Fruits and vegetables may be consumed as solids or juices. Eat 2 to 4 servings of fruits and 3 to 5 servings of vegetables per day (serving equals ½ cup).
- A healthy diet should consist of 20 percent milk, meat, and eggs, and 80 percent vegetables, fruits, and grains. (Fiber is found in grains, fruits, and vegetables.) This is similar to the recommendations that children receive 55 percent of their calories from carbohydrates, 30 percent from fats, and 15 percent from protein.

Eat Three Meals a Day—Breakfast (breaking the fast) is the most important meal of the day. Skipping breakfast can compromise performance at school. Research has shown that missing breakfast interferes with alertness, attention span, thinking, and memory. For dieters, skipping break-fast usually doesn't lead to weight loss. All meals should contain fruits or vegetables, and grains as well. Meat or milk should be included in two of the meals.

Eating snacks is largely a habit. Snacks are unnecessary for good nutrition but harmless unless your child is overweight. If your child likes snacks (and most children do), encourage fruits, vegetables, yogurt, dry cereal, corn chips, and crackers. Allow only 1 snack between meals, but don't give one if it is close to mealtime.

Decrease the Intake of Fat (Meat and Milk Products)—Americans eat excessive amounts of meat and dairy products. Although cholesterol is important for rapid growth, after age 2 it should be consumed in moderation (not eliminated). To decrease the intake of fat, follow these guidelines:

- Remember that one serving of meat per day is adequate for normal growth and development. (Don't serve meat more than twice a day.)
- Serve more fish and poultry and fewer red meats, since the latter have the highest cholesterol levels. Lean meats are lean ground beef, pork loin, veal, and lamb.
- Trim the fat off meats and remove the skin from poultry.
- Don't serve bacon, sausages, spareribs, pastrami, and other meats that have a high fat content. Cut back on hot dogs, lunch meats, and corned beef.
- Limit eggs to 3 or 4 per week.
- Use 1 or 2 percent or skim milk instead of whole milk (after 2 years of age).
- Decrease milk intake to 2 or 3 cups per day. (Encourage water for satisfying thirst.) On the other hand, teenage girls may need to be reminded to consume adequate milk products (the equivalent of 3 glasses of milk) to lay down the bone mass to prevent osteoporosis later in life.
- Use a vegetable oil spread (with no trans fats) instead of butter (butter is high in saturated fat).
- Keep in mind that red meats may be hard to give up because of the widespread misconception that red meat helps to build muscle mass and strength.

Increase the Intake of Fruits, Vegetables, and Grains—Children should consume 2 to 4 servings of fruits and 3 to 5 servings of vegetables per day. (50 percent of American children eat only one fruit or vegetable per day.)

- Try to serve a fruit at every meal.
- Offer fruits as dessert and snacks.
- Start every day with a glass of fruit juice. (Caution: Avoid excessive fruit juice, which can cause diarrhea or decrease the appetite for essential foods. The American Academy of Pediatrics recommends the following limits in fruit juice consumed per day: 6 ounces for children 6 months to 6 years, 12 ounces for children 7 to 18 years.)
- Serve 100 percent fruit juices, not fruit drinks. Fruit drinks mainly contain water and sugars. They don't count as a serving of fruit.
- Don't force children to eat vegetables they don't like. Offer ones they do like or substitute a fruit. From a practical standpoint, fruits and vegetables are interchangeable.
- When making casseroles, increase the amount of vegetables and decrease the amount of meat.
- Serve more soups.
- Encourage more cereals for breakfast.
- Use more whole-grain bread in making sandwiches.

Maintain an Adequate Iron Intake—Throughout our lives we need an adequate amount of iron in our diets to prevent anemia. Everyone should know which foods are good sources of iron. Red meats, fish, poultry, and eggs are best. Having 2 servings per day will provide adequate iron. Although liver is a good source of iron, it contains 16 times more cholesterol than beef and should be avoided. For those young children who refuse meats in general, some low-fat luncheon meats can be provided as an iron source. Adequate iron is also found in iron-enriched cereals, beans of all types, peanut butter, raisins, prune juice, sweet potatoes, spinach, and egg yolks. The iron in these foods is better absorbed if the meal also contains fruit juice or meat.

Maintain an Adequate Calcium Intake—Calcium is important for building strong bones, thereby preventing fractures in teens and soft bones (osteoporosis) in later adulthood. Most of the calcium that gives healthy bone density is laid down between ages 9 and 18 years. During this time calcium intake should be 1,200 mg per day. A cup (8 ounces) of milk contains 300 mg, so optimal intake is 4 servings of milk products per day. One cup of milk is equivalent to 8 ounces of yogurt, 1½ ounces of cheese (approximately 2 slices), or 1 cup of calcium-fortified fruit juice. Whole, 2 percent, 1 percent, and skim milk all contain the same amount of calcium per cup. Children age 1 to 4 years need 2 servings of calcium per day and those 4 to 9 years need 3 servings per day. If a child of any age doesn't like the taste of milk, intake can easily be improved by serving flavored milk.

Avoid Excessive Salt—Salt is not usually harmful for people without high blood pressure. However, we can discourage a taste for excessive salt in infants by not adding it to their foods. The salt shaker can be removed from the dinner table. Other herbs and spices (salt-free seasoning) can be used instead of salt. Salty foods such as potato chips and pretzels can be purchased sparingly.

Avoid Excessive Pure Sugars—See SUGAR AND SWEETS, page 189.

Eating Before Exercise—The best foods to consume before prolonged exercise are complex carbohydrates. These include bread, crackers, pasta (noodles), potatoes, and rice. These should be consumed 3 to 4 hours before the athletic event so they have passed out of the stomach. Water consumption continues to be important right up to the time of participation and every 20 to 30 minutes during the activity. Eating meat does not improve athletic performance.

Food Myths

Some Americans consider a faulty diet to be the cause of most health problems. If this were true the practice of medicine would become relatively easy. Unfortunately, most diseases do not respond to a change in the diet. The following misleading statements have received some attention in the media.

"Everyone Needs Vitamin Supplements"—In general in our society vitamins are overused (the "once a day" vitamin habit). Vitamins do not improve a child's appetite, prevent infections, or increase pep and energy. Added vitamins are unnecessary once your child has reached 1 year of age, if he consumes a regular balanced diet from all 4 food groups.

Keep in mind that vitamins and minerals are already present in foods. Vitamin supplements are helpful in special situations (for instance, if your child is a picky eater, is dieting, or has a chronic disease). Some vitamins taken in excess (mainly vitamins A and D) are stored in the body and can cause symptoms (such as headaches and kidney stones). The danger of overdosage is a good example of "more is not better." Any extra vitamin B or C is safe and is quickly passed in the urine.

"Natural Foods Are Better"—Natural or organic foods are those grown without pesticides or artificial fertilizers, and processed without preservatives, food colorings, or food additives. Natural foods have no nutritional advantages. They have no higher level of vitamins or minerals. Foods grown in worn-out soil are no different in food value from those grown in rich soil. Foods grown with chemical fertilizers are just as healthy as foods grown with natural fertilizers. The chemicals used to preserve food do not take away from its nutritional or health value. The main difference between these two types of foods is that natural foods are more costly.

"Fast Foods Are Bad"—Some people consider any meal served at a fast-food restaurant to be harmful. In truth these meals can contain foods from all four groups (although they may be heavy on fat and low on fiber). The main risk of eating fast foods is obesity. Fast-food meals are fine if they aren't eaten frequently and you avoid super-sized portions.

"Junk Foods Are Bad"—Junk foods are the source of some confusion. Some people define any sweet or dessert as a junk food. They claim that these foods "lack nutritional value." While that may be true for some sweets (e.g., candy) and not true for others (e.g., peach pie), eating sweets in moderation is not harmful. (See SUGAR AND SWEETS, page 189.)

CHOLESTEROL SCREENING OR TESTING

Everyone needs to have some cholesterol in their blood. Cholesterol is a fat that is essential for building hormones and cells. Cholesterol has become a health issue because high cholesterol levels carry an increased risk of coronary heart disease (CHD). A 1 percent decrease in blood cholesterol leads to a 2 percent decrease in risk of CHD in adults. Societies with low serum cholesterol usually have a low incidence of CHD. The amount of cholesterol and saturated fats we eat contributes to the level of cholesterol in our bloodsteam. The level of cholesterol in childhood tends to persist (track) into adulthood in about 50 percent of children. This ability of the child's level of cholesterol to predict the adult level increases in adolescence. Furthermore, reducing the cholesterol and saturated fat in the diet does reduce the level of cholesterol in the bloodstream. One major goal of preventive medicine is to lower cholesterol to healthy levels.

Types of Cholesterol—Cholesterol is composed of high-density lipoproteins (HDL) and low-density lipoproteins (LDL). HDL and LDL transport cholesterol in the bloodstream. HDL is called "good" cholesterol because it carries cholesterol away from the arteries and to the liver for elimination. LDL is referred to as "bad" cholesterol because an excess of LDL deposits cholesterol on the inner walls of the arteries over time. As a result, the arteries become clogged. In addition to reducing total cholesterol levels, we would like to see you increase your HDL and decrease your LDL. A 1 percent rise in HDL may give a 3 percent reduction in CHD in adults.

Normal and Abnormal Cholesterol Levels

	NORMAL	BORDERLINE	ABNORMAL
Total Cholesterol	< 170	170–200	> 200
LDL Cholesterol	< 100	100–130	> 130
HDL Cholesterol	> 60	40–60	< 40

(National Cholesterol Expert Panel, 2003)

High-Risk Children: At What Age to Test?—The American Academy of Pediatrics and the American Heart Association are in complete agreement that all children who have risk factors for CHD should be screened soon after age 2. The reason children aren't tested before age 2 is that during this period of rapid growth and development, the diet needs to be high in fat. Two main risk factors should be considered: (1) a family history of high blood cholesterol and (2) a family history of CHD. The first factor includes an early history of heart attack (less than 50 years of age in men or less than 60 years of age in women), angina, stroke, or bypass surgery. The family history is considered positive if these diseases have occurred in parents, grandparents, aunts, or uncles. Information must be obtained about the grandparents, since the parents are often too young to have entered the high-risk age group for CHD. By screening these high-risk children, over 50 percent of children with high cholesterol are identified.

All Other Children: At What Age to Test?—The practice of performing cholesterol testing on all children is controversial. The main reason for universal testing is to identify all children with high cholesterol. Good eating and exercise patterns in children need to be established early if these patterns are to be followed throughout life. The main arguments against testing all children are that testing is costly, high cholesterol levels do not persist into adulthood 50 to 60 percent of the time, and healthy diets and an active lifestyle can be started on all children without knowing cholesterol levels. If routine testing is done, it's usually performed between ages 2 and 5 years, often upon school entry.

Retesting Children with High Cholesterol—If your child's cholesterol value is borderline high or high, the test will be repeated in one to two weeks to confirm that the value is high. There is some normal day-to-day variation in cholesterol levels. If the level remains high, it's assumed to be accurate. Children with confirmed high total cholesterol—greater than 200 (the 95th percentile)—will then have blood drawn for a lipid profile or panel. This test measures not only total cholesterol but also LDL, HDL, and triglycerides. Depending on the results, treatment will be initiated and the level retested in approximately 2 to 4 months.

If your child has a total cholesterol level between 170 and 199 (75th to 95th percentiles), treatment can be started without additional tests. The test for total cholesterol will probably be repeated yearly. The reason we don't obtain routine lipid panels on all children is that it requires fasting for at least 12 hours and the test costs much more than a total-cholesterol test. In addition, the lipid panel requires drawing blood from a vein (which can be a more difficult procedure in children) rather than a simple fingerstick.

Retesting Children with Normal Cholesterol—Children with normal total cholesterol—below 170 (the 75th percentile)—do not need their cholesterol rechecked until they reach adolescence. Most physicians who monitor adult levels repeat tests for cholesterol every 5 years as long as the levels remain within normal range.

Testing Family Members—If your child's value is high (greater than the 95th percentile), we recommend that you have everyone else in your family tested for total cholesterol. If a child has a high level, other family members also have high values in over 80 percent of cases. This will provide you with additional reasons to start your family on a healthier diet and exercise program. If your child's cholesterol level is high or high-normal, see Treating High Cholesterol Levels, below.

TREATING HIGH CHOLESTEROL LEVELS

If your child's cholesterol level is high or borderline high, start the programs listed below. (If your child's cholesterol level is normal, it still would be a good idea to place your family on the same programs.) High cholesterols are not the only risk factor for coronary heart disease (CHD). The following risk factors are just as harmful as being on a high cholesterol diet: physical inactivity, obesity, and smoking. The more risk factors that you and your child have, the higher the risk of CHD. Living a long and healthy life requires healthy eating and exercise patterns. It is easier to start these habits as a child than to have to adopt them as an adult. Review with your family the following checklist of ways to reduce cholesterol levels. If you already are carrying out the majority of these recommendations, you are protecting your child's heart and blood vessels.

Low-Fat Diet

The American Heart Association recommends that all children over age 2 be on a low-cholesterol, low-saturated-fat diet. Currently most Americans take in 40 percent of their daily calories as fat. A healthy (prudent) diet keeps fat to 30 percent of total calories. The goal is eating fat in moderation, not eliminating fat entirely. Lowering your child's fat intake to 30 percent of daily calories carries no risk for children over age 2. (None of the following recommendations applies to children under age 2.)

Foods of plant origin such as fruits, vegetables, and grains do not contain cholesterol. Foods of animal origin such as meats, eggs, and milk products do contain cholesterol. Our blood cholesterol is raised by consuming cholesterol itself, or by eating saturated fats that stimulate the production of cholesterol. Even without any fat intake, the liver produces a small amount of cholesterol each day. Therefore we will always have some cholesterol in the blood.

Serving a low-fat diet in your house is rather easy:

- Serve more fish, turkey, and chicken, since they have less fat than red meats. Buy lean ground beef for hamburgers. Use lean ham or turkey for sandwiches.
- Trim the fat from meats and remove the skin from poultry before eating.
- Avoid meats with the highest fat content, such as bacon, sausages, salami, pepperoni, and hot dogs.
- Limit the number of eggs eaten to 3 or 4 per week. Although egg yolks are rich in cholesterol, eating eggs does not increase serum cholesterol as much as eating saturated fats, found in bacon, sausage, and fatty meats. A recent study from Harvard showed that adults who consume 1 egg per day do not have an increased risk for heart attacks.
- Limit the amount of all meats to portions of moderate size.
- Use 1 percent or skim (0.5 percent) milk instead of whole milk (which is 3.5 percent).
- Use a margarine product (vegetable oil spread without the trans fats) instead of butter.
- Avoid deep-fat fried food or food fried in butter or fat. If you prefer to fry meats, use special margarine or nonstick cooking sprays.
- Increase your child's fiber intake. Fiber is found in most grains, vegetables, and fruits.

Family Exercise Program

Exercise is the best way to raise your HDL level. Your goal should be at least 20 to 30 minutes of vigorous exercise three times per week. Vigorous exercise must involve the large muscles of the legs and cause your heart to beat faster (aerobic exercise). Vigorous exercise also improves your heart's response to work. A child is much more likely to exercise if you exercise with him. Try the following forms of exercise:

- Encourage walking or biking instead of riding in a car.

- Encourage using stairs instead of elevators.
- Encourage taking the dog for a walk, jumping rope, or playing ball if your child appears to be bored.
- Encourage your child to join a team (e.g., soccer) or learn a new sport (e.g., roller-skating) that requires vigorous (aerobic) activity. Swimming, jogging, and basketball are sports that burn lots of calories. Sports such as baseball and football do not give the heart much of a workout.
- Encourage exercising to a videotape or music on TV.
- Limit TV and video game time to 2 hours or less per day. These sitting activities interfere with physical fitness.
- Encourage using an exercise bike, dancing, or running in place while watching TV.
- Support better physical education programs and aerobics classes in your schools.

Ideal Body Weight

Children who are overweight tend to have a low HDL and a high LDL. Helping your child return to ideal body weight will improve his blood cholesterol levels. When people decrease the fat in the diet, they automatically decrease the calories they consume each day because fat has twice as many calories as the same amount of protein or carbohydrates. A low-fat diet *and* exercise are the key ingredients for losing weight. If your child is overweight, also see the guideline on overweight (page 203).

Smoke-Free Home

A good way to raise your HDL level is to stop smoking. Also avoid exposing your child to passive smoking. If someone in your home smokes, see the guideline on passive smoking (page 229).

Set a Good Example

If your child needs to lower his cholesterol level, he will need help from his family. You cannot put him on a special diet without putting the entire family on it. You cannot put him on a special exercise program without having other family members participate. Eat healthy foods and snacks so your child will eat similarly. Play more sports and watch less TV sports—as you would like your child to do.

Statin Drugs to Lower Cholesterol

Statins are rarely used in children unless they have a rare form of high cholesterol, relating to disease rather than diet. If your child's level remains high despite your initial efforts, request a consultation with a nutritionist regarding special diets. Also, join an exercise program at a local gym or fitness center. These additional steps will usually help your child.

When to Recheck Your Child's Cholesterol Level

Generally, for high cholesterol (above the 95th percentile) the level is rechecked approximately 2 to 4 months after starting a program to lower it. If the cholesterol level is borderline high (above the 75th percentile), it is usually rechecked yearly.

SUGAR AND SWEETS

A popular misconception suggests that eating sugar is harmful or demonstrates poor self-control. Many well-educated parents worry needlessly about sugar, candy, and desserts. Sweets are not bad. They just need to be eaten in moderation. If you want to protect your child's health, get after the Cholesterol Monster, not the Sugar Monster and the Cookie Monster.

The Normal "Sweet Tooth"—Soon after birth, infants show a preference for sweet solutions (such as breast milk) over unsweetened solutions. Most humans are born with a "sweet tooth," which probably has a genetic basis. Most adults also naturally seek out and enjoy sweets. Giving candy as a gift for holidays or birthdays is a common symbol of affection. Many members of the animal kingdom also show a craving for sweets.

People forget that the recommended daily amount of calories from carbohydrates (sugar and starches) is 55 percent. The amount from refined sugars (sucrose) should not exceed 10 percent of daily calories. Sugar is present in most foods except the meat group.

Lactose is the sugar present in milk, fructose is the sugar present in fruits, and maltose is the sugar present in grain products. Sucrose, the sugar in sugarcane and sugar beets, has no greater adverse effect on body functioning than any of the other sugars.

Side Effects of Sugar—The main risk of sugar is its ability to increase tooth decay. This is the only permanent harm from consuming too much sugar. This risk can be greatly reduced if the teeth are brushed after sugar-containing foods are eaten. The foods causing the most dental cavities (caries) are those that stick to the teeth (e.g., raisins carry considerable risk). The greatest risk factor for causing severe dental caries is falling asleep or walking around with a bottle of sugar solution in the mouth. The solution can be fruit juice, Kool-Aid, or milk. This type of tooth decay is called "baby-bottle caries." Constant access to a sippy cup filled with a sugary solution also can accentuate "tooth rot."

A temporary side effect may be seen 2 hours after excessive sugar consumption. A withdrawal reaction consisting of sweating, hunger, dizziness, tiredness, or sleepiness may be felt. This reaction to a sugar binge is brief, harmless, and can be relieved by eating some food. The sleepiness is caused by serotonin, a calming neurochemical produced by the body in response to the high level of blood sugar that follows eating refined sugar (sucrose).

Myths About Sugar—Eating sugar is basically not harmful. Candy does not cause cancer, heart disease, or diabetes mellitus. The following facts address some common myths: (1) Obesity is due to overeating in general and not specifically to eating sugars. Fatty foods have twice the calories per amount as sugar and are much more related to obesity. (2) Extensive research has shown that sugar does not cause hyperactivity. In fact, 10 teaspoons of refined sugar (as found in the usual 12 ounces of soft drink) usually causes drowsiness one or two hours later. (3) The term "junk food" has led to considerable confusion in our country. Some people define any sweet or dessert as a "junk food." Others define fast foods as "junk foods." Let's junk this negative term, which implies that if a food is sweet or purchased from a fast-food chain, consuming any of it is bad for your health.

Recommendations for the Safe Use of Sugar

- *Allow sugar in moderation.* In general, eating foods in moderation is healthy, but eating foods in excess is unhealthy. One precaution is to avoid sweets if possible during the first year of life. If they are introduced too early, they may interfere with a willingness to try new nonsweet foods. (Note: These guidelines about sugar in moderation may not apply to children with diabetes mellitus.)

- *Don't try to forbid sugar.* Some parents do this in hopes of preventing a preference for sweet foods. Since this preference is present at birth, we have little influence over it. If we forbid sweets entirely, children may become fascinated with them and engage in candy binges. With candy and other sweets so readily available in stores and vending machines, a sugar embargo cannot be monitored and becomes unenforceable as a child grows up. If we make an issue of it, this becomes an unnecessary battleground.

- *Limit the amount of sweets you buy.* The more sweets there are in the house, the more your child will eat.

- *Limit how much sweets are eaten.* While one candy bar is fine, eating an entire bag of candy at one time is unacceptable. Try to eliminate bingeing on candy or other sweets. Do this mainly by setting a good example. Exceptions of allowing extra candy can be on Halloween, other holidays, birthday parties, and other parties. The worst that could happen is that your child could become extra sleepy or have a mild stomachache.

- *Allow sweets for desserts.* As stated earlier, sweets cause symptoms only if they are eaten in excess. As long as they follow a well-balanced meal, they cause no symptoms. An acceptable dessert, therefore, can be just about anything—cookies, cake, or even a candy bar.

- *Discourage sweets for snacks.* Candy, soft drinks, or other sweets are not a good choice for a snack. Since very little else is eaten with the snack, consuming mainly refined sugar can cause a withdrawal reaction one or two hours later. Teach your child that if he does take a soft drink or Kool-Aid as a snack, he should eat something else from the grain or fruit food groups along with it. An occasional sweet drink with a sugar substitute is fine. Stock up on nutritious snacks (such as juices), and set a good example by what you eat for snacks.

- *Insist that the teeth be brushed after sweets are eaten.* Unless you encourage this good habit, a "sweet tooth" will become a decayed tooth.

Special Benefits of Sugar—Using candy occasionally as a reward is not habit-forming. The joy of eating sweets is a natural preference, not enhanced by this practice. Candy and other sweet treats are a powerful incentive. Whether we like it or not, the best motivators are always items that children crave. In addition, candy is inexpensive and easy to purchase. Because of the many types of candy, the child also has many choices. Candy may bring about a breakthrough in behavior with a negative child who has not responded to other approaches. Star charts and praise should be used simultaneously for improved behavior and continued after the candy has been phased out.

Second, sugar can be useful in helping a finicky eater try an essential new food. Some children who have breast-fed until almost a year of age will not accept any cow's-milk products. One way of helping them make this transition is by sweetening the cow's milk temporarily with honey or other flavorings. (Caution: Avoid giving honey before 1 year of age because of the small risk of botulism for this age group.) After the child is drinking adequate amounts of milk the sweetener can be gradually phased out.

Third, some children will take bitter medicines more readily when they are mixed with a sweet flavoring such as Kool-Aid powder, chocolate pudding, or pancake syrup.

Call Your Child's Physician During Office Hours If

• You think your child has a problem with sugar.
• You have other questions or concerns.

BABY BOTTLE TOOTH DECAY: PREVENTION

Symptoms and Characteristics

Baby bottle tooth decay (BBTD) is the main type of tooth decay in infants. Infants who are allowed to have a bottle in bed or older toddlers who are allowed to carry around a bottle during the day are at risk for this type of tooth decay.

Although the decay can start soon after your child's baby teeth appear, the problem is often not noticed until about 1 year of age. The earliest sign is white spots on the baby teeth. The upper front teeth (incisors) are usually damaged first.

Causes—Tooth decay occurs when sugar in liquids is in contact with the teeth for a prolonged time. Milk, formula, juice, Kool-Aid, and soft drinks all contain sugar. If a child falls asleep with a bottle in the mouth or constantly drinks from a bottle during the day, the sugar coats the upper teeth. The normal bacteria in the mouth change the sugar to an acid.

The enamel (protective coating) of baby teeth is only half the thickness of an eggshell. The acid gradually dissolves the enamel and allows decay to occur in the teeth.

The availability of plastic bottles instead of glass bottles has led many parents to be less concerned about giving their infant a bottle. Leaving a baby with a bottle of formula or juice may be used as a quick way to help a child go to sleep at night or deal with middle-of-the-night crying. The bottle may also come in handy when dealing with fussiness during the day. Many parents are unaware that these kinds of bottle habits can lead to tooth decay problems.

Expected Outcome—Dental repair of BBTD requires general anesthesia. If the problem is detected at an early level, the teeth can be covered with stainless-steel caps. If the decay is severe, the decayed teeth will need to be pulled out.

If BBTD is not discovered and treated, decay will eventually destroy the teeth and they will break off at the gumline. The decay will continue to destroy the root of the tooth and cause ongoing pain.

If the child has teeth pulled, he may have the following problems:

• The child will then have to chew with the teeth on the side of the mouth.

• He may get teased about the missing teeth.

• The permanent teeth may come in crooked or be crowded because the baby teeth are no longer there to save the appropriate space.

How to Prevent Baby Bottle Tooth Decay

Never Give Your Infant a Crib Bottle—Don't bottle-feed your baby until he falls asleep. This is the most common cause of bottle dependency and will eventually cause sleep problems because your child will expect a bottle as a transition into sleep, even following normal awakenings during the night. Separate the last bottle-feeding of the evening from bedtime. Even though baby teeth don't start coming in until 6 months, don't start a bad habit. In general, don't allow your infant to ever think that the bottle belongs to him. He won't voluntarily give it back.

Don't Allow Your Infant to Have a Tote or Companion Bottle During the Day—Don't substitute a bottle for a pacifier, security object, toy, or being held. Give a bottle only during mealtimes.

Introduce a Cup by 6 Months of Age—Introducing a cup is the best way to prevent bottle dependency. Don't expect a child to start weaning himself unless he has been exposed to a cup. Also don't expect weaning to occur in 1 day or 1 week. It takes gradual exposure to a cup over 3 months or longer for a child to learn to prefer the cup over the bottle.

Substitute Water—If your infant has developed a bottle habit, continue to give him the bottle, but fill it only with water. Water cannot harm tooth enamel. Water is also boring and will help your child eventually give up the bottle. The bottle itself is not harmful.

Call Your Child's Physician During Office Hours If

- Your child cannot give up the bottle.
- You see white spots on the baby teeth.
- You think your child might have BBTD.
- You have other questions or concerns.

TOOTH DECAY PREVENTION

Tooth decay causes toothaches, lost teeth, malocclusion, and costly visits to the dentist. With present knowledge, 80 to 90 percent of tooth decay can be prevented. Here are some tips for raising a cavity-free generation.

Fluoride

- Fluoride builds strong, decay-resistant enamel. Fluoride is needed from 6 months to 16 years of age. By 16 years, the enamel formation on the 3rd molars is completed. Drinking fluoridated water (containing 0.7 to 1.2 parts per million) or taking a prescription fluoride supplement is the best protection against tooth decay, reducing cavities by 70 percent.
- If fluoride is consumed in drinking water, a child must take at least 1 pint per day (preferably 1 quart per day by school age).
- If your city's water supply doesn't have fluoride added or you are breast-feeding, ask your physician for a prescription for fluoride drops or tablets during your next routine visit. The dosage of fluoride is 0.25 mg per day in the first 3 years, 0.5 mg from 3 to 6 years of age, and 1.0 mg over

age 6. Try to give fluoride on an empty stomach, because mixing it with milk reduces its absorption to 70 percent.

- Bottled water usually doesn't contain adequate fluoride. Call the bottler for information. If your children drink bottled water containing less than 0.7 ppm of fluoride, ask your child's physician for a fluoride supplement.

- Fluoride is safe. The American Dental Association has recommended fluoridation of water supplies since 1950. Over 70 percent of all Americans drink fluoridated water. *Consumers Report* states: "The simple truth is that there is no scientific controversy over the safety of fluoridation. The practice is safe, economical and beneficial. The survival of any controversy is one of the major triumphs of quackery over science in our generation."

- One concern about fluoride is white spots or mottling on the teeth (called fluorosis). This can occur when a child ingests 2 mg or more per day. The preventative dose is 1 mg or less. Children can ingest excessive fluoride if they receive supplements when it is already present in the city water supply. Occasionally they ingest it by eating their toothpaste. A ribbon of toothpaste contains about 1 mg of fluoride. Therefore, people of all ages should use only a drop of toothpaste the size of a pea. This precaution and encouraging your child not to swallow most of the toothpaste will prevent fluorosis.

Tooth-Brushing and Flossing

The purpose of tooth-brushing is to remove plaque from the teeth. Plaque is the invisible scum that forms on the surface of teeth. Within this plaque, mouth bacteria change sugars to acids, which in turn etch the enamel.

- Tooth-brushing or wiping with a damp cloth should begin before 1 year of age.

- Try to brush after each meal, but especially after the last meal or snack of the day.

- Brush the molars (back teeth) extra carefully. Decay usually starts in the pits and crevices of the molars.

- To prevent the mouth bacteria from changing food caught in the teeth into acid, tooth-brushing must occur within the first 5 to 10 minutes after meals.

- Help your child brush the teeth at least until age 6. Most children don't have the coordination or strength to brush their own teeth adequately before then.

• If your child is negative about tooth-brushing, have him brush your teeth first before you brush his.

• A fluoride toothpaste is beneficial at all ages starting at 1 year. Adults and children tend to use too much toothpaste; an amount the size of a small pea is all that is needed.

• If your child is in a setting where he can't brush his teeth, teach him to rinse his mouth with water after meals instead. Chewing on sugar-free gum (or even regular gum) for 10 minutes after meals gets the saliva flowing enough to clean the teeth.

• Dental floss is essential for cleaning between the teeth where a brush can't reach. This should begin when your child's molars start to touch. In the early years, most of the teeth have spaces between them. As my dentist says, floss only the teeth you want to keep.

Diet

A healthy diet from a dental standpoint is one that keeps the sugar concentration in the mouth at a low level. The worst foods contain sugar and also stick to the teeth.

• Prevent baby bottle tooth decay by not letting your infant sleep with a bottle of milk, juice, or any sweetened liquid in the mouth (see page 193). Once the teeth erupt, if your baby must have a bottle at night, it should contain only water.

• Avoid allowing the child to carry around a bottle or sippy cup during waking hours. Young children who use milk, juice or other sweetened liquid to comfort themselves are prone to severe dental decay.

• Discourage prolonged contact with sugar (e.g., hard candy) or any sweets that are sticky (e.g., caramels or raisins).

• Avoid frequent snacks. Grazing on snack foods is bad for the teeth.

• Give sugar-containing foods only with meals.

• Since we can't keep children away from candy completely, try to teach your child to brush after eating candy.

Dental Visits

The American Dental Association recommends that dental checkups begin at age 3 (sooner for dental symptoms or abnormal-looking teeth).

Dental Sealants

The latest breakthrough in dental research is dental sealing of the pits and grooves (fissures) of the biting surfaces of the molars. Fluoride does little to prevent decay on these surfaces. A special plastic seal can be applied to the top surfaces of the permanent molars at about age 6, when the first molars erupt. The seal may protect against decay for 10 to 20 years without needing replacement. Ask your child's dentist about the latest recommendations.

FOOD ALLERGIES

While food allergies tend to be overdiagnosed, about 5 percent of children have true reactions to foods. Suspect that your child may have a food allergy if the following three characteristics are present:

• Your child has allergic symptoms after eating certain foods. The most common reactions involve the mouth (swelling), GI tract (diarrhea), or skin (hives). Rarely a child has a severe allergic reaction (anaphylactic reaction) that may be life-threatening. Common anaphylactic symptoms are a rapid onset (within 2 hours) of difficulty breathing, difficulty swallowing, weakness from a fall in blood pressure (shock), or confused thinking.

• Your child has other allergic conditions, such as eczema, asthma, or hay fever. Children with these conditions have a much higher rate of associated food allergies than nonallergic children.

• Other family members (parents or siblings) have food allergies. Food allergies are often inherited.

Cause—Allergic children produce antibodies against certain foods. When these antibodies come in contact with the allergic foods, the reaction releases numerous chemicals (such as histamine) that cause the symptoms.

The tendency to be allergic is inherited. If one parent has allergies, about 40 percent of the children will develop allergies. If both parents have allergies, about 75 percent of the children will. Sometimes the child is allergic to the same food as the parent.

Expected Outcome—At least half of the children who develop a food allergy during the first year of life outgrow it by age 2 or 3. Some food reactions (e.g., to milk) are more commonly outgrown than others. Whereas 3 percent to 4 percent of infants have a cow's-milk allergy, less than 1 percent of them develop a lifelong allergy to cow's milk. Allergies to peanuts, tree nuts, fish, and shellfish (shrimp, crab, and lobster) often persist for life.

Common Symptoms of Food Allergies

The following symptoms are all commonly seen with food allergies:
- Lips, tongue, or mouth swelling
- Diarrhea or vomiting
- Hives
- Itchy red skin (especially with underlying eczema)

Some less common symptoms are:
- Sore throat or constant throat-clearing
- Nasal congestion, runny nose, sneezing, or sniffing (especially with underlying hay fever)

An occasional child with asthma, migraine headaches, colic, or recurrent abdominal pain may have some attacks triggered by food allergies. These children, however, also have some of the typical symptoms (listed above) that occur with food reactions. Attention-deficit/hyperactivity disorder (ADHD) and behavioral disorders have not been scientifically linked to food allergies.

Common Allergenic Foods—Overall, the most allergenic food is the peanut. In infants, however, allergies to egg and milk products are more common. The following 4 foods account for over 80 percent of food reactions: peanuts (and peanut butter), eggs, cow's-milk products, and soybeans (and soy formula). Eight foods (fish, shellfish, tree nuts, wheat, and the preceding 4 foods) account for over 95 percent of food reactions. Four foods (chocolate, strawberries, corn, and tomatoes) are highly overrated as triggers of symptoms. While commonly mentioned, they rarely cause any allergic symptoms.

Diagnosing a Food Allergy

Keep a Diary of Symptoms and Recently Eaten Foods—If the ingestion of a particular food is clearly the cause of particular symptoms, go directly to step 2. Otherwise be a good detective and keep a symptom/food diary for 2 weeks. Any time your child has symptoms, write down the foods he ate during the preceding meal. After 2 weeks, examine the diary for foods that were repeatedly consumed on days your child had symptoms. Expect some inconsistency, depending on the amount of food consumed. While anaphylactic reactions can be triggered by small amounts of allergenic foods, other symptoms (e.g., diarrhea) usually increase as the amount of the allergenic food increases, but not to the point of being serious. Reactions to food may be worse when a child is also reacting to other substances in the environment such as pollens. Therefore, food allergies may flare up during pollen season.

Eliminate the Suspected Food from the Diet for 2 Weeks—Record any symptoms that occur during this time. If you have eliminated the correct food, all symptoms should disappear. Most children improve within 2 days, and almost all of them improve after a week of avoiding the allergic food.

Rechallenge Your Child with the Suspected Food—(Caution: This step should never be carried out if your child has experienced a severe or anaphylactic reaction to a food.) The purpose of rechallenging is to prove that the suspected food is definitely the cause of your child's symptoms. Give your child a small amount of the suspected food. The same symptoms should appear 10 minutes to 2 hours after the food is consumed. Discuss a food challenge with your child's physician before doing it.

Treatment of Food Allergies

If confirmed by your child's physician:

Avoid the Allergenic Food—This should keep your child free of symptoms. If you are breast-feeding, eliminate the food your child is allergic to from your diet until breast-feeding is discontinued. Food allergens can be absorbed from your diet and enter your breast milk. Talk to a nutritionist if you have questions.

Consider Avoiding Other Foods in That Food Group—Some children are allergic to 2 or more foods. Occasionally the foods belong to the same food group. The most common cross-reaction involves children allergic to ragweed pollen. They commonly react to watermelon, cantaloupe, musk-melon, honeydew melon, or other foods in the gourd family. Children allergic to peanuts may rarely cross-react with soybeans, peas, or other beans. Surprisingly, most tree nuts are unrelated to each other and also do not cross-react with peanuts.

Provide a Substitute for Any Missing Vitamins or Minerals—Eliminating single foods usually does not cause a nutritional deficiency. If a major food group (such as milk products) is eliminated, however, your child may develop a vitamin or mineral deficiency unless he receives appropriate supplements. Talk to your physician or a nutritionist about this.

Give Benadryl for Hives—If hives or itching are the only symptom, give Benadryl 4 times a day in the appropriate dosage until the hives have been gone for 12 hours.

Join the Food Allergy and Anaphylaxis Network—This national organization can help with any food allergy questions you might have. Contact them at 11781 Lee Jackson Highway, Fairfax, VA 22033 or www.foodallergy.org.

Preventing Food Allergies in High-Risk Children—High-risk or allergy-prone children have parents or siblings with asthma, eczema, severe hay fever, or documented food allergies. The risk is highest if both parents are allergic to foods. The onset of allergies in these children may be delayed by being somewhat careful about their diet. If possible they should breast-feed during the first year of life. The mother should avoid milk products, peanuts, and eggs in her diet during this time. If the mother cannot breast-feed, there are two choices: a formula made from protein hydrolysate (known as an elemental formula) or a soy protein formula. The allergy-prone child should avoid all solid foods until 6 months (instead of 4). Try to avoid milk products, eggs, peanut butter, soy protein, fish, wheat, and citrus fruits during the entire first year of life. Try to avoid the most allergenic foods (peanuts and fish) until age 2.

Call an Emergency Rescue Squad (911) Immediately If

- Your child develops any serious symptoms such as wheezing, croupy cough, difficulty breathing, passing out, tightness in the chest or throat.

Call Your Child's Physician

Immediately If
- Widespread hives, swelling, or itching occur.
- Other mild symptoms occur within 30 minutes of eating a suspected food.

During Office Hours If
- You suspect your child has a food allergy.
- You want to rechallenge your child with a food you suspect.
- You think your child needs to be seen.

OVEREATING: PREVENTION OF

The main cause of overweight is overeating. Overeating means consuming more calories each day than are needed for normal activity and growth. Overeating is mainly a bad habit, and it's learned during the early years of life. Currently 10 percent of 2- to 5-year-old children in the United States are overweight. Any child in a family with a strong tendency toward overweight needs to learn healthy eating habits at an early age. Don't wait to make changes in feeding/eating until your child shows signs of becoming overweight. Prevention is far easier than trying to lose weight.

Feeding Precautions to Prevent Overeating

If your family has a problem with easy weight gain, consider the following feeding precautions to help your child:
- From the beginning, try to teach your child to stop eating before she reaches a point of satiation. Help her stop before she feels completely full and is reluctant to eat another bite.
- Avoid any grazing. Grazing is eating at frequent intervals instead of when the child is hungry. Since grazers rarely experience hunger, when they do they become very upset.
- Only feed for hunger. Help your child recognize hunger and eat only when he's hungry. Teach him not to eat for other cues, such as when he's bored, lonely, stressed, watching TV, etc.

- Don't deny your child food if she is hungry. Parents have control over what they serve but not over the amount eaten. Research has shown that if parents try to control the child's food intake, the child usually develops poor self-control.
- Try to breast-feed. Breast-feeding teaches infants to monitor their intake. Because overfeeding by breast is unusual, breast-fed babies tend to be leaner than bottle-fed kids.
- If you are breast-feeding and your milk has come in, don't allow your infant to graze. Grazing is nursing at frequent intervals, sometimes hourly. Such infants learn to eat when they are upset and to use food for comfort.
- If you are bottle-feeding, don't allow your child to keep a bottle as a companion during the day or night. Children who are allowed to carry a bottle or sippy cup around with them learn to eat frequently and use food as a comforting device.
- Don't feed your baby every time he cries. Most crying babies want to be held and cuddled or may be thirsty and just need some water.
- Also teach your infant to use human contact (rather than food) to relieve stress and discomfort.
- Don't assume a sucking baby is hungry. Your baby may just want a pacifier or help with finding her thumb.
- Don't mistake thirst for hunger. Fussing in hot weather may mean that your baby is thirsty and needs some water.
- Don't insist that your baby finish every bottle. Unless your baby is underweight, he knows how much formula he needs.
- Don't enlarge the hole in the nipple of a baby bottle. The formula will come out of the bottle too fast.
- If you bottle-feed, try to feed your infant no more often than every 2 hours at birth, and no more often than every 3 hours from 2 to 6 months of age.
- Feed your child slowly rather than rapidly.
- Avoid solids until your child is 4 months old.
- Change to 3 meals and 2 snacks a day by 6 months of age.
- Don't insist that your child clean his plate or finish a jar of baby food.
- Don't encourage your child to eat more after she signals she is full by turning her head or not opening her mouth.

- Discontinue breast- and bottle-feeding by 12 months of age.
- Avoid sweets until at least 12 months of age.
- Don't give your child food as a way to distract him or keep him occupied. Instead, give him something to play with when you need free time.
- Avoid giving children bottles, sippy cups, or other snacks while they are in car seats or strollers. They need to learn to entertain themselves at these times.
- Use praise and physical contact instead of food as rewards for good behavior. Use food for rewards only in solving special problems such as difficult toilet training.
- Caution: Don't put your baby on 2 percent milk or skim milk before 2 years of age. Your baby's brain is growing rapidly and needs the fat content of whole milk.

OVERWEIGHT: A WEIGHT-REDUCTION PROGRAM

Symptoms and Characteristics
- Your child has an overweight appearance.
- Weight is more than 20 percent over the ideal weight for your child's height.
- Your teen's skin fold thickness of her arm's fat layer is more than 1 inch (25 millimeters).
- Obesity is defined as weight-to-height ratio (body mass index or BMI) above the 95th percentile.
- Obesity occurs in 10 percent of American children ages 2 to 5 and 15 percent of those ages 6 to 19.

Causes—The tendency to be overweight is usually inherited. If one parent is overweight, 50 percent of the children will have a risk for becoming overweight. If both parents are overweight, 80 percent of the children will be at risk for being overweight. If neither parent is overweight, less than 10 percent of the children will be at risk for overweight. Heredity alone (without overeating) accounts for most mild weight problems (less than 30 pounds over ideal weight as an adult).

Moderate weight problems are usually due to a combination of heredity, overeating, and underexercising. However, some overeating is normal in our society. People like to eat because it makes them feel good. But only those who have the tendency to be overweight will gain weight. It is therefore not reasonable to blame your child for being overweight. The family environment (how much they exercise, how much they watch TV and what foods they serve) is equally important. Perhaps 10 percent of overweight adults eat excessively because they are depressed.

Less than 1 percent of obesity has a physical cause. Your physician can easily determine this by a simple physical examination and a review of your child's growth chart. While being overweight is not your child's fault, something can be done about it.

Health Risks—There are health risks as well as social problems that may occur in overweight children. These include high blood pressure, type 2 diabetes, obstructive sleep apnea from severe snoring, exercise intolerance, lower self-esteem, and depression.

Expected Course—Losing weight is very difficult. Keeping the weight off is also a chore. The best age for losing weight is over 15 years, or whenever appearance becomes critical to your child. The self-motivated teenager has the willpower to change to a healthier diet and lose weight. The best age for slowing the rate of weight gain is any age. The younger your child, the more control you have over what foods are being served. However, the diet must be acceptable to your child at any age. During the first 2 years of life, it is not healthy to lose weight but slowing down the rate of gain is helpful.

How to Help Older Children and Teenagers Lose Weight

Readiness and Motivation— Children are most motivated if the healthier diet and exercise program is undertaken by the entire family. Competing with a parent to see who can lose weight faster can be helpful. Teenagers can be helped with motivation by joining a weight-loss club such as TOPS (Take Off Pounds Sensibly), Weight Watchers, or Overeaters Anonymous. Sometimes schools have a special class or gym class for helping with weight loss. Often the school nurse will talk with overweight children both in groups and individually once a week, as well as weigh them.

Weight loss is not healthy during the rapid growth spurt of the first 2 years of life or early adolescence. During these years any attempt to change weight should try to slow down the rate of gain without actually losing any weight.

Protecting Your Child's Self-Esteem—Self-esteem is more important than an ideal body weight. If your child is overweight, he is probably already disappointed in himself. He needs his family to support him and accept him as he is. Self-esteem can be reduced or destroyed by parents who become overconcerned about their child's weight. Avoid the following pitfalls:

• Don't tell your child he's "fat." Use terms such as "big," "solid," or "a little on the heavy side." Don't discuss his weight unless he brings it up.

• Never try to put your child on a strict diet. Diets are unpleasant and should be self-imposed.

• Never deprive your child of food if he says he is hungry. Offer a healthy snack. Withholding food from a hungry child eventually leads to overeating.

• Don't nag him about his weight or eating habits.

Setting Weight-Loss Goals—Pick a realistic target weight, depending on your child's bone structure and degree of overweight. The loss of ½ pound per week is usually an attainable goal for a teenager. Your child will have to work quite hard to maintain this rate of weight loss for several weeks. Weigh your child once per week at the most. Daily weighings generate too much false hope or false disappointment. When losing weight becomes a strain, have your child take a few weeks off. During this time, help your child hold his or her weight constant.

Once your child has reached the target weight, the long-range goal is to try to maintain that weight within 5 pounds in either direction. Staying at a particular weight is possible only through a permanent moderation in eating. The tendency to gain weight easily will probably be with your child for a lifetime. It's important for your child to understand this.

Healthy Eating Program: Decreasing Calorie Consumption— Your child should eat 3 well-balanced meals a day and average-sized portions. There are no forbidden foods. Your child can have a serving of anything his family or friends are eating. However, there are forbidden amounts. While your child is reducing, he must leave the table a bit hungry. Your child can't eat until he's satiated (full) and hope to lose weight. Shortcuts such as fasting, crash dieting, or diet pills rarely work and may be dangerous. Calorie-counting is helpful for some people but it is too time-consuming for many. Consider the following guidelines on what to eat:

- Fluids: Mainly use low-calorie drinks such as fruit juice diluted with an equal amount of water, diet drinks, or flavored mineral water. Have your child take all milk as skim, 1 percent, or 2 percent milk. Limit milk to 16 ounces per day, as it has lots of calories. If your teen can't give up soda, offer diet soda. Encourage drinking 6 glasses of water per day.
- Meals: Encourage average portions. Discourage seconds.
- Desserts: Encourage smaller-than-average portions. Encourage more Jell-O and fresh fruits as desserts. Avoid rich fatty desserts such as ice cream. No seconds.
- Snacks: Limit snacks to 2 or fewer per day. Serve only low-calorie foods such as raw vegetables (carrot sticks, celery sticks, raw potato sticks, pickles, etc.), raw fruits (apples, oranges, cantaloupe, etc.), popcorn, or diet soft drinks.
- Types of food: Serve fewer fatty foods. Fat has twice as many calories as the same portion of protein or carbohydrate. Trim the fat off meats. Serve more baked, broiled, boiled, or steamed foods and fewer fried foods. Serve more fruits, vegetables, salads, and grains. While no food is a particularly good appetite suppressant, many low-calorie fruits, vegetables, and salads are filling.
- Vitamins: Give your child one multivitamin tablet per day while reducing.

Healthy Eating Habits—Most overeating is due to bad habits. In order to counteract the tendency to gain weight, your youngster must learn healthy eating tips and habits that will last for a lifetime. The following habits can make keeping off pounds easier:

- Discourage skipping any of the 3 basic meals.
- Encourage drinking a glass of water before meals.
- Serve smaller portions. Don't serve adult helpings to children before adolescence.

- Suggest chewing the food slowly, paying more attention to flavors and textures.

- Offer second servings only if your child has waited for 10 minutes after finishing the first serving. It takes at least 20 minutes from the start of the meal for the sensation of fullness to occur.

- Discourage the expectation that all of the food that has been prepared must be eaten. Leftovers can be placed in the refrigerator.

- Don't purchase high-calorie snack foods such as potato chips, candy, or regular soft drinks.

- Do purchase and keep available diet soft drinks, fresh fruits, and vegetables.

- Leave only low-calorie snacks out on the counter—fruit, for instance. Put away the cookie jar. You can buy small amounts of high-calorie treats for special occasions.

- Store food only in the kitchen. Keep it out of other rooms.

- Offer no more than 2 snacks per day. Strongly discourage your child from continual snacking ("grazing") throughout the day. The number of snacks we eat each day is a matter of habit. A person can learn to go through a day with no snacks without developing symptoms.

- Allow eating in your home only while sitting at the kitchen or dining room table.

- Discourage mindless eating while watching TV, at the movie theater, studying, riding in a car, or shopping in a store. Once eating becomes associated with these events, the body learns to expect it.

- Discourage eating alone.

- When eating out, avoid supersize and value meals.

- Help your child reward herself for hard work or studying with a movie, TV, music, or book, rather than food.

- Put up reminder cards on the refrigerator and bathroom mirror that state EAT LESS.

Exercise: Increasing Calorie Expenditure—Small changes in activity level will burn up a surprising number of calories. Daily exercise to the point of breathing hard will have a major impact on the rate of weight loss as well as the sense of physical well-being. Diet and exercise together are the only effective way to lose weight and maintain your new weight.

As your child loses weight, exercise will become less tiring because he or she will be in better condition and have less weight to move about. Try the following forms of exercise:

• Walk or bike instead of riding in a car.

• Use stairs instead of elevators.

• Learn new sports such as roller-skating or jumping rope. Swimming and jogging are the sports that burn the most calories. Your child's school may have an aerobics class.

• Spend more time outdoors.

• Walk 30 minutes per day (e.g., take the dog for a long walk).

• Limit TV sitting time to 2 hours or less per day.

• Use exercise equipment while watching TV.

• Dance to music on TV.

Social Activities: Keeping the Mind off Food—The more outside interests your child participates in, the easier it will be for him or her to lose weight. Spare time fosters nibbling in everyone. Most snacking occurs between 3:00 and 6:00 P.M. Help your child fill after-school time with activities such as music, drama, sports, Scouts, or other clubs. A part-time job after school may help. If nothing else, encourage your child to call or visit a friend. An active social life almost always leads to weight reduction.

EATING PROBLEMS: OTHER STRATEGIES

Doesn't Eat Enough—See APPETITE SLUMP IN TODDLERS, page 171, and PICKY EATERS, page 175.

Stands Up in the High Chair

Rule: "Don't stand up in your chair. Stay seated until the meal is over." This is an important safety issue.

Discipline technique: Some children can be confined to their high chair with the safety strap; others can wiggle out of it. Logical consequences of being put down and having the meal end can teach your child not to stand up.

Praise your child: For staying in his chair at future meals.

Plays with Food

During the early months of learning self-feeding, many children will make a mess of their high-chair tray and of themselves. They may also make a mess because they mix their food with hand or spoon. Children should not be punished for this normal behavior.

Rule: "Don't throw or drop your food. Don't put food on your body. Eat without making a mess."

Discipline technique: When your child throws food, take him out of the high chair and put him in time-out in the playpen for 2 minutes. Then let him return to the table. If he repeats the misbehavior, assume he has had enough to eat and put him down permanently. To deal with some of the normal sloppiness of young eaters, put down newspapers and offer your child small amounts of food at any one time. A dog also comes in handy for cleanup.

Praise your child: For eating without making a mess.

Eats Too Slowly

Some of these children are not hungry. Others are being negative. The problem arises when a child has not finished eating but the rest of the family has completed their meal.

Rule: "The meal is over when everyone else is done eating, because we have to clean up."

Discipline technique: Natural consequences. Clear away your child's plate and put her down after a reasonable amount of time. Don't give her any between-meal snacks if she only eats part of her meal. Serve her smaller portions next time.

Praise your child: For not playing or wasting time during meals.

Eats Too Fast

Most of these children are in a hurry to go back to their play. They may gulp their food in an unsavory manner.

Rule: "Mealtime lasts for at least ten minutes [or whatever length of time the parents decide on] whether you're done earlier or not. Mealtime is a special time when our family gets together."

Discipline technique: Logical consequences. Children will learn that finishing quickly does not allow them to leave the dinner table sooner.

Praise your child: For eating slowly, chewing food with the mouth closed, and eating with good manners.

Demands Frequent Snacks

Some children want a snack, fruit juice, or soda pop every 30 minutes. Frequent snacking leads to tooth decay, is disruptive, and can't be continued when the child enters school.

Rule: "Don't ask for a snack until snack time. We only have one snack in the morning and one snack in the afternoon."

Discipline technique: Ignore your child's requests for snacks before snack time. If he persists, send him to time-out.

Takes Food from the Refrigerator or Cupboards

Rule: "You're not permitted to open the refrigerator until you're five years old. Ask a grown-up if you need something out of the refrigerator."

Discipline technique: If your child opens the refrigerator without your permission, send her to time-out. Put a stop sign on the refrigerator door as a reminder. If your child gets into food cupboards, also send her to time-out. With a persistent child, you may need to put locks on the doors or move snack foods to higher cupboards.

Leaves the Kitchen a Mess

Rule: "Whoever makes a mess in the kitchen cleans it up."

Discipline technique: Logical consequences. If you find the kitchen messy, call your child to clean it up. If your child is not at home, cancel the snack privilege for the next day. As a reminder, put up a sign in the kitchen: EVERYONE CLEAN UP AFTER YOURSELF.

Praise your child: For cleaning up the kitchen.

Model: Clean up after yourself in the kitchen area.

Messes Up the Rest of the House with Food

Rule: "We only eat in the kitchen."

Discipline technique: Logical consequences. If you find crumbs or dirty dishes outside the kitchen area, call your child to clean it up. If your child starts to walk around the house eating food, send your child back to the kitchen.

Model: Don't take food outside the kitchen yourself.

DEVELOPMENT AND SAFETY

DEVELOPMENTAL STIMULATION

Normal Development

The most rapid changes in development occur during the first year of life. Your baby will go from a helpless, unresponsive little bundle to a walking, talking, unique personality. Almost all parents worry about whether their baby is developing fast enough, especially if a sibling or neighbor's child is progressing differently. Keep in mind that there is a wide variation in normal development. While the average child walks at 12 months of age, the normal range for walking is any time between 9 and 16 months of age. All of these children are normal. Motor development occurs in an orderly sequence, starting with lifting the head, then rolling over, sitting up, crawling, standing, and walking. Although the sequence is predictable and follows the maturation of the spinal cord downward, the rate varies from one child to another and it can't be accelerated.

Again, for speech development the sequence goes from cooing and gurgling at birth to vowel sounds (ah and ooh) by 3 months, babbling (bah-bah) by 6 months, imitating speech sounds by 9 months, first spontaneous words (mama) by 12 months, and using words together (go bye-bye) at 18 months. The rate, however, can vary considerably and still be normal. The most reassuring characteristics of normal development are the presence of alert eyes, alert facial expressions, and curiosity about the environment.

Ways to Stimulate Your Child's Development

From birth on, the main determinant of an infant's social, emotional, and language development is the amount of positive contact he has with his parents and other caregivers. His strong attachment to you (which begins at 3 or 4 months of age) will make him eager to learn from you. Experiences during the first 3 years of life determine the permanent "wiring" of the brain. Your role in stimulating your child's mind should be fun for both of you. The following recommendations may be helpful:

Hold Your Baby as Much as Possible—Touching and cuddling are good for your baby. Give him or her lots of eye contact, smiles, and affection at these times. Use feedings to emphasize these warm personal contacts.

Talk to Your Baby—Babies enjoy being talked and sung to from birth onward. Talk while you're doing chores. Put a name on everything your child touches or does. Sing silly songs with your child. Babies must first receive language before they are able to express language. You don't need a scriptwriter—just put into words whatever you are thinking and feeling.

Play with Your Baby—If this doesn't come easily for you, try to loosen up and rediscover your free spirit. Respond to your baby's attempts to initiate play. Provide your baby with various objects of interest. Toys need not be expensive; try mobiles, rattles, spools, pots and pans, and various packages that things come in. Encourage your baby's efforts at discovering how to use his or her hands and mind.

Read to Your Baby—Even 6-month-olds enjoy looking at pictures in a book. Cut out interesting pictures from old magazines and put them in a scrapbook for your baby. Look at the family photo album. Move on to nursery rhymes. Reading to your child correlates better with later school success than anything else you can do. Never let the sun set without having read at least 1 book to your child.

Teach Your Baby to Communicate with Elementary Sign Language—This can be done starting at 7 or 8 months old. Books and classes are available. Within 1 to 2 months, your child will be signing many words.

Show Your Baby the World—Enrich his or her experience. Babies don't need to visit a museum yet. They need a guide to point out the leaves, clouds, stars, and rainbows. Don't forget trains, airplanes, and fire trucks. Help your child describe what he or she is experiencing. Provide your own running commentary about the world as it passes by. These first encounters can be exhilarating and unforgettable.

Pretend with Your Child—Many children talk more freely while they are pretending. Choose 2 stuffed animals, give 1 to your child, hold the other, and pretend they talk to each other. Pretend you're in a spaceship. Make up stories about anything.

Give Your Child Social Experiences with Other Children by Age 2—If he or she is not in day care, consider starting a play group. Young children can learn wonderful lessons from one another, especially the give-and-take of how to get along with other people.

Avoid Formal Teaching Until Age 4 or 5—Some groups in our country have recently overemphasized academic (cognitive) development of young children. Trying to create "superkids" through special lessons, drills, computer programs, and classes has put undue pressure on many young children and may result in early burnout. Old-fashioned creative play and spontaneous learning are much more beneficial during the early years. If it's not fun, your child won't follow through the way you would like.

Symptoms Requiring a Developmental Evaluation

The following developmental milestones (reprinted with the permission of William K. Frankenburg, M.D.) are listed by the age at which 80 to 90 percent of normal children are able to perform them. If your child has reached the listed age (corrected for any prematurity by subtracting the number of months the child was born early from his actual age) and is not able to perform the listed tasks, he or she should be seen by your child's physician for a developmental checkup. While failing one of these items does not mean that your child's development is abnormal, it is a warning sign that deserves attention.

3 Months
- When your baby is lying on his back, he can move each of his arms as easily as the other and each of his legs as easily as the other. If your child makes jerky or uncoordinated movements with one or both of his arms or legs, this is abnormal.
- Your child can make sounds such as gurgling, cooing, babbling (such as bah-bah), or other noises, in addition to crying.

6 Months
- Your child plays with his hands by touching them together.
- When you hold your baby under his arms, he tries to stand on his feet and supports some of his weight on his legs.

9 Months
- When your child is playing and you come up quietly behind him, he turns his head as though he heard you. He responds to quiet sounds or whispers in this manner. (Loud sounds do not count.)

- Your child has rolled over at least two times from stomach to back or from his back to his stomach. (This occurs later than it used to because of sleeping on the back.)

12 Months

- When you hide behind something (or around a corner) and then reappear again, your baby eagerly looks for you to reappear.
- Your baby makes "mama" or "dada" sounds.

18 Months

- Your child uses a regular cup or glass without help and drinks from it without spilling.
- Your child walks all the way across a large room without falling or wobbling from side to side.

24 Months

- Your child can say at least three specific words (other than "dada" and "mama") that mean the same thing each time they are said.
- Your child can take off clothes such as pajamas or pants. (Diapers, hats, and socks do not count.)

36 Months

- Your child can name at least one picture when you look at animal books together.
- Your child can throw a ball overhand (not sidearm or underhand) toward your stomach or chest from a distance of five feet.

4 Years

- Your child can pedal a tricycle at least 10 feet forward.
- Your child can play hide-and-seek or other games where he takes turns and follows rules.

5 Years

- Your child can button some of his clothing or his doll's clothes. (Snaps do not count.)
- Your child is comfortable when you leave him with a baby-sitter. (He does not become overly upset.)

6 Years

- Your child can dress himself completely without help.
- Your child can catch a small ball (such as a tennis ball) using only his hands. (Large balls do not count.)

INJURY PREVENTION

Infant Safety

During the first 3 years of life, children have little sense of danger or self-preservation. They are totally dependent on adults to look after their safety. They cannot be left unattended on a table or bed; they may roll off it and strike their head. For the same reason, crib railings must always be kept in the raised position. A small child cannot be given toys with small parts, because of the danger that the child may put them in his or her mouth and choke on them. Mattresses should not be covered with pieces of thin plastic, because children may get the plastic caught on the face and be smothered by it. Children cannot be left alone in a bathtub while a parent answers the doorbell, because they could drown. Talcum powder should not be used on them because they may breathe it in and develop severe chemical pneumonia. A pacifier or teething ring should not be tied about the neck because it could catch on something and strangle them. And babies should not be left to sleep in a car, because they could develop life-threatening heatstroke.

Unfortunately this is only a partial list of the unexpected injuries that can befall a young child. Adult supervision and vigilance are essential.

Injury Prevention Overview

The prevention of various injuries is discussed throughout this book, along with the appropriate first aid. For details on the prevention of any of the following injuries, turn to the appropriate pages.

CAR SAFETY SEATS

The number 1 killer and crippler of children in the United States is motor vehicle crashes. More than 600 children under the age of 5 years are killed each year, and about 270,000 are injured. Proper use of car safety seats can reduce traffic fatalities by at least 80 percent. All 50 states have passed laws that require children to ride in approved child safety seats.

A parent cannot protect a child by holding him or her tightly. In a 30-mile-per-hour crash, the child will either be crushed between the parent's body and the dashboard or ripped from the parent's arms and possibly thrown from the car. Car safety seats also help to control a child's misbehavior, prevent motion sickness, and reduce the number of accidents caused by a child distracting the driver.

Types of Car Safety Seats

Before you buy a car safety seat, look at several different models. Make sure that the car seat will fit in your car and that your seat belts will work with the seat. There are several types of car safety seats:

Infant-Only Seats—These are rear-facing-only seats. They can be used from birth until a child weighs approximately 20 pounds (depending on the model). They are small and portable.

Some of these seats come with a detachable base. You attach the base to the seat of the car. This allows you to easily snap the car seat in and out of the car without reinstalling the car seat each time. If the base does not attach tightly to your car, it is better to attach the seat each time and not use the base.

Convertible Safety Seats—These seats can be used in both rear- and forward-facing positions. The seat needs to stay in the rear-facing position until your child is over 1 year old and has reached the highest weight allowed for the rear-facing position (usually about 30 pounds, but may be more or less depending on the car seat). They can then be used in the forward-facing position until the child has reached 40 pounds.

Combination Seats—These seats are forward-facing seats that can be used after your child has reached 20 pounds and is at least 1 year old. Your child must wear the 5-point harness until he or she has reached 40 pounds. When your child is over 40 pounds, you can use this seat as a booster seat by correctly positioning the car's lap/shoulder belt across your child. It can be used as a booster seat until your child is about 80 pounds (depending on the model).

Booster Seats—These are forward-facing seats that lift the child higher so your car's lap/shoulder belt will fit correctly over the child. A booster seat is for children over 40 pounds and should be used until the child is 56 inches tall, a height usually reached between 9 and 12 years of age.

Travel Vests—Travel vests are used if you have only lap belts in your car. They vary in weight ranges depending on the model, but are typically used for children at least 2 years old and up to 100 pounds. The lap belt fits through a backrest or loops and the shoulder straps come over your child and buckle.

Built-in Seats (Integrated Seats)—Some cars and vans come with built-in child safety seats. These may be used by children who are over 1 year of age and weigh at least 20 pounds. Weight and height requirements vary depending on the car manufacturer. Check with the maker of the car to find out the specific height and weight requirements.

Tethers and Anchors

Starting in 2002, most new vehicles and car safety seats will have a new system called LATCH (lower anchors and tethers for children). This system may be an easier way to attach safety seats. It allows you to attach the car seat without using a seat belt. However, you will need to continue attaching the car safety seat with a seat belt unless you have both a new car seat and a new car with the LATCH system.

Tether straps are found on most new forward-facing car seats. A tether strap hooks the top of a car safety seat to a permanent anchor in the car to provide extra protection. Tethers reduce the amount of forward movement of the car seat in a crash. Check your car to see if it has an anchor. Cars made since September 2000 are required to have tether anchors. Cars made since 1989 can be retrofitted with tether straps. Most anchors are on the rear window ledge, back of the seat, floor, or ceiling of the car. There are tether kits available for older car seats. Check with your car seat and car manufacturer.

Backseat Versus Front Seat

Whenever possible and at any age, put the safety seat in the backseat of the car, which is much safer than the front seat.

Air bags are standard equipment in most new cars. They have saved many lives. However, they are very hazardous to infants in rear-facing child safety seats and have caused death from brain injury. If your car has air bags, take the following precautions:

• Infants riding in rear-facing child safety seats should never be placed in the front seat of a car or truck with a passenger-side air bag. They must be in the car's rear seat or not ride in that vehicle.

• Children in forward-facing child safety seats should also ride in a car's rear seat until 12 years of age.

• If the vehicle does not have a rear seat, children riding in the front seat should be positioned as far back as possible from the air bag. Move the seat all the way back so that the child is as far as possible from the dashboard. Some cars come with air bag on/off switches. Turn the air bag off only if your car has no backseat.

Switching to a Regular Seat Belt

Keep your child in a booster seat as long as possible. Your child could be ready for a regular seat belt anywhere between 9 and 12 years old depending on height and weight. Your child should be about 57 inches tall and at least 60 to 80 pounds to properly fit in an adult seat belt. When your child is ready for a regular seat belt, use a lap belt low across the thighs. If your child is using a shoulder belt, it should cross your child's chest, not the neck or throat. Never put the shoulder belt under the arm or behind the back.

Safety Standards for Car Seats

Since January 1981, all manufacturers of child safety seats have been required to meet stringent federal government safety standards, including crash-testing. The American Academy of Pediatrics (AAP) publishes a list of infant/child safety seats that have met the federal motor vehicle standards. The list is updated yearly. To get this list, write to the AAP or visit their Web site:

American Academy of Pediatrics (AAP)
Division of Public Education
PO Box 927
Elk Grove Village, Illinois 60007
www.aap.org/family/carseatguide.htm

Each state has its own seat belt laws and safety standards. Although all states require that children be buckled in, not all states require that children travel in the safest way possible. Using a car safety seat correctly is very important. Follow the safety seat instructions and make sure you are keeping your child as safe as possible.

Tips for Using a Car Seat Properly

If used consistently and properly, your child's car seat can be a lifesaver. Your attitude toward safety belts and car seats is especially important. If you treat buckling up as a necessary, automatic routine, your child will follow your lead and also accept car seats and seat belts. To keep your child safe and happy, follow these guidelines from the American Academy of Pediatrics:

• Always use the safety seat. Use the safety seat on the first ride home from the hospital, and continue using it for every ride.

• Everyone buckles up. Allow no exceptions for older kids and adults. If adults ride unprotected, the child quickly decides that safety is just kid stuff.

• Give frequent praise for appropriate behavior in the car.

• Remember that a bored child can become disruptive. Keep a supply of favorite soft toys on hand. Use munchies as a last resort, since they contribute to the unhealthy habit of grazing and overeating.

• Never let a fussy child out of the car seat or safety belt while the car is in motion. If your child needs a break, stop the car. Responding to complaints by allowing your child to ride unprotected is a disastrous decision that will make it harder to keep him or her in the seat on the next ride.

• Similarly, parents should never take off their seat belt to reach into the backseat to attend to a child while the car is in motion. Too many parents have been seriously injured when their car was struck during those few seconds.

• Some infants begin crying at 4 or 5 months (possibly from separation anxiety) when placed in their rear-facing car seats in the backseat. Try distracting them with soothing words, music, and toys. Also give them practice time in the car seat at home, using it for pleasant activities such as playing or eating.

• If a child tries to get out of the seat, stop the car and firmly but calmly explain that you won't start the car until he or she is again buckled in the car seat.

• Booster seats must be used with a lap/shoulder belt.

- When your child travels in another person's car (such as a baby-sitter's or grandparent's car), insist that the driver also use the safety seat.
- For long-distance trips, plan for frequent stops and try to stop before your child becomes restless. Cuddle a young child. Let an older child run around for 10 to 15 minutes. Offer a snack if he hasn't eaten in over 2 hours.

SHOES

The following information may help you make more practical decisions about buying shoes for your young infant.

Shoes Versus Barefoot

- The only purpose of shoes is to protect feet from injury, cold, or burns (from asphalt surfaces). No shoes are needed until your child begins to walk in rough terrain. Children who are walking inside a house or outside on sand or grass do not require shoes.
- Before the age of walking, keep your child's feet warm with booties or socks during the winter.
- Once your child begins to walk, he will prefer to walk barefooted because it gives him a better sense of where his feet are and enables him to use his toes for balance. Shoes may interfere with learning to walk.

Types of Shoes

- When your child finally needs a shoe, buy tennis shoes (sneakers) or some other shoe with a softer flexible sole, such as moccasins, which allow free movement of the foot. Sneakers have the advantage over leather shoes of being comfortable, ventilated, easy to wash, inexpensive, and good for traction. During the first year of walking, moccasins are usually better. Toddlers in sneakers may have too much traction, catch the rubber sole on things, and fall.
- Hand-me-down shoes are fine if they are still in good condition (the sole is still skidproof) and fit. The suggestion that shoes with a previous wear pattern on the heels will cause leg or foot pains is a myth.
- Expensive shoes have no advantage at any age for 99 percent of children. Arches do not "fall." Save your money for something more important.

- Heels are not essential at any age, and they can cause tripping during the first 2 years.
- High-top shoes are not useful, and children who wear them are often teased. Occasionally a toddler will need high-top sneakers because his or her feet continually slip out of low-cut ones.
- Even children with flat feet rarely need a special shoe or heel. Tennis shoes are fine for most of these children.

Shoe Size and Fit

- With a little practice, most parents can determine whether or not a shoe fits. Check proper fit with your child putting weight on the shoes. The length should be approximately ½ inch (an index finger) longer than the big toe. The width should allow you to grasp a small piece of shoe at the widest portion of the foot (the pinch test). The heel area should be snug enough to keep the shoe from flopping up and down during walking. Also, maximum flex should be where the foot flexes and not in the middle of the shoe.
- In young, growing children, shoes commonly become too tight before they wear out.
- During the second and third year of life, shoe size can change three times a year, so check the fit every few months.

PREVENTING INFECTIONS

THE PREVENTION OF INFECTIONS

Public health measures have had the greatest impact in preventing the spread of infectious diseases. Proper sewage disposal and safe water supplies have largely eliminated major epidemics such as typhoid fever and cholera. Immunizations and vaccinations constitute another success of modern medicine and have controlled infectious diseases like smallpox and polio. Precautions within the home can limit the spread of gastrointestinal illnesses. Unfortunately, controlling the spread of colds, coughs, and sore throats within a family unit is impractical if not impossible.

How Different Infectious Diseases Are Spread

Diseases are mainly spread by touching something (e.g., a toy, doorknob, or child's hand) that is contaminated with viruses or bacteria and getting them on your fingers. The second step in transmission is touching your nose or mouth, giving the germs a chance to move in and start a new infection. Here are some specifics:

• Nose, mouth, and eye secretions are the most common sources of respiratory infections. These secretions are usually spread by contaminated hands or occasionally by kissing. Toddlers are especially prone to spreading these infections because of their habits of touching or mouthing everything.

• Droplets in the air spread by coughing or sneezing is a less common means of transmission of respiratory infections. Droplets can travel up to 6 feet.

• Fecal contamination of hands or other objects accounts for the spread of most diarrhea, as well as infectious hepatitis. Unlike urine, which is usually sterile, bowel movements are composed of up to 50 percent bacteria.

- The discharge (fluid or pus) from sores such as chicken pox and fever blisters is contagious. However, most red rashes without any fluids coming out of them are not contagious if you touch them.

- Contaminated food or water accounted for many epidemics in earlier times. Even today, some foods frequently contain bacteria that cause diarrhea. (For example, over 50 percent of raw turkey or chicken contains campylobacter or salmonella bacteria. By contrast, only 1 percent of raw eggs are contaminated with salmonella. Also, ground beef may be contaminated with E. coli.)

- Contaminated utensils such as bottles and dishes can occasionally be a source of respiratory or intestinal infections.

- Contaminated objects such as combs, brushes, and hats can lead to the spread of lice, ringworm, or impetigo.

How to Prevent or Reduce the Spread of Infectious Diseases

The following preventive actions can help reduce the spread of disease within your household.

- Encourage hand washing. Hand washing is critical to preventing the spread of gastrointestinal infections. Scrubbing the hands vigorously with plain water is probably as effective as using soap and water. Hand washing is especially important after using the toilet, changing diapers, and contact with turtles or aquarium water. Choose a day-care center where the staff practices good hand washing after changing diapers. Young children must be supervised in their use of toilets and sinks. A surprising finding of recent studies was that hand washing is also the mainstay in preventing the spread of respiratory disease. (Therefore wash the hands after blowing or touching the nose.)

- Clean off a public toilet seat before sitting on it, if it appears wet or soiled. Use a wet paper towel or wet wipe. For additional protection, line the toilet seat with toilet paper or a seat cover. Sitting on toilet seats does not spread infection if you teach your child always to wash the hands afterward.

- Discourage habits of touching the mouth and nose. Again, this is extremely helpful in preventing the spread of respiratory infections to others. Also, touching the eyes after touching the nose is a common cause of eye infections.

- Don't smoke around your children. Passive smoking increases the frequency and severity of colds, coughs, croup, sinus infections, ear infections, asthma, wheezing, etc. (See PASSIVE [INVOLUNTARY] SMOKING, page 229.)

- Discourage kissing pets. Pets (especially puppies) can transmit bloody diarrhea, worms, and more. Pets are for petting. Don't let your pet lick your child on the face or mouth.

- Cook all poultry thoroughly. Undercooked poultry is a common cause of diarrhea. If it is frozen, thaw it in the refrigerator rather than at room temperature to prevent multiplication of the bacteria. After preparation, carefully wash your hands and any object that comes in contact with raw poultry (such as the knife and cutting board) before using them with other foods. Never serve chicken that is still pink inside (a common problem with outdoor grilling). Don't place the cooked meat on the same platter that the uncooked meat was removed from.

- Use a plastic cutting board. Germs can't be completely removed from wooden cutting boards.

- Avoid eating raw eggs. Don't undercook your eggs. If you make your own eggnog or ice cream, use pasteurized eggs.

- Choose in-home child care over a large child-care center. Day care provided in private homes has a lower rate of infections. Children who are cared for in their own homes by baby-sitters have the lowest rate of infection. Since colds have more complications during the first year of life, try to arrange for home-based day care if your child is in this age group.

- Clean contaminated areas with disinfectants. These products kill most bacteria, including staph. Disinfecting the diaper-changing area, cribs and strollers, play equipment, and food service items is effective in limiting intestinal diseases at home and in day-care centers.

- Don't share cups. When playing team sports, tell your child to use a disposable cup. Don't drink directly from a community water bottle.

- Don't share towels. In public places, use paper towels.

- Contact your child's physician if your child is exposed to meningitis or hepatitis. Antibiotics are useful in preventing some types of bacterial meningitis in exposed children. An injection of immune globulin is helpful in preventing hepatitis in those who have had intimate or extended contact (i.e., greater than 4 hours) with someone having this disease.

- Keep your child's immunizations up-to-date (see below).
- Don't attempt to isolate your child. Isolation is mentioned last because its value within a family unit is questionable. By the time a child shows symptoms of a cold, he or she has already shared the germs with the family. Also, from a practical standpoint, isolation at home is impossible to enforce.

IMMUNIZATIONS FOR PREVENTION

Immunizations protect your child against many serious, life-threatening diseases. Your child should receive shots according to the American Academy of Pediatrics schedule, which is updated yearly. If your child's shots are not up to date, call your child's medical office for an appointment. Ask for an immunization card, keep it up to date, and bring it with you to health checkups and school enrollment.

Reasons Not to Vaccinate

If any of the following conditions apply to your child, talk to your child's physician before getting your child vaccinated.

- Your child had an allergic reaction to a previous vaccine.
- Your child has a serious neurologic disease. The pertussis vaccine (DTaP) should not be given. Your child can still have the tetanus and diphtheria vaccine without the pertussis vaccine.
- Your child has immune system problems. Children with immune systems that are weakened by certain diseases or medicines should not get live-virus vaccines (for example, chicken pox, oral polio, or MMR). A live-virus vaccine can cause the actual disease if the immune system is very weak.
- Your child has egg allergies. Children who have a severe allergy to eggs should not receive the influenza vaccine. However, children who are allergic to eggs can receive all other routine immunizations. Although the measles and mumps vaccines are grown in chick cells, the egg proteins are removed from these vaccines and the vaccines can be given without having your child skin-tested for an egg allergy.

Unwarranted Reasons Not to Vaccinate

Many children in the United States have not received all of the recommended immunizations. Unnecessary precautions have led parents to postpone or cancel scheduled immunizations. The following list of conditions are *not* routine reasons for postponing or canceling immunizations.

Your child *can* still get immunizations if:

- Your child had soreness, redness, or swelling at the injection site after a previous DTaP shot.
- Your child had a fever of less than 105°F (40.5°C) after a previous DTaP shot.
- Your child has a mild illness such as a cold, cough, or diarrhea without a fever.
- Your child is recovering from a mild illness such as a cold, cough, or diarrhea.
- Your child has recently been exposed to an infectious disease.
- Your child is taking antibiotics.
- Your child was premature.
- Your child is breast-feeding.
- Your child has allergies (unless it is an egg allergy).
- Your family has a history of convulsions or sudden infant death syndrome (SIDS).

IMMUNIZATION REACTIONS

Reactions to vaccines are common and almost always harmless. Severe allergic (anaphylactic) reactions to any vaccine are possible, but they are extremely rare or have never been reported. Keep in mind that after careful thought, almost all physicians have decided to immunize themselves and their own children.

Call 911 Immediately If

You notice any of the following severe allergic reactions within 2 hours of receiving the vaccine:

- Difficulty breathing
- Weakness

- Wheezing
- Fast heartbeat
- Hives
- Dizziness or fainting
- Swelling of the throat

Call Your Child's Physician Immediately If

- Your child develops a fever over 104°F, or 40.0°C (0.4 percent).
- Crying continues for more than 3 hours (1 percent).
- Your child's cry is high-pitched or unusual (0.1 percent).
- You suspect any other unusual reaction.

The percentage listed next to each reaction shows the percentage of children who have this reaction.

Possible Reactions to Specific Immunizations

Diphtheria-Tetanus-Pertussis (DTaP)

- Pain, tenderness, swelling, or redness at the injection site for 24 to 48 hours (25 to 45 percent). Giving your child ibuprofen or acetaminophen and placing a cold, wet washcloth over the tender area may provide some relief.
- Fever for 24 to 48 hours (15 to 25 percent). Give your child ibuprofen or acetaminophen if the fever is over 102°F (38.9°C). The next time your child gets a DTaP shot, give your child acetaminophen at your health care provider's office and continue the medicine every 4 to 6 hours for 24 hours.
- Mild drowsiness (15 percent), fretfulness (40 percent), or poor appetite (10 to 15 percent) for 24 to 48 hours.
- Painless lump at the injection site 1 or 2 weeks later. The lump is harmless and will disappear in about 2 months. Call your child's doctor within 24 hours if it turns red or is tender.

Measles, Mumps, Rubella (MMR)

These reactions may begin 7 to 10 days after getting the vaccine.

- Fever of 101 to 103°F (38.3 to 39.5°C) for 2 or 3 days (10 percent). Give your child ibuprofen or acetaminophen if the fever is over 102°F (38.9°C). Call your doctor within 24 hours if the fever lasts over 72 hours or is over 104°F (40°C).

- A mild pink rash mainly on the body (5 percent). No treatment is necessary. The rash will last 2 to 3 days. Call your doctor immediately if the rash changes to purple spots. Call within 24 hours if the rash becomes itchy or the rash lasts more than 3 days.

Polio Vaccine (IPV)

- Sore injection site (rare). No treatment is necessary. Giving your child ibuprofen or acetaminophen and placing a cold, wet washcloth over the tender area may provide some relief.
- Fever (1 to 4 percent). Give your child ibuprofen or acetaminophen if the fever is over 102°F (38.9°C).

Pneumococcal Vaccine

- Fever, usually mild (10 percent). Give your child ibuprofen or acetaminophen if the fever is over 102°F (38.9°C).
- Redness, tenderness, or swelling at the shot site (30 percent). Giving your child ibuprofen or acetaminophen and placing a cold, wet washcloth over the tender area may provide some relief.

Hemophilus Influenza Type B Vaccine (HIB)

- Sore injection site (up to 25 percent) or mild fever (5 percent). Giving your child ibuprofen or acetaminophen and placing a cold, wet washcloth over the tender area may provide some relief.

Hepatitis B Vaccine

- Sore injection site (10 to 25 percent). Giving your child ibuprofen or acetaminophen and placing a cold, wet washcloth over the tender area may provide some relief.
- Fever (up to 7 percent). Give your child ibuprofen or acetaminophen if the fever is over 102°F (38.9°C).

Chicken Pox Vaccine

- Never give your child aspirin for any symptom within 6 weeks of receiving the vaccine. (Reye's syndrome has been linked with the use of aspirin to treat fever or pain caused by a virus.) For fever or pain, give ibuprofen or acetaminophen.
- The chicken pox vaccine may cause pain or swelling at the injection site for 1 to 2 days (20 percent).
- Some children (15 percent) may have a fever that begins 2 to 4 weeks

after the vaccination and lasts 1 to 3 days. Give your child ibuprofen or acetaminophen if the fever is over 102°F (38.9°C).

- A few children (3 percent) develop a mild rash at the injection site or elsewhere on the body. The rash begins 5 to 26 days after the vaccine, looks like a few (2 to 10) chicken pox sores, and usually lasts a few days.

Children with these rashes can go to day care or school. If the vaccine rash contains fluid, cover it with clothing or a Band-Aid. Avoid school if there are widespread, weepy sores (because this may be real chicken pox).

Hepatitis A Virus Vaccine

- Sore injection shot site (20 to 50 percent). Giving your child ibuprofen or acetaminophen and placing a cold, wet washcloth over the tender area may provide some relief.
- Headache or fatigue (less than 10 percent).

Influenza Virus Vaccine

- Pain, tenderness, or swelling at the injection site within 6 to 8 hours (10 percent). Giving your child ibuprofen or acetaminophen and placing a cold, wet washcloth over the tender area may provide some relief.
- Fever of 101 to 103°F or 38.3 to 39.5°C (18 percent). Fevers mainly occur in young children. Give your child acetaminophen or ibuprofen for fever over 102°F (38.9°C).

PASSIVE (INVOLUNTARY) SMOKING

Nonsmoking children who live in homes with smokers are involuntarily exposed to cigarette smoke. The smoke comes from two sources: secondhand smoke and sidestream smoke. Secondhand smoke is exhaled by the smoker. Sidestream smoke rises off the end of a burning cigarette and accounts for most of the smoke in a room. Sidestream smoke contains two or three times more harmful chemicals than secondhand smoke because sidestream smoke does not pass through the cigarette filter. At its worst, a child in a very smoky room for 1 hour with several smokers inhales as many bad chemicals as he would by smoking 10 or more cigarettes. In general, children of smoking mothers absorb more smoke into their bodies than children of smoking fathers because the children spend more time with their mothers. Children who are breast-fed by a smoking mother are at the greatest risk because chemicals are found in the breast milk as well as in the surrounding air.

Harmful Effects of Passive Smoking on Children

Children who live in a house where someone smokes have an increased rate of all respiratory infections. Their symptoms are also more severe and last longer than those of children who live in a smoke-free home. The impact of passive smoke is worse during the first five years of life, when children spend most of their time with their parents. The more smokers there are in a household and the more they smoke, the more severe a child's symptoms. Passive smoking is especially hazardous to children who have asthma. Exposure to smoke causes more severe asthma attacks, more emergency-room visits, and increased admissions to the hospital. These children are also less likely to outgrow their asthma. The following conditions are worsened by passive smoking:

- Ear infections
- Middle-ear fluid and blockage
- Coughs or bronchitis
- Croup or laryngitis
- Wheezing or bronchiolitis
- Asthma attacks
- Pneumonia
- Influenza
- Colds or upper-respiratory infections
- Sinus infections
- Sore throats
- Eye irritation
- School absenteeism for all of the above
- Crib deaths (SIDS)

How to Protect Your Child from Passive Smoking

Give Up Active Smoking—Sign up for a smoking cessation class or program. Giving up smoking is even more urgent if you are pregnant, because your unborn baby has twice the risk for prematurity and complications of the newborn if you smoke during pregnancy. It is also important to avoid smoking if you are breast-feeding, because harmful smoke-related chemicals get into your breast milk. You can stop smoking if you get help. The American Lung Association at 1-800-586-4872 or lung usa.org is dedicated to preventing lung disease. Contact them for free self-help materials (written or audio cassettes) and the location of Freedom from Smoking clinics. If you want your child not to smoke, set a good example.

Never Smoke Inside Your Home—Some parents find it difficult to give up smoking, but all parents can change their smoking habits. Restrict your smoking to times when you are away from home. If you feel you have to smoke when you are home, smoke only in your garage or on the porch. If these options are not available to you, designate a smoking room within your home. Keep the door to this room closed, and periodically open the window to let fresh air into the room. Wear a special overshirt in this room to protect your underlying clothing from collecting the smoke. Never allow your child inside this room, and don't smoke in other parts of the house. Apply the same rules to visitors.

Never Smoke While Holding Your Child—If you feel your smoking habit cannot be controlled to the degree mentioned above, at a minimum protect your child from smoking when you are close to him. This precaution will reduce his exposure to smoke and protect him from cigarette burns. Never smoke in a car when your child is a passenger. Never smoke when you are feeding or bathing him. Never smoke in your child's bedroom. Even doing this much will help your child to some degree.

Avoid Leaving Your Child with a Caretaker Who Smokes—Inquire about smoking when you are looking for day-care centers or babysitters. If your child has asthma, this safeguard is crucial.

CONTAGIOUS DISEASES AND INCUBATION PERIODS

Young children are afflicted with infectious diseases 10 to 15 times per year. The attack rate decreases with age because with each new infection we build up antibodies against future ones. Most of these infections are due to viruses or bacteria, but occasionally fungi or parasites are involved. Your child's symptoms are probably due to an infection if fever is present or the illness spreads to others. The following information is intended to improve your understanding of contagious diseases. (See pages 233–34 for details.)

The Incubation Period

The incubation period is defined as the time interval between exposure to an infectious disease and the onset of symptoms. This information should help answer the questions (1) "When will my child come down with it?" and (2) "Should we cancel our weekend plans?"

If the outer time limit of the incubation period passes and your child is still well, he or she has probably escaped that infection for now (or has previous antibodies against it).

The Contagious Period

The contagious period is defined as that time interval during which a sick child's disease is contagious to others. Knowing the period of contagion helps answer the question "How long does my child have to stay home from school or day care?"

For major illnesses (such as hepatitis), a child will need to remain in isolation at home or in the hospital until all chance of spread has passed. For minor illnesses (like the common cold) restrictions are minimal. Most physicians would agree that a child should stay home at least until he feels well enough to return to school and the fever has been gone for 12 hours.

DISEASE	INCUBATION PERIOD (DAYS)	CONTAGIOUS PERIOD (DAYS)
Skin Infections/Rashes:		
Chicken pox	10–21	2 days before rash until all sores have crusts (6–7 days)
Fifth disease (erythema infectiosum)	4–14	7 days before rash until rash begins
Hand, foot, and mouth disease	3–6	Onset of mouth ulcers until fever gone
Impetigo (strep or staph)	2–5	Onset of sores until 24 hours on antibiotic
Lice	7	Onset of itch until 1 treatment
Measles	8–12	4 days before until 4 days after rash appears
Roseola	9–10	Onset of fever until rash gone (2 days)
Rubella (German measles)	14–21	7 days before until 5 days after rash appears
Scabies	30–45	Onset of rash until 1 treatment
Scarlet fever	3–6	Onset of fever or rash until 24 hours on antibiotic
Shingles (contagious for chicken pox)	14–16	Onset of rash until all sores have crusts (7 days) (note: no need to isolate if sores can be kept covered)
Warts	30–180	Minimally contagious
Respiratory Infections:		
Bronchiolitis	4–6	Onset of cough until 7 days
Colds	2–5	Onset of runny nose until fever gone
Cold sores (herpes)	2–12	See note 1 (page 234)
Coughs (viral) or croup (viral)	2–5	Onset of cough until fever gone
Diphtheria	2–5	Onset of sore throat until 4 days on antibiotic
Influenza	1–2	Onset of symptoms until fever gone
Sore throat, strep	2–5	Onset of sore throat until 24 hours on antibiotic
Sore throat, viral	2–5	Onset of sore throat until fever gone
Tuberculosis	6–24 months	Until 2 weeks on drugs (note: most childhood TB is not contagious)
Whooping cough (pertussis)	7–10	Onset of runny nose until 5 days on antibiotic
Intestinal Infections:		
Diarrhea, bacterial	1–5	See note 2 for diarrhea precautions
Diarrhea, giardia	7–28	See note 2 for diarrhea precautions
Diarrhea, traveler's	1–6	See note 2 for diarrhea precautions
Diarrhea, viral (rotavirus)	1–3	See note 2 for diarrhea precautions
Hepatitis A	14–50	2 weeks before until 1 week after jaundice begins
Pinworms	21–28	Minimally contagious, staying home is unnecessary
Vomiting, viral	2–5	Until vomiting stops
Other Infections:		
Infectious mononucleosis	30–50	Onset of fever until fever gone (7 days)
Meningitis, bacterial	2–10	7 days before symptoms until 24 hours on IV antibiotics in hospital
Mumps	12–25	5 days before swelling until swelling gone (7 days)
Pinkeye without pus (viral)	1–5	Mild infection, staying home is unnecessary
Pinkeye with pus (bacterial)	2–7	Onset of pus until 1 day on antibiotic eyedrops

Notes

1. Cold sores: Less than 6 years old, contagious until cold sores are dry, 4–5 days (no isolation if sores are on part of body that can be covered); more than 6 years old, no isolation necessary if beyond touching/picking stage.

2. Diarrhea precautions: Contagious until stools are formed. A toilet-trained child should stay home until fever is gone, diarrhea is mild, blood and mucus are gone, and child has control over loose BMs. Non-toilet-trained children should stay home until stools are formed. Shigella and E. coli 0157 require extra precautions. Consult your day-care provider regarding attendance restrictions.

Infections That Are Not Contagious

Try not to become preoccupied with infections. Some of the more serious ones are not even contagious (e.g., encephalitis). Some infections are due to blockage of a passageway followed by an overgrowth of bacteria. Examples of these are ear infections and sinus infections. Urinary tract infections are not contagious. Lymph node and bloodstream infections are also rarely contagious. Pneumonia is a complication of a viral respiratory infection in most cases and is usually not contagious. While exposure to meningitis requires consultation with your child's physician, most children exposed to this disease do not become infected. Venereal (genital) diseases are usually noncontagious unless there is sexual contact or shared bathing arrangements.

FREQUENT COLDS AND OTHER INFECTIONS

Some children seem to constantly have the sniffles. They get one cold after another. Many a parent wonders: "Isn't my child having too many colds?" Children start to get colds after about 6 months of age. During infancy and the preschool years, they average 7 or 8 colds a year. School-age children average 5 or 6 colds a year. During adolescence they finally reach an adult level of approximately 4 colds a year. Colds account for more than 50 percent of all acute illnesses with fever. A young child who has 8 colds a year (each lasting 10 to 14 days) actually is sick almost a third of that year.

In addition, children can have diarrhea illnesses (with or without vomiting) 2 or 3 times per year. Some children are especially worrisome to their parents because they tend to get high fevers with most of their colds or they have a sensitive gastrointestinal (GI) tract and develop diarrhea with the majority of their colds. These repeatedly ill children cause their parents a great deal of consternation.

Similar Condition: Allergies—If your child is over age 3, sneezes a lot, has a clear nasal discharge that lasts over a month, doesn't have a fever, doesn't spread the symptoms to other people, and especially if these symptoms occur during pollen season, your child probably has a nasal allergy and you should refer to the guidelines on HAY FEVER, page 556. Allergies are much easier to treat than frequent colds because medicines are effective at controlling symptoms.

Causes—The main cause of frequent colds is that your child is being exposed to new viruses. There are at least 200 different cold viruses. The younger the child, the less the previous exposure and subsequent protection. Your child is exposed more if he or she attends day care, a play group, a church nursery, or a preschool. Your child has more indirect exposures if he has older siblings in school. Therefore, colds are more common in large families. The rate of colds triples in the wintertime, when people spend more time crowded together indoors breathing recirculated air. In addition, smoking in the home increases your child's susceptibility to colds.

What Doesn't Cause Frequent Infections

Most parents are worried that their repeatedly ill child has some serious underlying disease. Children with immune system diseases (inadequate antibody or white blood cell production) don't experience any more colds than the average child. Instead, they have two or more bouts per year of serious infections such as pneumonia, sinus infection, draining lymph nodes, or boils. They also heal slowly from these infections. In addition, most children with serious disease neither gain weight adequately nor appear well between bouts of infection. Tell your physician if your family is worried about a particular diagnosis so your physician can discuss this concern with you. Also, recurrent ear infections don't mean that your child has a serious health problem, only that his eustachian tubes don't drain properly.

Other parents worry that they have neglected their child or done something wrong to cause frequent colds. On the contrary, having all these colds is an unavoidable part of growing up. Colds are the one infection we can't prevent yet. From a medical standpoint, colds are an educational experience for your child's immune system.

Dealing with Frequent Infections

Look at Your Child's General Health—If your child is vigorous and gaining weight, you don't have to worry about his or her basic health. Your child probably is no sicker than the average child of her age. Children get over colds by themselves. While you can do something to reduce the symptoms, you can't shorten the course of each cold (see COLDS, page 550). Your child will just have to muddle through like every other child. The long-term outlook is good. The number of colds will decrease over the years as your child's body builds up a good antibody supply to the various viruses. To help put infections in perspective, a recent survey found that on any given day, 10 percent of children have a cold, 8 percent have a fever, 5 percent have diarrhea, and 3 percent have an ear infection.

Send Your Child Back to School as Soon as Possible—The main requirement for returning your child to school or day care is that the fever is gone and the symptoms are not excessively noisy or distracting to classmates. It doesn't make sense to keep a child home until we can guarantee that he or she is no longer shedding any viruses (as this could take 2 or 3 weeks). If isolation for respiratory infections were taken seriously, insufficient days would remain to educate children. Also the "germ warfare" that normally occurs in schools is fairly uncontrollable. Most children shed germs during the first days of their illness before they even look sick or have symptoms. In other words, contact with respiratory infections is unavoidable in group settings, such as schools or day care. Also, as long as your child's fever has cleared, there is no reason not to attend parties, play with friends after school, and go on scheduled trips. The overexertion of gym and team sports may need to wait a few extra days.

Try Not to Miss Work—When both parents work, these repeated colds are extremely inconvenient and costly. Since the complication rate is low and the improvement rate is slow, don't hesitate to leave your child with someone else at these times. If your baby-sitter is willing to accept the care of a child with a fever, take advantage of the offer. If your child is in day care or preschool, send him or her back once the fever is gone. There's no need to prolong the recovery at home if you need to return to work. Early return of a child with a respiratory illness won't increase the complication rate for your child or the exposure rate for other children.

Likewise, you don't need to cancel an important social engagement because your child has a minor acute illness. There will be many more of these. You also don't need to take your child out of preschool or day care permanently because of the nuisance aspect of all these repeated illnesses. Consider switching to a small, home-based day care if your child is less than 2 years old. Also find another day-care center if someone on the staff smokes on site.

What Doesn't Help

There are no instant cures for recurrent colds and other viral illnesses. Antibiotics are not helpful unless your child develops complications such as an ear infection, sinus infection, or pneumonia. Since the colds are not caused by bad tonsils, having your child's tonsils removed is not helpful (see TONSIL AND ADENOID SURGERY, page 576). Colds are not caused by poor diet or lack of vitamins. They are not caused by bad weather, air conditioners, or wet feet. Again, the best time to have these infections and develop immunity is during childhood.

Related Topic

PREVENTION OF COLDS (see page 554)

MEDICINES

NONPRESCRIPTION DRUG DOSAGE TABLES

Determine your child's dosage by finding his or her weight in the top row of each of the tables that follow.

ACETAMINOPHEN DOSAGE (FOR FEVER AND PAIN)									
Child's weight more than (pounds)	7	14	21	28	42	56	84	112	lbs
Total amount (mg)	40	80	120	160	240	325	480	650	mg
Infant drops 80 mg/0.8 ml	0.4	0.8	1.2	1.6	2.4	—	—	—	ml
Syrup 160 mg/5 ml (1 tsp)	—	½	¾	1	1½	2	3	4	tsp
Chewable 80 mg tablets	—	—	1½	2	3	4	5–6	8	tabs
Chewable 160 mg tablets	—	—	—	1	1½	2	3	4	tabs
Adult 325 mg tablets	—	—	—	—	—	1	1½	2	tabs

- Repeat every 4–6 hours as needed. Don't give more than 5 times a day.

- Note: Acetaminophen also comes in 80, 120, 325, and 650 mg suppositories (the rectal dose is the same as the dosage given by mouth).

- Don't use under 3 months of age (reason: fever during the first 12 weeks of life needs to be documented in a medical setting; if fever is present, your infant needs a complete evaluation).

BENADRYL DOSAGE (ANTIHISTAMINE)

Child's weight more than (pounds)	20	25	38	50	100	lbs
Total amount (mg)	10	12.5	19	25	50	mg
Liquid 12.5 mg/5 ml (1 tsp)	3/4	1	1½	2	—	tsp
Chewable 12.5 mg	—	1	1½	2	4	tablets
Capsules 25 mg	—	—	—	1	2	caps

- Repeat every 6–8 hours as needed.
- Don't use under 1 year of age without consulting your child's physician (reason: it's a sedative).

CHLORPHENIRAMINE DOSAGE (ANTIHISTAMINE)

Child's weight more than (pounds)	22	33	44	55	66	77	88	lbs
Total amount (mg)	1	1½	2	2½	3	3½	4	mg
Liquid 2 mg/5 ml (tsp)	½	3/4	1	1	1½	1½	2	tsp
Tablets 4 mg	—	—	½	½	½	1	1	tablets

- 6–12 years: 8 mg long-acting tablet every 12 hours as needed.
- 12 years and older: 12 mg long-acting tablet every 12 hours as needed.
- Don't use under 1 year of age (reason: it's a sedative).

DEXTROMETHORPHAN (DM) DOSAGE (COUGH SUPPRESSANT)

Child's weight more than (pounds)	16	32	48	64	80	96	130	lbs
Total amount (mg)	2.5	5	7.5	10	12.5	15	20	mg
Liquid 5 mg/5 ml (1 tsp)	½	1	1½	2	2½	3	—	tsp
Liquid 7.5 mg/5 ml (1 tsp)	—	—	1	1	1½	2	3	tsp
Liquid 10 mg/5 ml (1 tsp)	—	—	—	1	1	1½	2	tsp

- Repeat every 6–8 hours as needed.
- Don't use under 1 year of age (reason: cough is a protective reflex).

IBUPROFEN DOSAGE (FOR FEVER AND PAIN)

Child's weight more than (pounds)	12	18	24	36	48	60	72	96	lbs
Total amount (mg)	50	75	100	150	200	250	300	400	mg
Infant drops 50 mg/1.25 ml	1.25	1.875	2.5	3.75	5.0	—	—	—	ml
Liquid 100 mg/5 ml (1 tsp)	1/2	3/4	1	1 1/2	2	2 1/2	3	4	tsp
Chewable 50 mg tablets	—	—	2	3	4	5	6	8	tabs
Junior-strength 100 mg tablets	—	—	—	—	2	2 1/2	3	4	tabs
Adult 200 mg tablets	—	—	—	—	1	1	1 1/2	2	tabs

- Repeat every 6–8 hours as needed.
- Infant drops come with a syringe.
- Don't use under 6 months of age (reason: safety not established and doesn't have FDA approval).

PSEUDOEPHEDRINE DOSAGE (DECONGESTANT)

Child's weight more than (pounds)	18	27	36	54	72	140	lbs
Total amount (mg)	7.5	12	15	22	30	60	mg
Infant drops 7.5 mg/0.8 ml	0.8	1.2	1.6	—	—	—	ml
Liquid 15 mg/5 ml (1 tsp)	1/2	3/4	1	1 1/2	2	—	tsp
Chewable 15 mg	—	—	1	1 1/2	2	4	tabs
Tablet 30 mg	—	—	—	—	1	2	tabs
Tablet 60 mg	—	—	—	—	—	1	tabs

- Repeat every 6 hours as needed.
- Don't use under 6 months of age (reason: risk of dosage error).

MEDICINES: OVERUSE

We are a greatly overmedicated society. Many people believe that there is a drug for every symptom. Some physicians prescribe a drug during every office visit. These habits can convey to our young people that drugs are the answer to life's discomforts. More than $6 billion per year is spent on nonprescription drugs for fever, colds, and coughs—many of them unnecessary. Drugs for vomiting and diarrhea are largely ineffective, and these symptoms respond best to dietary changes. Remember that mild symptoms do not require any medication, and moderate symptoms often respond to home remedies. Drugs are not essential to recovery from most illnesses. Life is not a drug-deficient state.

Common Symptoms and Nonprescription Medicines

- When your child is sick with a viral illness, your goal is to make him as comfortable as possible.
- If your child is playing and sleeping normally, nonprescription medicines are not needed.
- Give medicines only for symptoms that are causing discomfort, disrupting sleep, or really bothering your child—coughing spasms, for instance.
- Medicines for symptoms can only partially relieve those symptoms (e.g., a fever will be lowered but not to normal).
- Medicines for symptoms do not shorten the course of an illness.
- Nonprescription (over-the-counter) medicines also can have side effects.

ANTIBIOTICS: PREVENTING UNNECESSARY USE

Antibiotics are strong medicines that can kill bacteria. Antibiotics have saved many lives and prevented many serious complications. However, antibiotics have no impact on viral infections. One of the more important decisions made daily by every physician is whether a child's infection is viral or bacterial. Parents can learn to make some of these decisions themselves.

Viral Infections

Viruses cause most infections in children, including:

- All colds
- All croup
- 99 percent of coughs
- 95 percent of fevers
- 90 percent of sore throats
- 99 percent of diarrhea and vomiting

Bacterial Infections

Bacterial infections are much less common than viral infections. Bacteria cause:

- Most ear infections
- Most sinus infections
- 10 percent of sore throats (strep throat)
- Whooping cough (pertussis)
- Some pneumonia (lung infection)

Common Myths About Symptoms

These symptoms are sometimes misinterpreted as signs of bacterial infection:

- Yellow nasal discharge. Yellow discharge is more likely to be a normal part of the recovery from a cold than a clue to a sinus infection.
- Yellow phlegm (sputum). This is a normal part of a viral tracheitis or bronchitis, not necessarily a sign of pneumonia.
- High fevers. A fever can be caused by a virus or bacteria.

Reasons Not to Overuse Antibiotics

Some people think that children with colds need antibiotics to prevent ear or sinus infections. Following a cold, about 10 percent of children will develop an ear infection and 1 percent will develop a sinus infection. Giving antibiotics to the other 89 percent who don't need them can cause the bacteria to become more resistant and your child to have unnecessary side effects. It is better to wait and give antibiotics to children who really have a bacterial infection.

Bacterial Resistance—When bacteria become resistant to an antibiotic, that medicine can no longer kill that type of bacteria. The more antibiotics that are used, the more bacteria become more resistant to the medicine. Research shows that half of the prescriptions for antibiotics are not necessary. This makes future treatment of bacterial infections more difficult. Many bacteria are now resistant to antibiotics that used to control them. When we turn to newer and more expensive antibiotics, bacteria develop resistance to them as well. In the battle between antibiotics and bacteria, the bacteria seem to be winning.

Side Effects—All antibiotics have side effects. Unless your child really needs an antibiotic, there is no reason to risk the side effects of the medicine. Some children taking antibiotics develop diarrhea, nausea, vomiting, or a rash. The diarrhea is often due to the loss of healthy intestinal bacteria. If your child gets a rash, your doctor must decide if the rash is an allergic reaction to the drug or if it is an unrelated viral rash (such as roseola). Because it's difficult to be sure, your child may be considered allergic to a family of antibiotics when he really isn't. Then your child can't take that type of antibiotic again.

Summary

Don't pressure your child's doctor to prescribe an antibiotic. If your child has a viral illness, an antibiotic will not shorten the course of the fever or help the other symptoms. Antibiotics will not get your child back to school or you back to work sooner. If your child develops side effects to the antibiotic, he will feel worse instead of better.

Let's save antibiotics for ear infections, sinus infections, strep throat and other bacterial infections. Let's not waste them on yellow nasal discharge, yellow phlegm, high fevers, and other normal symptoms associated with coughs and colds. Treat your child's symptoms with over-the-counter medicines or home remedies. Many just need extra TLC (tender loving care) until they feel better. Fortunately the body's normal antibodies, once produced, can kill future viruses. Call the doctor if your child develops any new signs that suggest a bacterial illness. Usually antibiotics are not the answer when your child becomes sick.

MEDICINES: SAFE USE

- Most medicines can cause poisoning. Keep them out of reach of children. Keep the child-proof caps on.

- Give the correct amount (dosage) for your child. Read the directions on the label carefully. Measure the dose out exactly. Use a measuring spoon or device. A 1-teaspoon measuring spoon should hold 5 ml (or 5 cc). Tableware teaspoons hold varying amounts (2 to 7 ml) and should not be used.

- Give the medicine at the correct time intervals. If you forget a dosage, give it as soon as you remember it, and give the next one at the correct interval following the late dosage. Generally, "4 times a day" does not mean you have to awaken your child in the middle of the night unless he sleeps more than 8 hours.

- "Do not take with food" means food will partially interfere with drug absorption. Give the medicine either 1 hour before or 2 hours after meals.

- If you think your child is having a reaction to the medicine, call your physician before discontinuing it. Drug allergies tend to be overdiagnosed (see AMOXICILLIN RASH, page 445). Many drug symptoms, such as nausea or jitteriness, disappear when the dosage is reduced.

- Continue antibiotics until the bottle is empty. Your physician will prescribe the correct amount of antibiotic to kill all the bacteria. Stopping the antibiotic early can result in a flare-up.

- Give symptomatic medicines only when your child is having lots of symptoms (e.g., hacking cough) or is uncomfortable (e.g., fever over 102 or 103°F). These medicines do not need to be given continuously. If you decide to use them continuously, however, be certain to stop them once the symptoms have cleared for more than 12 hours.

- Don't give a prescription medicine to anyone except the person it was prescribed for—not to brothers or sisters, for instance. Some adult medicines are never prescribed for children because of their special side effects on the growing body, such as staining the teeth.

- Don't use outdated medicines. They lose their strength over time and some may be harmful. Most liquid antibiotics are worthless after 4 weeks, so discard them if any is left. Most other medicines are potent for 1 to 4 years. While pills usually last longer than liquid medicines, check the label for an expiration date.

Related Topics

Giving ear drops—see under SWIMMER'S EAR, page 545
Giving eye drops—see under RED OR PINKEYE WITH PUS, page 527
Giving nose drops—see under COLDS, page 550

MEDICINES: HELPING CHILDREN SWALLOW THEM

A Preventive Approach

When your child is sick, he may need to take some medicines. For liquid medicines, a plastic syringe or oral dropper is easier to use than a spoon with infants or struggling children. If you have only a spoon, keep a towel handy for spills.

Approach your child in a matter-of-fact way with an expectation that he will take it without resistance. Some children will respond better to an enthusiastic "Mary Poppins" approach.

Position your child sitting up and pour or drip the medicine onto the back of the tongue or into the pouch inside the cheek. Some young children become cooperative if you let them hold the syringe and place it in the mouth. Then all you have to do is push the plunger. If your child is uncooperative, however, you must place the liquid beyond the teeth or gumline. Also, if you're using a syringe, don't squirt it forcefully into the back of the throat, because of the danger of its going into the windpipe and causing choking. If you drip the medicine in slowly, you can avoid gagging or choking.

Medicines That Taste Bad: Disguising the Taste

Bitter medicines will often lead to refusal unless some of the following preventive steps are taken:

- Have your child suck on a Popsicle beforehand to numb the mouth partially.
- Serve the medicine cold to reduce the taste.
- Mix it with a strong flavor (such as Kool-Aid powder or chocolate syrup) to hide the bad taste.
- Dilute the medicine as much as possible (e.g., 1 dose mixed in 2 glasses of cold apple juice) if you're certain your child can drink it all.
- Mix crushed pills with one of your child's favorite foods that doesn't require chewing. Consider ice-cream toppings (especially chocolate syrup), honey, pancake syrup, applesauce, ice cream, sherbet, or yogurt. Before adding the medicine, have your child practice swallowing the food alone without chewing it, since chewing would bring out the bad taste of the medicine.
- Have a glass of your child's favorite cold drink ready to rinse his mouth afterward—a sort of "chaser."
- Praise and hug your child for all cooperation.
- The older your child is, the more you can ask for his or her suggestions.
- Some respond to being given complete control of the spoon or syringe.

Refusal of Liquid Medicines

Some 1- to 4-year-old children vigorously refuse to take medicines, even after you have tried to hide the taste. If the medicine is not essential to recovery (such as most nonprescription medicines for coughs, colds, and fever), discontinue it. If you are uncertain of the importance of the medicine, call your physician for advice. If the drug is essential (such as most antibiotics), apply the following recommendations:

- Be honest and sympathetic ("I'm sorry it tastes bad. We can mix it with anything you like").
- Be firm and give a reason ("You have to take it, or you won't get well").
- Give your child a time-out in the corner to think about it. Every 5 minutes, ask him, "Are you ready yet?" If 15 minutes pass, take action.
- Immobilize your child. Two people are usually needed. Have your friend position your child on the lap, holding the arms with one hand and the head with the other. You can use one hand to hold the medicine and the other to open your child's mouth. If you are alone, first wrap your child with a sheet. Ask the office nurse to show you how this is done.
- Be sure your child is not lying flat, to prevent choking.
- Open your child's mouth by pushing down the chin or running your finger inside the cheek and pushing down on the lower jaw.
- Insert the syringe between the teeth and drip the medicine onto the back of the tongue.
- Keep the mouth closed until your child swallows. Gravity can help if you have your child in an upright position. However, swallowing can't occur if the head is bent backward.
- Afterward, apologize and review the alternative: "I'm sorry we had to hold you. If you cooperate next time, we won't have to."
- Give your child a hug.
- Forcing your child in this way to take an important medicine will teach him you mean business and will eventually bring cooperation.
- Don't attack self-esteem—for instance, by saying, "You're acting like a baby."
- Don't punish, as with spanking or yelling.
- If your child vomits or spits out the medicine, estimate the amount lost and repeat it.

Refusal of Pills or Capsules

Some children have difficulty swallowing pills and capsules. If so, try some of the following approaches:

- The easiest approach is to convert it to a liquid form. Empty out the capsules or crush the pills. This approach is acceptable unless the product is a slow-release or enteric-coated pill. (Check with your physician if you are uncertain what you can do.)
- Slow-release capsules can be emptied as long as the contents are swallowed without chewing. Since capsules usually contain medicines with a bitter taste, the contents need to be mixed with a sweet food.
- Pills are usually made as a convenient alternative to the liquid form, and they may not taste bad. Pills can be crushed between two spoons. Crushing is made easier by first moistening the pill with a few drops of water and letting it soften for 15 minutes.
- Place the pill or capsule far back on the tongue and have your child quickly drink water or Kool-Aid through a straw. If your child concentrates on swallowing (even gulping) the liquid, the pill will follow downstream without a hitch. Sometimes coating the pill with butter helps.
- If your child is over 7 or 8 years old and unable to swallow pills, he should practice this skill when he's not sick or cranky. (Some children can't accomplish pill-swallowing until age 10, however.) Start with mini M&M's and progress to plain M&M's. This technique works well because children are not intimidated by M&M's, and if the child has difficulty swallowing them, they will melt. If necessary, first coat them with butter.

Use the liquid and straw technique. Once candy pellets are mastered, pills will usually be manageable. For extra confidence, split the pill into halves or quarters.

Call Your Child's Physician If

- Your child vomits the medicine more than once.
- You are unable to get your child to take an essential medicine.

The next time your physician prescribes a medicine, be sure to mention that your child has this common problem. He may be able to prescribe one that tastes better.

FIRST AID KIT

The first aid kit may be needed at home, on a vacation, or while hiking or camping. Therefore, the contents should be kept in a small box that is portable. Medicines are usually not included for short hikes.

- Band-Aids
- Sterile gauze pads—both regular and nonstick type
- Adhesive tape, ½-inch wide
- Steristrips or butterfly Band-Aids (for closing minor lacerations)
- Soap—small sample bar (note: hydrogen peroxide solution is unnecessary, as it's no better than soap and water for cleaning wounds)
- Alcohol wipes (individually wrapped packets)
- Elastic bandage (for sprained ankle)
- Triangular bandage (for arm injury)
- Tourniquet (can use the triangular bandage)
- Needle and tweezers without teeth (for removing slivers or ticks)
- Small scissors
- Meat tenderizer powder for bee stings
- Insect repellent (30 percent DEET)
- Sunscreen with SPF of 30 or higher
- Adrenaline and syringes (optional; needed if family member has a severe bee-sting allergy) (See ALLERGIC REACTION, SEVERE, page 13, for details.)
- Optional medicines for camping: antibiotic ointment, hydrocortisone cream, antihistamines, acetaminophen, ibuprofen
- Extra supplies for hiking or camping: compass, whistle, flashlight, matches

HOME MEDICINE CHEST
(Nonprescription Medicines)

This list of nonprescription drugs and supplies will be sufficient to relieve symptoms in the majority of acute illnesses that affect every family. Since these medicines will not shorten the course of the illnesses, give them only when symptoms are really bothering your child. See the specific guidelines for more details on using these drugs. (Caution: Keep these medicines locked up and away from children.)

- Acetaminophen: for fever or pain
- Ibuprofen: for fever or pain
- Thermometer, appropriate type for age (see page 436)
- Rubber suction bulb: for stuffy, blocked nose, after using saline or warm water nose drops
- Butterscotch hard candies: for sore throat
- Cough drops: for mild coughs
- Dextromethorphan-containing (cough-suppressant) cough syrup: for severe coughs
- Humidifier: for coughs or croup
- Ice bag or cold pack: for injured muscles, bones, and joints
- Antibiotic eye drops: for bacterial eye infections with a yellow discharge (note: this is the only prescription item on this list)
- Cotton balls: for cleaning infected eyes
- Sunscreen (cream and lip balm)
- Hydrocortisone, 1 percent: for itchy skin conditions such as mosquito bites and poison ivy
- Antibiotic ointment: for skin infections
- Acetone (nail polish remover): for removing tape from the skin
- Rubbing alcohol (70 percent isopropyl alcohol): for sterilizing the skin or needles
- Antihistamine medicine: for hives, hay fever, and eye allergies
- Dramamine tablets: for motion sickness (optional; if family member has this condition)
- Glucose-electrolyte solution (also called oral rehydration solution): if you have a child less than 1 year old, keep a bottle handy for severe vomiting or diarrhea
- Gastrointestinal medicines: Vomiting and diarrhea respond best to dietary changes, and the numerous nonprescription medicines that are available are unnecessary or harmful. Acute constipation may occasionally require some milk of magnesia, but most children, again, respond to dietary change.

- Tincture of time: cures the majority of self-limited illnesses
- TLC (tender loving care): makes the time pass more quickly for most symptoms

ANTIBIOTICS, FAILURE TO IMPROVE ON

If your child is taking an antibiotic for an ear infection, sinus infection, pneumonia, urinary tract infection, etc., he should begin to improve between 24 and 72 hours. If not, he may have a complication or a resistant bacteria.

Call Your Child's Physician

Immediately If
- The fever continues for more than 72 hours despite use of the antibiotics.
- Your child develops a stiff neck.
- Your child starts to look or act very sick.
- You think your child needs to be seen.

During Office Hours If
- The fever goes away for 24 hours or more and then returns.
- Symptoms other than fever (e.g., headache or earache) have not improved after 72 hours on the antibiotic.
- You have other questions or concerns.

Home Care
Bacterial infections usually do not respond to the first dose of antibiotics. While some infections (such as strep) respond fast, most take 48 to 72 hours before we see any improvement.

V. Behavior: Preventing and Solving Problems

SLEEP PROBLEMS

CRYING BABY (Colic)

Characteristics of Fussy Crying (Colic)
- Unexplained crying
- Healthy child (not sick or in pain)
- Well-fed child (not hungry)
- Usually cries 1 to 2 hours at a time
- Cries once or twice per day
- Acts fine (happy or contented) between bouts of crying
- Usually consolable when held and comforted
- Onset usually under 2 weeks of age (crying that begins after 4 weeks of age usually is not colic)
- Resolution by 3 months of age

If your child's symptoms are different, call your physician for help.

Cause—Normally infants do some crying during the first months of life. When babies cry excessively and without being hungry, overheated, or in pain, we call it colic. About 10 percent of babies have colic. While no one is certain what causes colic, these babies seem to want to be soothed so they can go to sleep. Colic tends to occur in babies with a sensitive, active temperament. Keep in mind that all babies are not the same, and you have one with extra energy and persistence. Ask your mother if you were that way as a baby because temperament tends to be genetic. These traits will be an asset someday.

Let's review some misconceptions about what causes colic. Colic is not the result of bad parenting, so don't blame yourself. Colic is also not due to excessive gas, so don't bother with extra burping or special nipples. Colic is not due to inadequate breast-feeding. Cow's-milk allergy may cause crying in a few babies, but only if your baby also has eczema, diarrhea, and/or vomiting. Colic is not caused by abdominal pain. The reason the belly muscles feel hard is that a baby needs these muscles to cry. Drawing up the legs is also a normal posture for a crying baby, as is flexing the arms.

Expected Course—This fussy crying is harmless for your baby. The hard crying spontaneously starts to improve at 2 months and is gone by 3 to 4 months. Although the crying can't be eliminated, the minutes of crying per day can be dramatically reduced with treatment. In the long run, these children tend to remain more alert and responsive to their surroundings.

Call Your Child's Physician

Immediately If
- It seems to be a painful cry rather than a fussy one.
- Your baby has been crying constantly for more than 3 hours.
- You can't find a way to soothe your baby (inconsolable crying).
- Your baby is under 2 months old *and* acts sick.
- You are afraid you might hurt your baby.
- You have shaken your baby. (Note: Shaking an infant can cause severe bleeding in the brain.)

During Office Hours If
- The colic-type crying occurs 3 or more times per day.
- The crying began after 1 month of age.
- Your baby is over 4 months old.
- Diarrhea, vomiting, or constipation occur with the crying.
- Your baby is not gaining weight and may be hungry.
- You are exhausted from all this crying.
- Your baby mainly cries when you're trying to sleep.
- You have other questions.

Home Care for a Crying Baby

Hold and Soothe Your Baby Whenever He Cries Without a Reason—A soothing, gentle activity is the best approach to helping a baby relax, settle down, and go to sleep. You can't spoil a baby during the first 3 or 4 months of life. Consider using the following:

- Cuddling your child in a rocking chair
- Rocking your child in a cradle
- Swaddling in a light blanket
- Placing your child in a baby carrier or sling (which frees your hands for housework)
- A wind-up swing or a vibrating chair
- A stroller (or buggy) ride—outdoors or indoors (instead of a ride in the car)
- A monotonous type of sound, such as running a washing machine or a vacuum cleaner. CDs of such sounds are available.
- Anything else you think may be helpful (e.g., a pacifier, a warm bath, or massage)

Swaddle Your Baby in a Blanket—Snug swaddling is extremely helpful for calming crying babies. It also reduces awakenings caused by the startle reflex and increases the length of sleep. To swaddle your baby use the 3-step "burrito-wrap" technique. Start with your baby lying on the blanket and the arms at the sides. Then (1) pull the left side of the blanket over the body and tuck, (2) pull the bottom up, and (3) pull the right side over and tuck. It is a useful technique from birth to 4 months of age. For more details, consult Dr. Harvey Karp's book *The Happiest Baby on the Block*.

A Last Resort: Let Your Baby Cry Himself to Sleep—If none of these measures quiets your baby after 30 minutes of trying and he has been fed recently, your baby is probably trying to go to sleep. He needs you to minimize outside stimuli while he tries to find his own way into sleep. Wrap him up tightly (swaddled) and place him on his back in his crib. He will probably be somewhat restless until he falls asleep. Close the door, go into a different room, turn up the radio, and do something you want to do. Even consider earplugs or earphones. Save your strength for when your baby definitely needs you. But if he cries for over 15 minutes, pick him up and again try the soothing activities.

Prevent Later Sleep Problems—Although babies need to be held when they are crying, they don't need to be held all the time. If you overinterpret the advice for colic and rock your baby every time he goes to sleep, you will become indispensable to your baby's sleep transition process. Your baby's crying during the night won't resolve at 3 months of age. To prevent this from occurring, when your baby is drowsy but not crying, place him in the crib and let him learn to self-comfort and self-induce sleep. Don't rock or nurse him to sleep at these times. While colic can't be prevented, secondary sleep problems can be.

Promote Nighttime Sleep (Rather than Daytime Sleep)—Try to keep your infant from sleeping excessively during the daytime. If your baby has napped 3 hours, gently awaken him and entertain or feed him, depending on his needs. In this way, the time when your infant sleeps the longest (often 5 hours) will occur during the night.

Try These Feeding Strategies—Don't feed your baby every time he cries. Being hungry is only one of the reasons babies cry. It usually takes about 2 hours for the stomach to empty, so wait that long between feedings unless you're convinced your baby is hungry. For breast-fed babies, however, nurse them every time they cry until your milk supply is well established and your baby is gaining weight (usually 2 weeks). Babies who feed too frequently during the day become hungry at frequent intervals during the night. If you are breast-feeding, avoid drinking or taking excessive coffee, tea, colas, and other stimulants (2 servings per day are usually fine).

Suspect a cow's-milk allergy if your child also has diarrhea, vomiting, eczema, wheezing, or a strong family history of milk allergy. If any of these factors are present, try a soy formula for 1 week. Soy formulas are nutritionally complete and no more expensive than regular formula. If you are breast-feeding, avoid all forms of cow's milk in your diet for 1 week. If the crying dramatically improves when your child is on the soy formula, call your child's physician for additional advice about keeping him on the formula. Also, if you think your child is allergic but he doesn't improve with soy formula, call about the elemental formulas (e.g., Alimentum).

Get Rest and Help for Yourself—While the crying can be reduced, what's left must be endured and shared. Avoid fatigue and exhaustion. Get at least one nap a day, in case the night goes badly. Ask your partner, a friend, or a relative for help with other children and chores. Caring for a colicky baby is a two-person job. Hire a baby-sitter so you can get out of the house and clear your mind. Talk to someone every day about your mixed feelings. The screaming can drive anyone to desperation.

Common Mistakes—If you are breast-feeding, don't stop. If your baby needs extra calories, talk with a lactation consultant about ways to increase your milk supply. Never place your baby on a water bed or sheepskin rug. While these surfaces can be soothing, they also run the risk of suffocation. A young infant may not be able to lift the head adequately to breathe. The available medicines for colic are ineffective and some (especially those containing phenobarbital) are dangerous for children of this age. The medicines that slow intestinal activity (the anticholinergics) can cause fever or constipation. The ones that remove gas bubbles have been shown not to help the crying in most studies, but they are harmless. Inserting a thermometer or suppository into the rectum to "release gas" does nothing except irritate the anal sphincter. Stay with TLC (tender loving care) for best results.

Call Your Child's Physician Later If

- The crying continues after your baby reaches 4 months of age.
- Your baby seems to be in pain.
- Your baby cries constantly for more than 3 hours.
- You can't find a way to soothe your baby.

Recommended Reading

Harvey Karp, *The Happiest Baby on the Block* (New York: Bantam Dell, 2002).

PREVENTION OF SLEEP PROBLEMS: BIRTH TO 6 MONTHS

Parents want their children to sleep through the night, giving the parent 7 or 8 hours of uninterrupted sleep. Newborns, however, are not born able to sleep through. They have a limit to how many hours they can go without a nighttime feeding, usually 4 or 5. By 2 months of age, some 50 percent of bottle-fed infants can sleep through the night. By 4 months, most bottle-fed infants have acquired this capacity. Most breast-fed babies can sleep through the night by 5 or 6 months of age. Good sleep habits may not develop, however, unless you have a plan.

Consider the following guidelines if you want to teach your baby that nighttime is a special time for sleeping, that her crib is where she stays at night, and that she can put herself back to sleep following normal awakenings that don't relate to hunger. It is far easier to prevent sleep problems before age 6 months of age than it is to treat them later.

Newborns

Help Your Baby Fall Asleep Using Any Technique That Works—
During the first month of life, survival is the main agenda. If your baby
falls asleep at the breast or bottle, so be it. If he needs skin-to-skin contact to fall asleep, fine, we can fix that later. But if your baby is on the
brink of falling asleep and calm, try to put him in his crib and try to introduce self-initiation of sleep into his repertoire. (Note: The safe sleep
position for healthy babies is on the back.)

Swaddle Your Baby in a Blanket—Snug swaddling reduces awakenings
caused by the startle reflex and increases the length of sleep. Swaddling
also helps babies fall asleep. Swaddling should be done before your baby is
put down in the crib. To swaddle your baby use the 3-step "burrito-wrap"
technique. Start with your baby lying on the blanket and the arms at the
sides. Then (1) pull the left side of the blanket over the body and tuck it
in, (2) pull the bottom up, and (3) pull the right side over and tuck. It is
a useful technique from birth to 4 or 6 months of age. For more details,
consult Dr. Harvey Karp's book *The Happiest Baby on the Block.*

Try Different Techniques to Calm Your Baby—If your baby is tired
but irritable, try holding and gentle rocking to calm her. If that doesn't
work, try swaddling her, which is comparable to being hugged. Try hum-
ming, singing lullabies, or white noise. Try massage or patting. Even try a
pacifier. Different babies respond to different calming techniques.

Do Not Use a Pacifier to Help Your Baby Fall Asleep—While it's
okay to use a pacifier to calm a crying infant if holding does not work,
don't use a pacifier when your child is drowsy. Your infant will not be able
to locate and reinsert the pacifier until at least 10 months of age. Therefore, don't let it become part of the falling-to-sleep process. If you do,
you will need to be present following all normal awakenings.

**Keep Daytime Feeding Intervals to at Least 2 Hours for
Newborns—**More frequent daytime feedings (such as hourly) lead to
frequent awakenings for small feedings at night. (Exception: the first
week, when breast milk is still coming in.) Demand feedings are appropriate, but only if your baby is hungry. Crying is the only form of communication newborns have. Crying does not always mean your baby is hungry.
He may be tired, bored, lonely, or too hot. Hold your baby at these times
or put him down to sleep. Don't let feeding become a pacifier (called

comfort nursing). For every time you nurse your baby, there should be 4 or 5 times that you snuggle your baby without nursing. Don't let him get into the bad habit of nursing every time you hold him (called grazing).

Give the Last Feeding at Your Bedtime (10 or 11 P.M.)—The reason for this advice is even when your baby is 4 months old, he will only be able to fast for 7 or 8 hours (i.e., until 5 or 6 A.M.). Try to keep your baby awake for the 2 hours before this last feeding. Going to bed at the same time every night helps your baby develop good sleeping habits. Look after your sleep needs by sleeping when your baby sleeps.

Do Not Let Your Baby Sleep for More than 3 Consecutive Hours During the Day—Try to awaken him gently and entertain him. In this way, the time when your infant sleeps the longest will occur during the night. (Note: Many newborns can sleep 5 consecutive hours once during the 24-hour clock, and you can teach them to sleep for this longer period at night.)

Don't Let Your Baby Sleep in Your Bed—Once your baby is used to sleeping with you, a move to his own bed will be extremely difficult. In addition, the risk of SIDS during the first 8 months is 20 times higher sleeping in an adult bed than in a crib. So teach your child to prefer his crib. For the first 2 or 3 months, you can keep your baby in a crib or bassinet next to your bed.

1-Month-Old Babies

Learn to Recognize the Signs of Drowsiness—These include droopy eyelids, tired eyes not interested in the surroundings, yawning, decreased body movement, decreased facial expression, and quietness. When these occur, put your baby in the crib. If you miss these signs and your baby becomes overtired, he may become irritable and harder to put down. Therefore if your child has been awake longer than 2 hours, assume he needs some sleep.

Place Your Baby in the Crib When He Is Drowsy but Partially Awake—This step is very important. Without it, the other preventive measures will fail. Your baby's last waking memory should be of the crib, not of being held or of being fed. He must learn to put himself to sleep without you. Don't expect him to go to sleep as soon as you lay him down. It often takes 10 to 20 minutes of restlessness and fussiness for a baby to go to sleep. If he is crying, hold him and try to calm him. But when he settles down, try to place him in the crib before he falls asleep. Handle naps in the same way. This is how your child will learn to put himself back to sleep after normal awakenings during the night. Don't help your infant when he doesn't need any help.

Comfort Your Baby for All Crying, but Not for Normal Fussiness—All new babies cry some during the day and night. Always respond to a crying baby. Babies can't be spoiled during the first 6 months of life. But by 1 month of age, hold your baby just for crying, not for normal fussiness. Soothe him until he's calm, not until he's asleep. (Note: Even colicky babies have a few times each day when they are drowsy and not crying. On these occasions, place your child in the crib and let him learn to comfort himself and put himself to sleep.)

Make Middle-of-the-Night Feedings Brief and Boring—You want your baby to think of nighttime as a special time for sleeping. When he awakens at night for feedings, don't turn on the lights, talk to him, or rock him. Feed him quickly and quietly in the dark. Provide extra rocking and playtime during the day. This approach will lead to longer periods of sleep at night. By contrast, during the day don't try to make his bedroom too quiet or too dark. Normal levels of background noise may keep him from oversleeping during the day.

2-Month-Old Babies

Move Your Baby's Crib to a Separate Room—By 3 months of age, your baby should be sleeping in a separate room. This will help parents who are light sleepers sleep better. Also, your baby may forget that her parents are available if she can't see them when she awakens. Also close the bedroom door so your child becomes accustomed to sleeping that way. If separate rooms are impractical, at least put up a screen or cover the crib railing with a blanket so that your baby cannot see your bed.

Try to Stretch Daytime Feeding Intervals to 3 Hours—Over the next 2 months gradually lengthen the interval between daytime feedings. The ability to fast for 3 hours during the day increases your infant's potential for sleeping through the night. Going beyond the 3-hour mark during the day is not important. In fact, it may build up a caloric deficit that will leave your child more hungry during the night. Therefore, if

4 hours passes during the day and your infant doesn't give any signals of being hungry, offer a feeding anyway.

Try to Delay Middle-of-the-Night Feedings—By now, your baby should be down to 1 feeding during the night (2 for some breast-fed babies). Before preparing a bottle, try holding your baby briefly to see if that will satisfy her. Never awaken your baby at night for a feeding except at your bedtime.

4-Month-Old Babies

Try to Discontinue the 2 A.M. Feeding Before It Becomes a Habit— By 4 months of age, your bottle-fed baby does not need to be fed formula more than four times a day. Breast-fed babies do not need more than 5 or 6 nursing sessions a day. If you do not eliminate the night feedings by 6 months of age, they will become more difficult to stop as your child gets older. Remember to give the last feeding at 10 or 11 P.M. Include extra baby food with this feeding. If your child cries during the night, try to comfort him with a back rub and some soothing words instead of with a feeding.

Don't Allow Your Baby to Hold His Bottle or Take It to Bed with Him—Babies should think that the bottle belongs to the parents. A bottle in bed leads to middle-of-the-night crying for refills because your baby will inevitably reach for the bottle and find it empty or on the floor.

Make Any Middle-of-the-Night Contacts Brief and Boring—All children have 4 or 5 partial awakenings each night. They need to learn how to go back to sleep on their own at these times. If your baby cries for more than a few minutes, visit him but don't turn on the light, play with him, or take him out of his crib. Comfort him with a few soothing words and stay for a less than 1 minute. If the crying continues for more than 10 minutes, calm him and stay in the room until he goes to sleep. (Exceptions: You feel your baby is sick, hungry, or afraid.)

PREVENTION OF SLEEP PROBLEMS: 6 MONTHS TO 2 YEARS

If you followed the previous advice, your 6-month-old baby should be sleeping through the night. Hopefully he's been doing it for several months.

The rest is easy. Help him become the best sleeper that he can be. Well-rested children behave better and learn faster.

6-Month-Old Babies

Continue to Place Your Baby in the Crib When Drowsy but Partially Awake—The ability to self-initiate sleep is a critical skill.

Provide a Friendly Soft Toy for Your Child to Hold in Her Crib— At the age of 6 months, children start to be aware and sometimes fearful of separation from their parents. A stuffed animal, doll, or blanket can be a security object that will give comfort to your child when she wakes up during the night. Exception: If your baby can't easily roll over both ways, don't place any soft objects in the crib until she can.

During the Day, Respond to Any Separation Fears by Holding and Reassuring Your Child—This lessens nighttime fears and is especially important for mothers who work outside the home.

For Middle-of-the-Night Fears, Make Contacts Prompt and Reassuring—For mild nighttime fears, check on your child promptly and be reassuring, but keep the interaction as brief as possible. If your child panics when you leave, or vomits with crying, stay in your child's room until she either is calm or goes to sleep. Do not take her out of the crib, but provide whatever else she needs for comfort, keeping the light off and not talking too much. At most, sit next to the crib with your hand on her. These measures will calm even a severely upset infant.

1-Year-Old Children

Establish a Pleasant and Predictable Bedtime Ritual—Bedtime rituals, which can start in the early months, become very important to a child by 1 year of age. Children need a familiar routine. Both parents can be involved at bedtime, taking turns with reading or making up stories. Both parents should kiss and hug the child goodnight. Make sure that your child's security objects are nearby. Finish the bedtime ritual before your child falls asleep.

Encourage Naps—Naps are important to young children, but keep them less than 2 hours long. Children stop having morning naps between 18 months and 2 years of age and give up their afternoon naps between 3 and 6 years of age.

Don't Worry About Noises or Movements During Your Child's Sleep—During dreams, children often display face-twitching, fist-clenching, or even eye-rolling. It doesn't mean it's a bad dream. Many people also have muscle jerks while dozing off to sleep. Keep in mind how a dog acts as it chases a rabbit during its dream state. Overall, anything short of not breathing is probably normal sleep behavior.

2-Year-Old Children

Switch from a Crib to a Bed at Age 2—Change sooner if your child learns how to climb out of a crib with the mattress at the lowest position. Climb-proofing a crib can't be done. The next attempt at climbing out could result in a serious head injury. Until you find a bed, put the mattress on the floor, use a sleeping bag, or keep the crib railing down and place a chair next to the crib so your child can descend safely. Don't buy bunk beds. They have a terrible injury rate with children of all ages. A good first bed is a mattress placed on the floor without a frame.

Once Put to Bed, Your Child Should Stay There—Some toddlers have temper tantrums at bedtime. They may protest about bedtime or even refuse to lie down. You should ignore these protests and leave the room. You can ignore any ongoing questions or demands your child makes. Once your child is in a regular bed, you must enforce the rule that your child can't leave the bedroom. If your child comes out, return him quickly to the bedroom and avoid any conversation. If you respond to his protests in this way every time, he will learn not to try to prolong bedtime.

If Your Child has Nightmares or Bedtime Fears, Reassure Him—Never ignore your child's fears or punish him for having fears. Everyone has 4 or 5 dreams a night. Some of these are bad dreams. If nightmares become frequent, try to determine what might be causing them, such as something your child might have seen on TV. R-rated movies (especially horror movies) are a significant risk factor at any age.

Don't Worry About the Amount of Sleep Your Child Is Getting—Different people need different amounts of sleep at different ages. The best way you can know that your child is getting enough sleep is that he is not tired during the day.

TRAINED NIGHT FEEDER (Night Awakenings from Feeding Until Asleep)

Characteristics

- Your child is over 4 months old and wakes up and cries one or more times a night to be fed.

- Your child can only return to sleep if you hold and feed him.
- Your child is breast-fed or bottle-fed until asleep at bedtime and for naps.
- Your child has been awakened to be fed at night since birth.

Normal Night Feedings—From birth to the age of 2 months, most babies awaken twice each night for feedings. Between the ages of 2 and 3 months, most babies need one feeding in the middle of the night. By 4 months of age, most bottle-fed babies sleep more than 7 hours without feeding. Most breast-fed babies can sleep through the night by 5 months of age. Normal children of this age do not need calories during the night to stay healthy.

Causes—Some common reasons that babies older than 4 months wake up at night to be fed include:

- Nursing or bottle-feeding the baby until asleep. If the last memory before sleep is sucking the breast or bottle, the bottle or breast becomes the baby's security object. The child does not learn to comfort himself and fall asleep without the breast or bottle. Therefore, when the child normally wakes up at night, the child has the habit of not being able to go back to sleep without feeding. Being brought to the parents' bed for a feeding makes the problem far worse.

- Leaving a bottle in the bed. Periodically during the night the child sucks on a bottle. When it becomes empty, the child awakens fully and cries for a refill. Bottles in bed, unless they contain only water, also can lead to severe tooth decay.

- Feeding often during the day. Some mothers misinterpret "demand feedings" to mean that they should feed the baby every time he cries. This misunderstanding can lead to feeding the baby every 30 to 60 minutes. The baby becomes used to being fed small amounts often instead of waiting at least 2 hours between feedings at birth and at least 4 hours between feedings at the age of 4 months. A pattern of feeding every hour or so is called grazing. This problem occurs more often in breast-fed babies if nursing is used as a pacifier. Bottle dependency leads to the bad habit of carrying a bottle around during the day. Also, giving a child a lot of liquid at night means your child will wake up more often because his diapers are soaked.

Expected Outcome—If you try the following recommendations, your child's behavior will probably improve in 2 weeks. The older your child is, the harder it will be to change your child's habits. Children over 1 year old will fight sleep even when they are tired. They will vigorously protest any change and may cry for hours. However, if you don't take these steps, your child won't start sleeping through the night until 3 or 4 years of age, when busy daytime schedules finally exhaust your child.

Helping a Trained Night Feeder

Try the following suggestions if your child is over 4 months old and wakes up and cries one or more times at night to be fed.

Gradually Lengthen the Time Between Daytime Feedings to 3 or 4 Hours—You can't lengthen the time between nighttime feedings if the time between daytime feedings is short. If a baby is used to frequent feedings during the day, he will get hungry during the night. Grazing often happens to mothers who don't separate holding from nursing. For every time you nurse your baby, there should be 4 or 5 times that you snuggle your baby without nursing. Gradually postpone daytime feeding times until they are more normal for your baby's age. If you currently feed your baby hourly, increase the time between feedings to 1¹/₂ hours. When your baby accepts the new schedule, go to 2 hours between feedings. When your baby cries, cuddle him or give him a pacifier. Your goal for a formula-fed baby is to give him 4 bottles a day by 4 months of age. Breast-fed babies often need 5 feedings each day until they are 6 months old, when solid foods are added to their diet. If your child is over 6 months old, also introduce cup feedings. Awaken your infant for a last feeding between 9 and 10 P.M. This is necessary until at least 8 months of age if you want your child to sleep until 6 A.M.

At Naps and Bedtime, Place Your Baby in the Crib Drowsy but Awake—When your baby starts to act sleepy, place her in the crib. If your baby is very fussy, rock her until she settles down or is almost asleep, but stop before she's fully asleep. If your baby falls asleep at the breast or bottle, it is best to wake her up. To help your baby not think of feeding at bedtime, consider feeding her 1 hour before bedtime or before a nap. Your baby's last waking memory needs to be of the crib and mattress, not of the breast or bottle. She needs to learn to put herself to sleep. Your baby needs to develop this skill so she can put herself to sleep when she wakes up at night.

• **If Your Baby Is Crying at Bedtime or Naptime, Visit Your Baby Briefly Every 5 to 15 Minutes**—Visit your baby before he becomes too upset. You may need to check babies younger than 1 year or more sensitive babies every 5 minutes. Gradually lengthen the time between your visits. Make your visits brief and boring but supportive. Don't stay in the room longer than 1 minute. Don't turn on the lights. Act sleepy. Whisper, "Shhh, everyone's sleeping." Do not remove your child from the crib. Do not feed, rock, or play with your baby, or bring him to your bed. This brief contact will not reward your baby enough for him to want to continue the behavior. Once you put your child in the crib, do not remove him.

For Crying During the Middle of the Night, Temporarily Hold Your Baby Until Asleep—Until your child learns how to put herself to sleep at naps and bedtime, make the middle-of-the-night awakenings as easy as possible. If she doesn't fuss for more than 5 or 10 minutes, respond as you do at bedtime. Otherwise, take your crying child out of the crib and hold her until she's asleep. However, don't turn on the lights or take her out of the room. Try not to talk to her very much. Often this works better if Dad goes in.

After the last feeding of the day, at 9 or 10 P.M., feed your baby only once during the night. Provide this nighttime feeding only if 4 or more hours have passed since the last feeding. Make this nighttime feeding boring and brief (no longer than 20 minutes). Stop it before your child falls asleep, and replace it with holding only.

Stop Giving Your Baby Any Bottle in Bed—If you feed your child at bedtime, don't let him hold the bottle. Also feed your child in a room other than the bedroom. Try to separate mealtime and bedtime. If your baby needs to suck on something to help him go to sleep, offer a pacifier or help him find his thumb.

Help Your Child Attach to a Security Object—A security (transitional) object is something that helps a waking child go to sleep. It comforts your child and helps your child separate from you. A cuddly stuffed animal, doll, other soft toy, or blanket can be a good security object. Sometimes covering a stuffed animal with one of the mother's T-shirts helps a child accept it. Include the security object whenever you cuddle or rock your child during the day. Also include it in your ritual before bedtime by weaving it into your storytelling. Tuck it into the crib next to your child. Eventually, your child will hold and cuddle the stuffed animal or doll at bedtime in place of you.

Later, Phase Out the Nighttime Feeding—Phase out the nighttime feeding only after the time between daytime feedings is more than 3 hours *and* your child can put herself to sleep without feeding or rocking. Then gradually phase out nighttime feedings over 2 weeks. Gradually reduce the amount you feed your baby at night. Decrease the amount of formula you give a bottle-fed baby by 1 ounce every 2 to 3 nights. Nurse a breast-fed baby on just one side and reduce the time by 2 minutes every 2 to 3 nights. After 1 to 2 weeks, your baby will no longer crave food at night and should be able to go back to sleep without holding or rocking.

Call Your Child's Physician During Office Hours If
- Your child is not gaining enough weight.
- You think the crying has a physical cause.
- Your child acts fearful.
- Someone in your family cannot tolerate the crying.
- The steps outlined here do not improve your child's sleeping habits within 2 weeks.
- You have other questions or concerns.

TRAINED NIGHT CRIER (Night Awakenings from Holding Until Asleep)

Characteristics
- Your child is over 4 months old and wakes up and cries one or more times a night.
- Your child can only return to sleep if you hold him.
- Your child is held, rocked, or walked until asleep at bedtime and for naps.
- Your child doesn't need to be fed in the middle of the night.
- Your child has awakened and cried at night since birth.

Normal Night Feedings—From birth to the age of 2 months, most babies awaken twice each night for feedings. Between the ages of 2 and 3 months, most babies need one feeding in the middle of the night. By 4 months of age, most bottle-fed babies sleep more than 7 hours without feeding. Most breast-fed babies can sleep through the night by 5 months of age. Normal children of this age do not need calories during the night and are capable of sleeping through the night without being rocked or held in the middle of the night.

Causes—Some common reasons babies over 4 months old wake up crying at night include:

- Holding or rocking your baby until asleep. All children normally wake up 4 or 5 times each night after dreams. Because they usually do not wake up fully at these times, most children can get back to sleep by themselves. However, children who have not learned how to comfort and quiet themselves cry for a parent. If your custom at naps and bedtime is to hold, rock, or lie down with your baby until asleep, your child will not learn how to go back to sleep without your help. Babies who are not usually placed in their cribs while they are still awake expect their mothers to help them go back to sleep when they wake up at night. Because they fall asleep away from their cribs, they don't learn to associate the crib and mattress with sleep. This is called poor sleep-onset association.

- Providing entertainment during the night. Children may awaken and cry more frequently if they realize they gain from it—for example, if they are walked, rocked, or played with, or enjoy other lengthy contact with their parents. Being brought to the parents' bed makes the problem far worse. Crying at night can also begin after situations that required the parents to give more nighttime attention to their baby for a while. Examples of such problems are colds, discomfort during hot summer nights, or traveling. Many babies quickly settle back into their previous sleep patterns after such situations. However, some enjoy the nighttime contact so much that they begin to demand it.

- Believing any crying is harmful. All young children cry when confronted with a change in their schedule or environment (called normal protest crying). Crying is their only way to communicate before they are able to talk. Crying for brief periods is not physically or psychologically harmful. The thousands of hours of attention and affection you have given your child will easily offset any unhappiness that may result from changing a bad sleep pattern.

Expected Outcome—If you try the following recommendations, your child's behavior will probably improve in 2 weeks. The older your child is, the harder it will be to change your child's habits. Children over 1 year old will fight sleep even when they are tired. They will vigorously protest any change and may cry for hours. However, if you don't take these steps, your child won't start sleeping through the night until 3 or 4 years of age, when busy daytime schedules finally exhaust your child.

Helping a Trained Night Crier

Try the following suggestions if your baby is over 4 months old and wakes up crying one or more times in the night.

Place Your Baby in the Crib Drowsy but Awake for Naps and Bedtime—It's good to hold babies and to provide pleasant bedtime rituals. However, when your baby starts to look drowsy, place him in the crib. Your child's last waking memory needs to be of the crib and mattress, not of you. If your baby is very fussy, rock him until he settles down or is almost asleep, but stop before he's fully asleep. He needs to learn to put himself to sleep. Your baby needs to develop this skill so he can put himself back to sleep when he normally wakes up at night.

If Your Baby Is Crying at Bedtime or Naptime, Visit Your Baby Briefly Every 5 to 15 Minutes—Visit your baby before she becomes too upset. You may need to check younger or more sensitive babies every 5 minutes. You be the judge. Gradually lengthen the time between your visits. Babies cannot learn how to comfort themselves without some crying. This crying is not harmful. If your child is fearful, hold him until he calms down. Then temporarily sit or lie down in his bedroom until he settles down. Try to leave before he falls asleep.

Make the Visits Brief and Boring but Supportive—Don't stay in your child's room longer than 1 minute. Don't turn on the lights. Keep the visit supportive and reassuring. Act sleepy. Whisper, "Shhh, everyone's sleeping." Add something positive, such as "You're a wonderful baby," or "You're almost asleep." Never show your anger or punish your baby during these visits. If you hug him, he probably won't let go. Touch your baby gently and help him find his security object, such as a doll, stuffed animal, or blanket.

Do Not Remove Your Child from the Crib—Once you put your child in the crib, do not remove her. Do not rock or play with your baby or bring her to your bed. Brief contact will not reward your baby enough for her to want to continue the behavior. Most young babies cry 30 to 90 minutes and then fall asleep.

For Crying During the Middle of the Night, Temporarily Hold Your Baby Until He Is Asleep—Until your child learns how to put himself to sleep at naps and bedtime, make the middle-of-the-night awakenings as easy as possible for everyone. If he doesn't fuss for more than 5 or 10 minutes, respond as you do at bedtime. Otherwise, take your crying child out of the crib and hold him until he is asleep. Don't turn on the lights or take him out of the room. Try not to talk to him very much. Often this works better if Dad goes in.

Help Your Child Attach to a Security Object—A security (transitional) object is something that helps a waking child go to sleep. It comforts your child and helps your child separate from you. A cuddly stuffed animal, doll, other soft toy, or blanket can be a good security object. Sometimes covering a stuffed animal with one of the mother's T-shirts helps a child accept it. Include the security object whenever you cuddle or rock your child during the day. Also include it in your ritual before bedtime by weaving it into your storytelling. Tuck it into the crib next to your child. Eventually, your child will hold and cuddle the stuffed animal or doll at bedtime in place of you.

Later, Phase Out the Nighttime Holding—Phase out nighttime holding only after your child has learned to quiet herself and put herself to sleep for naps and at bedtime. Then you can expect her to put herself back to sleep during normal middle-of-the-night awakenings. Go to her every 15 minutes while she is crying, but make your visits brief and boring. After your child learns to put herself to sleep at bedtime, awakening with crying usually stops in a few nights.

Other Helpful Hints for Sleep Problems

Move the Crib to Another Room—If the crib is in your bedroom, move it to a separate room. If this is impossible, cover one of the side rails with a blanket so your baby can't see you when he wakes up.

Avoid Long Naps During the Day—If your baby has napped for more than 2 hours, wake her up. If she has the habit of taking three naps during the day, try to change her habit to two naps each day.

Don't Change Wet Diapers During the Night—Change the diaper only if it is soiled or you are treating a bad diaper rash. If you must change your child's diaper, use as little light as possible (for example, a flashlight), do it quickly, and don't provide any entertainment.

Leave Your Child Standing in the Crib, if Necessary—If your child is standing up in the crib at bedtime, try to get your child to settle down and lie down. If he refuses or pulls himself back up, leave him that way. He can lie down without your help. Repeatedly helping your child lie down can soon become a game.

Keep a Sleep Diary—Keep a record of when your baby is awake and asleep. Bring it with you to your follow-up visit at your doctor's office.

Call Your Child's Physician During Office Hours If

- You think the crying has a physical cause.
- Your child acts fearful.
- Someone in your family cannot tolerate the crying.
- The steps outlined here do not improve your child's sleeping habits within 2 weeks.
- You have other questions or concerns.

BEDTIME RESISTANCE

Characteristics

- Children over age 2 refuse to go to bed or stay in the bedroom.
- These children come out of the bedroom because they no longer sleep in a crib.
- In the usual form, the child eventually goes to sleep while watching TV with the parent or in the parent's bed.
- In a milder form, the child stays in his bedroom but prolongs the bedtime interaction with ongoing questions, unreasonable requests, protests, crying, or temper tantrums.
- In the morning, these children sleep late or have to be awakened because they went to bed so late.

Cause—Bedtime resistance stems from a child's attempts to test the limits, not from fear. Your child has found a good way to postpone bedtime and receive extra entertainment and is stalling and taking advantage of your good nature. If given a choice, over 90 percent of children would stay up until their parents' bedtime. These children also often try to share the parents' bed at bedtime or sneak into their parents' bed during the middle of the night. By contrast, the child who comes to the parents' bed if he is frightened or not feeling well should be supported at these times.

Ending Bedtime Resistance

Clarify What a Good Sleeper Does—Tell your child what you want her to do: At bedtime a good sleeper stays in her bed and doesn't scream. During the night, a good sleeper doesn't leave her bedroom or wake up her parents unless it is an emergency. A good sleeper gets a sticker and a special treat for breakfast. A bad sleeper loses a privilege for the following day (for example, all TV or access to a favorite toy).

Start the Night with a Pleasant Bedtime Ritual—Provide a bedtime routine that is pleasant and predictable. Most pre-bedtime rituals last about 30 minutes and include taking a bath, brushing teeth, reading stories, talking about the day, saying prayers, and other interactions that relax your child. Try to keep the same sequence each night because familiarity is comforting for children. Try to have both parents take turns in creating this special experience. Never cancel this ritual because of misbehavior earlier in the day. Before you give your last hug and kiss and leave your child's bedroom, ask, "Do you need anything else?" Then leave and don't return. It's very important that you are not with your child at the moment of falling asleep; otherwise he will need you to be present following normal awakenings in the night.

If your child is fearful, tell her you will check on her every 15 minutes (instead of her checking on you). When you come in, tell her she's doing a good job of being quiet. Leave within 15 seconds. On one of your visits, you will find her asleep.

Establish a Rule That Your Child Can't Leave the Bedroom at Night—Enforce the rule that once the bedtime ritual is over and your child is placed in the bedroom, he cannot leave that room. Your child needs to learn to put himself to sleep for naps and at bedtime in his own bed. Do not stay in the room until he lies down or falls asleep. Parents can't force a child to fall asleep. Establish a set bedtime and stick to it. Make it clear that your child is not allowed to leave the bedroom between 8:00 at night and 7:00 in the morning (or whatever sleep time you decide upon). Usually, this change won't be accomplished without some crying or screaming for a few nights.

If your child has been sleeping with you, tell him, "Starting tonight, we sleep in separate beds. You have your room, we have our room. You have your bed, we have our bed. You are too old to sleep with us anymore."

Ignore Verbal Requests—Despite ongoing questions or demands from the bedroom, do not engage in any conversation with your child. All of these requests should have been dealt with during your pre-bedtime ritual. Don't return or talk with your child unless you think he is sick. Some exceptions: If your child says he needs to use the toilet, tell him to take care of it himself. If your child says his covers have fallen off and he is cold, promise him you will cover him up after he goes to sleep. You will usually find him well covered.

Close the Bedroom Door If Your Child Screams—For screaming from the bedroom, try to ignore it. If the screaming is disruptive, tell your child, "I'm sorry I have to close your door. I'll open it as soon as you're quiet." If he pounds on the door, you can open it after 1 or 2 minutes, and suggest that he go back to bed. If he does, you can leave the door open. If he doesn't, close the door again. For continued screaming or pounding on the door, reopen it approximately every 15 minutes and tell your child that if he quiets down the door can stay open. Never spend more than 30 seconds reassuring him. Although you may not like to close the door, you don't have many options. Rest assured that if your child is over 2 years old and has no daytime separation fears, it is quite reasonable to do this.

Close the Bedroom Door If Your Child Comes Out—If your child comes out of the bedroom, return him immediately to his bed. During this process, avoid any lectures and skip the hug and kiss. Get good eye contact and remind him again that he cannot leave his bedroom during the night. Warn him that if he comes out again, you're sorry but you will need to close the door. If he comes out, close the door. Tell him, "I'll be happy to open your door as soon as you're in your bed, and I'll leave it open as long as you stay in bed." If your child says he's in his bed, open the door. If he screams, every 15 minutes open the door just enough to ask your child if he's in his bed now.

Put Up a Gate or Lock the Bedroom Door If Your Child Repeatedly Leaves the Bedroom—If your child is very determined and continues to come out of the bedroom, consider putting a barricade in front of her door, such as a strong gate. A half-door or plywood plank may also serve this purpose. Sometimes the bedroom door will need to be closed temporarily to convince your child that staying in their room is not open to negotiation. Reassure your child you will open the door as soon as she falls asleep. Also, each night, give her a fresh chance to stay in the bedroom with the bedroom door open. (Caution: If your child has bedtime fears, don't close the door.)

If your child is a danger to himself or others, a full door may need to be kept closed until morning with a childproof handle cover, push-button lock, hook and eye screw, piece of rope, or chain lock. Although this step seems extreme, it may be critical to protect children less than 5 years old who wander through the house at night without an understanding of dangers, such as fire, hot water, knives, or going outside.

Return Him to His Bed If He Comes into Your Bed at Night—For middle-of-the-night attempts to crawl into your bed, unless your child is fearful, sternly order your child back to his own bed. If he doesn't move, escort him back immediately without any physical contact or pleasant conversation. If you are asleep when your child crawls into your bed, return him as soon as you discover his presence. If he attempts to come out again, lock his door until morning. If you are a deep sleeper, consider using some signaling device that will awaken you if your child enters your bedroom (such as a chair placed against your door or a loud bell attached to your doorknob). For children over age 5, some parents simply lock their bedroom door. Remind your child that it is not polite to interrupt other people's sleep. Tell him that if he awakens at night and can't go back to sleep, he can read or play quietly in his room, but he is not to bother his parents.

If She Awakens You at Night with Screaming or Demands, Visit Her Briefly—Reassure her that she is safe. If she needs blankets readjusted, help her do this. Then leave. On the following day teach her how to independently solve any complaints she makes during the night. (Remind your child that it is not polite to awaken people at night. Tell her that if she awakens at night and can't go back to sleep, she can read or play quietly in her room.)

Help Siblings Sleeping in the Same Bedroom—If the bedtime screaming wakes up a roommate, have the well-behaved sibling sleep in a separate room until the nighttime behavior has improved. Tell your child with the sleep problem that his roommate cannot return until he stays in his room quietly for 3 consecutive nights. If you have a small home, have the sibling sleep in your room temporarily; this will be an added incentive for your other child to improve.

Awaken Your Child at the Regular Time Each Morning—Even if he fought bedtime and fell asleep late, wake him up at the regular time so he will be tired earlier the next evening.

Start Bedtime Later If You Want to Minimize Bedtime Crying— The later the bedtime, the more tired your child will be and the less resistance he will offer. For most children, you can pick the bedtime hour. For children who are very stubborn and cry a lot, you may want to make bedtime 10:00 P.M. (or whenever your child naturally falls asleep). If the bedtime is 10:00 P.M., start the bedtime ritual at 9:30 P.M. After your child learns to fall asleep without fussing at 10:00 P.M., move the bedtime back by 15 minutes every week. In children who can't tell time, you can gradually (over 8 weeks or so) achieve an 8:00 P.M. bedtime in this way with many fewer tantrums. However, don't let your child sleep late in the morning or you won't be able to advance the bedtime.

Call Your Child's Physician During Office Hours If

- Your child is not sleeping well after trying this program for 2 weeks.
- Your child needs to he locked in the bedroom for more than 7 nights. (He probably needs some counseling.)
- Your child is frightened at bedtime.
- Your child has lots of nightmares.
- Your child also has several discipline problems during the day.
- You have other questions or concerns.

SLEEPING WITH THE PARENTS (Bed-Sharing)

In general, I don't recommend bed-sharing. During the first year of life, it can be harmful to sleep with your baby. If the adult mattress is soft, the infant can suffocate. In fact, the SIDS rate is 20 times higher sleeping in an adult bed compared to sleeping in a crib. In addition, there are about 100 deaths per year in our country from a parent rolling over onto the baby during sleep and causing suffocation. The risk is highest if one of the parents has a deep sleep disorder or drinks excessively.

While it's not harmful for your older children to sleep with you, it's unnecessary. And it may be bad for you. Once begun, it's rather hard to undo, so don't start until you have all the facts.

- Your child doesn't need this arrangement to be secure and happy. Children's fears and insecurities can be dealt with during the day. Children can turn out fine either way. The majority of children in our country sleep happily in their own bed. In poor countries, families sleep together by necessity.
- Bed-sharing is not quality time. If your child is asleep in your bed, it is neutral time. If your child is crying and keeping you awake, it is aggravating time. So there is really no quality time here.
- Several studies have shown that over 50 percent of children who sleep with parents resist going to bed and awaken several times at night. Most parents who bed-share have to lie down with their child for 30 to 60 minutes to get them to sleep. Most of these parents also do not get a good night's sleep and become sleep-deprived. Sleeping with your child is a bad choice if you are a light sleeper and need your sleep because you work outside the home.
- Bed-sharing is never a long-term solution to sleep problems. Your child will not learn to sleep well in your bed and then decide on his own to start sleeping in his bed. With every passing month, the habit becomes harder to change. Your child can no longer sleep alone.
- Bed-sharing is not harmful to children. There is no evidence that bed-sharing produces children who are more spoiled or dependent.

Prevention of Bed-Sharing

- Place your child in the crib drowsy but awake. In this way he will learn to put himself back to sleep following normal awakenings.
- Make middle-of-the-night feedings brief and boring. This is hard to do if you are sleeping with your child.
- Put your child in his own room by 3 or 4 months of age. Have a rule that he does not leave the crib at night, and after age 2, that he does not leave the bedroom. Most children in our country follow these guidelines and do just fine.
- If you must sleep in the same room with your infant, don't allow her to see you during her normal awakenings. If she does, it's an invitation to wake you to play. Instead, cover the side of her crib with something (e.g., a firmly attached blanket).
- Encourage a security object. After 6 months of age, encourage a soft toy or stuffed animal as a security object. Otherwise he may select you as his security object.

Putting an End to Bed-Sharing

If you are sleeping with your child and want to change it, here are some suggestions:

- Tell your child the new rule. "You are too old to sleep with us anymore. You have your bed, and we have our bed. Starting tonight, we want you to stay in your bed during the night."

- For being a "good sleeper" who sleeps in her bedroom all night, give her a treat with breakfast.

- If your child leaves his bedroom, return him immediately. If he does it again, close the door until he's in his bed.

- If he crawls into your bed during the night, order him back to his own bed, using a stern voice. If he doesn't move, escort him back immediately without any conversation.

- If you are asleep when he crawls into your bed, return him as soon as you discover him. If he attempts to come out again, temporarily close his door. If you are a deep sleeper, consider using some signaling device that will awaken you if your child enters your bedroom (such as a chair placed against your door or a loud bell attached to your doorknob). Some parents simply lock their bedroom door. Remind your child that "it is not polite to wake people who are sleeping unless it is an emergency."

- Expect some crying. Young children normally cry when they don't get their way.

NIGHTMARES

Definition—Nightmares are scary dreams that awaken a child. Occasional bad dreams are normal at all ages after about 6 months of age. When infants have a nightmare, they cry and scream until someone comes to them. When preschoolers have a nightmare, they usually cry and run into their parents' bedroom. Older children begin to understand what a nightmare is and put themselves back to sleep without waking their parents.

Cause—Everyone dreams 4 or 5 times each night. Some dreams are good, some are bad. Dreams help the mind process complicated events or information. The content of nightmares usually relates to developmental challenges. Toddlers have nightmares about separation from their parents, preschoolers have bad dreams about monsters or the dark, and school-age children are troubled by dreams about death or real dangers. Frequent nightmares may be caused by violent TV shows or movies.

Dealing with Nightmares

Reassure and Cuddle Your Child—Explain to your child that she was having a bad dream. Sit on the bed until she is calm. Offer to leave the bedroom door open (never close the door on a fearful child). Provide a night-light, especially if your child has fears of the dark. Most children return to sleep fairly quickly.

Help Your Child Talk About the Bad Dreams During the Day—Your child may not remember what the dream was about unless you can remind him of something he said about it when he woke up. If your child was dreaming about falling or being chased, reassure him that lots of children dream about that. If your child has the same bad dream over and over again, help him imagine a good ending to the bad dream. Encourage your child to use a strong person or a magic weapon to help him overcome the bad person or event in the dream. You may want to help your child draw pictures or write stories about the new, happier ending for the dream. Working through a bad fear often takes several conversations about it.

Protect Your Child Against Frightening Movies and TV Shows—For many children, violent or horror movies cause bedtime fears and nightmares. These fears can persist for months or years. Absolutely forbid these movies before 13 years of age. Between 13 and 17 years, the maturity and sensitivity of your child must be considered carefully in deciding when he is ready to deal with the uncut versions of R-rated movies. Be vigilant about slumber parties or Halloween parties. Tell your child to call you if the family he is visiting is showing scary movies.

Call Your Child's Physician During Office Hours If

- The nightmares become worse.
- The nightmares are not minimal after using this approach for 2 weeks.
- The fear interferes with daytime activities.
- Your child has several fears.
- You have other concerns or questions.

NIGHT TERRORS

Definition

- Your child is agitated and restless but cannot be awakened or comforted.

- Your child may sit up or run helplessly about, possibly screaming or talking wildly.
- Although your child appears to be anxious, he doesn't mention any specific fears.
- Your child doesn't appear to realize that you are there. Although the eyes are wide open and staring, your child looks right through you.
- Your child may mistake objects or persons in the room for dangers.
- The episode begins 1 to 2 hours after going to sleep.
- The episode lasts from 10 to 30 minutes.
- Your child cannot remember the episode in the morning (amnesia).
- The child is usually 1 to 8 years old.

Cause—Night terrors are an inherited disorder in which a child tends to have dreams during deep sleep from which it is difficult to awaken. They occur in 2 percent of children and usually are not caused by psychological stress. Getting overtired can trigger night terrors.

Expected Course—Night terrors usually occur within 2 hours of bedtime. Night terrors are harmless, and each episode will end of its own accord in deep sleep. The problem usually disappears by age 12 or sooner.

Dealing with Night Terrors

Try to Help Your Child Return to Normal Sleep—Your goal is to help your child go from agitated sleep to a calm sleep. You won't be able to awaken your child, so don't try to. Turn on the lights so he is less confused by shadows. Make soothing comments such as "You are all right. You are home in your own bed. You can rest now." Speak calmly and repetitively. Such comments are usually better than silence and may help your child re-focus. Some children like to have their hand held during this time, but most will pull away. Hold your child only if it seems to help him feel better. There is no way to shorten the episode abruptly. Shaking or shouting at your child will just cause him to become more agitated and will prolong the attack.

Protect Your Child Against Injury—During a night terror, a child can fall down a stairway, run into a wall, or break a window. Gently try to direct your child back to bed.

Prepare Baby-sitters or Other Caregivers for These Episodes— Explain to people who care for your child what a night terror is and what to do if one happens. Understanding this will prevent them from over-reacting if your child has a night terror.

Prevention of Night Terrors

Keep Your Child from Becoming Overtired—Sleep deprivation is the most common trigger for night terrors. For preschoolers, restore the afternoon nap. If your child refuses the nap, encourage a 1-hour "quiet time." Also avoid late bedtimes because they may trigger a night terror. If your child needs to be awakened in the morning, that means he or she needs an earlier bedtime. Make lights-out time 15 minutes earlier each night until your child can self-awaken in the morning.

Use Prompted Awakenings for Frequent Night Terrors—If your child has frequent night terrors and is over age 6, Dr. B. Lask of London has suggested a new way to eliminate this distressing sleep pattern in 90 percent of children. For several nights, note how many minutes elapse from falling asleep to the onset of the night terror. Then awaken your child 15 minutes before the expected time of onset. Remind your child at bedtime that when you do this, his job is "to wake up fast." Keep your child fully awake and out of bed for 5 minutes. Carry out these prompted awakenings for 7 consecutive nights. If the night terrors return, repeat this 7-night training program.

Call Your Child's Physician During Office Hours If

- Any drooling, jerking, or stiffening occurs.
- The episodes occur two or more times per week after doing the 7 prompted awakenings.
- Episodes last longer than 30 minutes.
- Your child does something dangerous during an episode.
- Episodes occur during the second half of the night.
- Your child has several daytime fears.
- You feel family stress may be a factor.
- You have other questions or concerns.

SLEEPWALKING

Definition

- Your child walks while asleep.
- Your child's eyes are open but blank.

- Your child is not as well coordinated as when awake.
- Your child may perform semipurposeful acts such as dressing and undressing, opening and closing doors, or turning lights on and off.
- The episode begins 1 to 2 hours after going to sleep.
- The episode may last 5 to 20 minutes.
- During this time the child cannot be awakened no matter what the parent does.
- The child is usually 4 to 15 years old.

Cause—Sleepwalking is an inherited tendency to wander during deep sleep. About 15 percent of normal children sleepwalk.

Expected Course—Sleepwalking usually occurs within 2 hours of bedtime. Children stop sleepwalking during adolescence.

Dealing with Sleepwalking

Gently Lead Your Child Back to Bed—First, steer your child into the bathroom, because he may be looking for a place to urinate. Then guide him to his bedroom. The episode may end once he's in bed. Don't expect to awaken him, however, before he returns to normal sleep.

Protect Your Child from Accidents—Although accidents are rare, they do happen, especially if the child wanders outside. Sleepwalkers can be hit by a car or bitten by a dog, or they may become lost. Put gates on your stairways and special locks on your outside doors (above your child's reach). Avoid having your child sleep in the upper part of a bunk bed.

Help Your Child Avoid Exhaustion—Fatigue and lack of sleep can lead to more frequent sleepwalking. So be sure your child goes to bed at a reasonable hour, especially when ill or exhausted. If your child needs to be awakened in the morning, that means she needs an earlier bedtime. Make lights-out time 15 minutes earlier each night until your child can self-awaken in the morning.

Try Prompted Awakenings to Prevent Sleepwalking—If your child has frequent sleepwalking and is over age 6, try to eliminate this distressing sleep pattern. For several nights, note how many minutes elapse from falling asleep to the onset of the sleepwalking. Then awaken your child 15 minutes before the expected time of onset. Remind your child at bedtime that when you do this, his job is "to wake up fast." Keep your child fully awake for 5 minutes. Carry out these prompted awakenings for

7 consecutive nights. If the sleepwalking returns, repeat this 7-night training program.

EARLY-MORNING RISER

Some children awaken before their parents do, usually between 5:00 and 6:00 A.M. The children are well rested and raring to go. They come out of their room or call out from the crib and want everyone to wake up. They are excited about the new day and want to share it with you. If the adults don't respond, they make a racket. Such a child is a morning person.

Causes—Most of these children have received plenty of sleep. They are no longer tired. They are not awakening early on purpose. Most of them were put to bed too early the night before, had too many naps, or had naps that were too long. Some of them have a reduced sleep requirement—one that is below the average of 10 to 12 hours a night. Such children often have a parent who needs only 6 hours or so of sleep at night. Other children may begin awakening early in the springtime because of sunlight streaming through their window. (This scenario is easily remedied with dark shades or curtains.) Finally, those children who are fed an early breakfast or allowed to come into their parents' bed early in the morning develop a bad habit that persists after the original cause is removed.

Home Care

Reduce Naps—Assume your child is getting too much sleep during the day. Most children over 1 year of age need only one nap (unless they are sick). If cutting back to one nap doesn't help, shorten the nap to 1½ hours maximum. Also make sure your child gets plenty of exercise after his nap, so he'll be tired at night.

Delay Bedtime Until 8:00 or 9:00 P.M.—These two steps should cure your child unless he has a below-average sleep requirement.

Establish a Rule—"You can't leave your bedroom until your parents are up. You can play quietly in your bedroom until breakfast." Also tell your child, "It's not polite to wake up someone who is sleeping. Your parents need their sleep."

If Your Child Is in a Crib, Leave Him There Until 6:00 A.M.—Put some toys in his crib the night before (but not ones he can stand on). If he cries, go in once to reassure him and remind him of the toys. Don't include any surprises or treats in his toy bag, or he'll awaken early, as children do on holiday mornings. If he makes loud noises with the toys, remove those particular toys. If he cries, ignore it. If crying continues, visit him briefly every 15 minutes to reassure him that all is well and most people are sleeping. Don't turn on the lights, talk much, remove him from his crib, or stay more than 1 minute.

If Your Child Is in a Floor-Level Bed, Keep Him in His Bedroom Until 6:00 A.M.—Get him a clock radio and set it for 6:00 A.M. Tell him he can't leave his bedroom until the music comes on. Tell him he can play quietly until then. Help him put out special toys or books the night before. If he comes out of his room, put up a gate or close the door. Tell him that you'll be happy to open the door as soon as he is back in his bed. If this is a chronic problem, put up the gate the night before.

If You Meet Strong Resistance, Change the Wake-up Time Gradually—Some children protest a great deal about the new rule, especially if they have been coming into your bed in the morning. In that case, move ahead a little more gradually. If he's been awakening at 5:00 A.M., help him wait until 5:15 for 3 days. Set the clock radio for that time. After your child has adjusted to 5:15, change the clock radio to 5:30. Move the wake-up time forward every 3 or 4 days.

Praise Your Child for Not Waking Other People in the Morning—A star chart or special treat at breakfast may help your child wait more cooperatively.

Change Your Tactics for Weekends—Many parents want their child to sleep in on Saturday and Sunday mornings. If this is your preference, keep your early-morning riser up an hour later the night before. If you are using a clock radio with your program, turn it off or reset the time for an hour later. As a last resort, put a breakfast together for your child the night before and allow him to watch a preselected videotape.

SLEEP PROBLEMS: OTHER STRATEGIES

Climbs Out of the Crib

Premise: Once a child climbs out of a crib with the mattress at the lowest level, he or she will definitely try to climb out again and eventually will fall and possibly get hurt.

Response: Correct this hazard on the same day your child climbs out. One solution is to put your child's mattress on the floor. Another is to leave your child in the crib with the crib railing down and a chair next to the bed so he or she can easily get out. When convenient, you should transfer your child to a floor-level bed.

Won't Take a Nap

Rule: "Don't leave your room during quiet time." Every day after lunch, you or your child's caretaker can expect him to spend 60 to 90 minutes resting in his room. During this time he may read or play quietly, but not turn on the radio or TV.

Discipline technique: Return your child to his room if he comes out before 60 to 90 minutes is up. If he comes out a second time, close the door temporarily.

Is Negative at Bedtime

Examples: Your child refuses to put on her pajamas, lie down, close her eyes, or stay in bed.

Rule: "Stay in your bedroom after we put you to bed."

Discipline technique: Natural consequences. Your child will eventually become tired and go to sleep. Your child can't be forced to fall asleep. Insisting on any of the actions mentioned above is unnecessary—it doesn't matter if your child sleeps on the floor in her daytime clothing.

Two Children Play and Talk in the Bedroom After Bedtime

Rule: "After bedtime you have to be quiet so that your mind will be able to go to sleep."

Discipline technique: Logical consequences. For every night that children stay up, fight, play, or make noise, they will be put to bed 15 minutes earlier the following night. If one child in particular tries to keep the other one up, that child can be sent to bed 1 hour earlier.

Praise your children: On the following morning, for going to sleep without a fuss.

Wanders or Prowls About During the Night

Examples: Some children awaken during the night and move about the house getting into trouble. They may raid the refrigerator or leave it open. They may watch TV or turn on the stove or water faucet. Unlike sleepwalkers, they are awake.

Rule: "If you wake up during the night, except for going to the bathroom, you have to stay in your room."

Discipline technique: Nighttime restriction to the bedroom. Because of the safety issues, until children are safety-conscious (at 4 or 5 years of age) they need a barricade to keep them in their bedrooms. This can be a gate, plywood plank, or locked door. A chain lock (hotel lock) on the outside of the door can keep your child in the room yet allow him to open the door partially in case he needs to cry out for someone. If your child is one who needs to urinate during the night, a potty chair can be placed in his room. After 4 years of age most children will stay in their rooms if they awaken early and have been told they're expected to stay and play quietly.

Wants to Choose His or Her Own Bedtime

Assumption: Adolescents should be able to take care of their own sleep requirements before going off to college.

Rule: "Stay up as late as you want, but it's your responsibility to get yourself up in the morning with an alarm clock and to get to school on time. Also, you can't make any noise after the rest of the family has turned in."

Discipline technique: Natural consequences.

TOILET-TRAINING PROBLEMS AND BEDWETTING

TOILET-TRAINING YOUR CHILD: THE BASICS

Definition

Your child is toilet-trained when, without any reminders, he walks to the potty, pulls down his pants, urinates or passes a bowel movement (BM), and pulls up his pants. Some children will learn to control their bladders first; others will start with bowel control. Both kinds of control can be worked on simultaneously. Bladder control through the night normally happens several years later than daytime control. The gradual type of toilet training discussed here can usually be completed in 1 to 3 months if your child is ready.

Toilet-Training Readiness

Don't begin training until your child is clearly ready. Readiness doesn't just happen; it involves concepts and skills you can begin teaching your child at 18 months of age or earlier. All children can be made ready for toilet training by 3 years, most by 2½ years, many by 2 years, and some earlier. Ways to help a child become ready include the following:

18 Months: Begin Teaching About Pee, Poop, and How the Body Works

- Teach the vocabulary (*pee, poop, potty,* etc.).
- Clarify that everyone makes pee and poop.
- Point out when dogs or other animals are going pee or poop.
- Clarify the body's signals when you observe them: "Your body wants to make some pee or poop."
- Praise your child for passing poop in the diaper.

- Don't refer to poop as "dirty" or "yucky" stuff.
- Make changing diapers pleasant for the child so he will come to you.
- Change your child frequently so he will prefer dry diapers.
- Teach the child to go to a parent whenever he is wet or soiled.

21 Months: Begin Teaching About the Potty and Toilet

- Teach what the toilet and potty chair are for ("The pee or poop goes in this special place"). Demonstrate by dumping poop from diapers into the toilet.
- Portray using the toilet and potty chair as a privilege.
- Have him observe toilet-trained children use the toilet or potty chair (having an older toilet-trained sibling can be very helpful).
- Give your child a potty chair. Help the child sit there with clothes on for fun activities (e.g., play, snacks, TV). Help the child develop a sense of ownership ("my chair").
- When your child is comfortable with the potty chair, put it in the bathroom. Have him sit on it (bare bottom) when you or others sit on the toilet.
- Don't allow diapers or pull-ups in the bathroom.

2 Years: Begin Using Teaching Aids

- Read toilet-learning books and watch toilet-learning videos.
- Help your child pretend she's training a doll or stuffed animal on the potty chair. It doesn't have to be a pricey doll that pees water.
- Present underwear as a privilege. Buy special underwear and keep it in a place where the child can see it.

Potty Chairs

Buy a floor-level-type potty chair. You want your child's feet to touch the floor when he sits on the potty. This provides leverage for pushing and a sense of security. He also can get on and off whenever he wants to. Take your child with you to buy the potty chair. Make it clear that this is your child's own special chair. Have your child help you put his name on it. Allow your child to decorate it or even paint it a different color. Then have your child sit on it fully clothed until he is comfortable with using it as a chair. Have your child use it while eating snacks, playing games, or looking at books. Keep it in the room in which your child usually plays. When your child clearly has good feelings toward the potty chair, move it to the bathroom.

Method for Toilet Training

Encourage Practice Runs to the Potty—A practice run (potty sit) is when you encourage your child to walk to the potty and sit there with his diapers or pants off. Your child can then be told, "Try to go pee-pee in the potty." Only do practice runs when your child gives a signal that looks promising, such as a certain facial expression, grunting, holding the genital area, pulling at his pants, pacing, squatting, squirming, etc. Other good times are after naps, 2 hours without urinating, or 20 minutes after meals. Say encouragingly, "The poop [or pee] wants to come out. Let's use the potty." If your child is reluctant to sit on the potty, you may want to read him a story. If your child wants to get up after 1 minute of encouragement, let him get up. Never force your child to sit there. Never physically hold your child there. Even if your child seems to be enjoying it, end each session after 5 minutes unless something is happening. Initially, keep the potty chair in the room your child usually plays in. This easy access markedly increases the chances that he will use it without your asking him. Consider owning two potty chairs. During toilet training, children need to wear clothing that's conducive to using the potty. That means one layer, usually the diaper. Avoid shoes and pants. (In the wintertime, turning up the heat is helpful.) Another option (though less effective) is loose sweatpants with an elastic waistband. Avoid pants with zippers, buttons, snaps, or a belt.

Praise or Reward Your Child for Cooperation or Any Success—All cooperation with these practice sessions should be praised. For example, you might say, "You are sitting on the potty just like Mommy," or "You're trying real hard to go pee-pee in the potty." If your child urinates in the potty, he can be rewarded with treats (e.g., animal cookies) or stickers, as well as praise and hugs. Although a sense of accomplishment is enough for some children, many need treats to stay focused. Big rewards (such as going to the toy store) should be reserved for when your child walks over to the potty on his own and uses it or asks to go there with you and then uses it. Once your child uses the potty by himself two or more times, you can stop the practice runs. For the following week, continue to praise your child frequently for using the potty. (Note: Practice runs and reminders should not be necessary for more than 1 or 2 months.)

Change Your Child After Accidents—Change your child as soon as it's convenient, but respond sympathetically. Say something like, "You wanted to go pee-pee in the potty, but you went pee-pee in your pants. I know that makes you sad. You like to be dry. You'll get better at this." If you feel a need to be critical, keep it to mild verbal disapproval and use it rarely (e.g., "Big boys don't go pee-pee in their pants") or mention the name of another child whom he likes and who is trained. Then change your child into a dry diaper or training pants in as pleasant and nonangry a way as possible. Avoid physical punishment, yelling, or scolding. Pressure or force can make a child completely uncooperative.

Introduce Underpants After Your Child Starts Using the Potty—
Regular underwear can spark motivation. Switch from diapers to underpants after your child is cooperative about sitting on the potty chair and passes urine into the toilet spontaneously 10 or more times. Take your child with you to buy the underwear and make it a reward for his success. Buy loose-fitting ones that he can easily lower and pull up by himself. Once you start using underpants, use diapers only for naps, bedtime, and travel outside the home.

The Bare-Bottom Weekend for Overcoming Toilet-Training Inertia (If Over 30 Months Old)

After your child has successfully used the potty a few times with your help and clearly understands the process, committing 6 hours or a weekend exclusively to toilet training can lead to a breakthrough. Avoid interuptions or distractions during this time. Younger siblings must spend the day elsewhere. Turn off the TV and don't answer the phone. Success requires monitoring your child during these hours of training.

The bare-bottom technique means not wearing any diapers, Pull-ups, underwear, or other clothing below the waist. This causes most children to become acutely aware of their body's plumbing. Children innately dislike pee or poop running down their legs. You and your child should stay in the vicinity of the potty chair—this can be in the kitchen or other room without a carpet. A gate may help your child stay on task. During bare-bottom times, supervise your child but refrain from all practice runs and most reminders, allowing the child to learn by trial and error with your support.

Create a frequent need to urinate by offering your child lots of her favorite fluids. Have just enough toys and books handy to keep your child playing near the potty chair. Keep the process upbeat with hugs, smiles, and good cheer. You are your child's coach and ally.

Call Your Child's Physician During Office Hours If

- Your child is over 2½ years old *and* negative about toilet training after using the methods described above for several months.
- Your child is over 3 years old and not yet daytime toilet-trained.
- Your child won't sit on the potty or toilet.
- Your child holds back bowel movements.
- The approach described here isn't working after 6 months.

TOILET-TRAINING RESISTANCE
(Encopresis and Daytime Wetting)

Definition

Children who refuse to be toilet-trained either wet themselves, soil themselves, or try to hold back their bowel movements (thus becoming constipated). Many of these children also refuse to sit on the toilet or will use the toilet only if the parent brings up the subject and marches them into the bathroom. Any child who is over 3 years old, healthy, and not toilet-trained after several months of trying can be assumed to be resistant to the process, rather than undertrained. Consider how capable your child is at delaying a bowel movement (BM) until she is off the toilet and has had a chance to hide. More practice runs (as you used in toilet training) will not help. Instead, your child now needs full responsibility and some incentives to re-spark her motivation.

The most common cause of resistance to toilet training is that a child has been reminded or lectured too much. Some children have been forced to sit on the toilet against their will, occasionally for long periods of time. A few have been spanked or punished in other ways for not co-operating. Many parents make these mistakes, especially if they have a strong-willed child.

Most children younger than 5 or 6 years of age with soiling (encopresis) or daytime wetting without any other symptoms are simply engaged in a power struggle with you. These children can be helped with the following suggestions. If your child holds back BMs and becomes constipated, medicines will also be needed (see ENCOPRESIS FROM STOOL-HOLDING, page 295).

Helping Children with Daytime Wetting or Soiling

Transfer All Responsibility to Your Child—Your child will decide to use the toilet only after she realizes that she has nothing left to resist. Have one last talk with her about the subject. Tell your child that her body makes "pee" and "poop" every day and it belongs to her. Explain that her "poop" wants to go in the toilet and her job is to help the "poop" come out. Tell your child you're sorry you forced her to sit on the toilet or reminded her so much. Tell her from now on she doesn't need any help. Then stop all talk about this subject ("potty talk"). Pretend you're not worried about this subject. When your child stops receiving conversation for nonperformance (not going), she will eventually decide to perform for attention.

Stop All Reminders—Let your child decide when she needs to go to the bathroom. Don't remind her to go to the bathroom nor ask if she needs to go. She knows what it feels like when she has to "poop" or "pee" and where the bathroom is. Reminders are a form of pressure, and pressure keeps the power struggle going. Stop all practice runs and never make her sit on the toilet against her will because this always increases resistance. Don't accompany your child into the bathroom or stand with her by the potty chair unless she asks you to. She needs to gain the feeling of success that comes from doing it her way.

Give Incentives—Your main job is to find the right incentive for using the toilet. Special incentives, such as favorite sweets or video time, can be invaluable. For using the toilet for BMs, intially err on the side of giving her too much (e.g., several sweets each time). The potency of these incentives also is increased by reducing baseline access to them. If you want a breakthrough, make your child an offer she can't refuse. In addition, give positive feedback, such as praise and hugs *every time* your child uses the toilet. On successful days consider taking 20 extra minutes to play a special game with your child or take her to her favorite playground.

Give Stars—Get a calendar for your child and post it in a conspicuous location. Have her place a star on it every time she uses the toilet. Keep this record of progress until your child has gone 1 month without any accidents.

Make the Potty Chair Convenient—Be sure to keep the potty chair in the room your child usually plays in. This gives her a convenient visual reminder about her options whenever she feels the need to pass urine or stool. For wetting, the presence of the chair and the promise of treats will usually bring about a change in behavior. Don't remind her even if she's squirming and dancing to hold back the urine.

Diapers, Pull-Ups, or Underwear—Whenever possible, replace Pull-Ups or diapers with underwear. Help your child pick out some underwear with favorite characters on them. Then remind her, "They don't like pee or poop on them." This usually precipitates the correct decision on the part of the child. Even if your child wets the underwear, persist with this plan. If your child holds back BMs, allow selective access to diapers or Pull-Ups for BMs only. Preventing stool-holding is very important.

Remind Your Child to Change Her Clothes—As soon as you notice that your child has wet or messy pants, tell her to clean herself up. The main role you have in this program is to enforce the rule "People can't walk around with messy pants." If your child is wet, she can probably change into dry clothes by herself. If your child is soiled, she will probably need your help with cleanup. If your child refuses to let you change her, ground her until she is ready.

Don't Punish or Criticize—Respond gently to accidents, and do not allow siblings to tease the child. Pressure will only delay successful training, and it could cause secondary emotional problems. Your child needs you to be her ally.

Get Help from Preschool or Day-Care Staff—Ask your child's teacher or day-care provider to allow your child to go to the bathroom any time she wants to. Keep an extra set of clean underwear at the school or with the day-care provider.

Call Your Child's Physician During Office Hours If:

- Your child holds back her bowel movements or becomes constipated.
- Pain or burning occurs when she urinates.
- Your child is afraid to sit on the toilet or potty chair.
- Resistance is not improved after 1 month on this program.
- Resistance has not stopped completely after 3 months.

INCENTIVES FOR MOTIVATING CHILDREN

Incentives are rewards for good behaviors. Incentives are especially helpful for overcoming resistance when children are "locked in" a power struggle (control battle) with their parent. Rewards give the child a reason to leave the power struggle.

How to Use Incentives

Four rules make incentives powerful:

- The incentive is strongly desired by the child. Ask your child for ideas (e.g., "What would help you remember to look after your poops?").
- It is given immediately after the child meets their goal (e.g., releases urine or stool in the toilet). Point systems for winning prizes are usually not too effective before age 6.
- The child is given access to the incentive for 30 to 60 minutes.
- It continues to be owned and controlled by the parent.

The fourth rule is essential. The child's access to a bike, costume, videotape, remote-control car, paint set, etc., needs to be time-limited. That way, your child earns a privilege, not another possession. That's the only way to maintain the incentive's value. None of these incentives is essential to normal child development and that is why they can be selectively withheld.

Incentives to Choose From

Access to New Toy or Favorite Toy

- Trike or bike time
- Train set time
- Star Wars toys time
- Lego project time
- Car and truck time
- Remote-control dog or car time
- Lion toys time
- Dinosaur toys time
- Creating jewelry time
- Art or drawing time
- Water pistol time
- Magic sword time

New Costume or Outfit
- Batman or Superman
- Snow White or Belle
- Nail polish
- Special shoes

Video or Movie
- New videos
- Videotape of favorite TV shows
- Go to the movie theater
- Computer or video games

Special Foods
- Candy or sweets
- Ice cream or popsicle
- Special cookies
- Favorite foods such as pizza or strawberries
- Go to the grocery store or favorite food place

Money (coins)

Grab Bag of Surprises (can write on pieces of paper)

Triple Rewards for Breakthroughs
- Go to fast-food place, then video store, and stay up late to watch the movie

Social Reinforcers Are Never Withheld

Social reinforcers include physical affection (e.g., hugs and kisses) and parent-child activities (e.g., going to the library or zoo, reading stories, or playing board games). Social reinforcers are never withheld or used as incentives because they are essential for the child's emotional growth and mental health. Nurturing also makes the child more receptive to parental rules and requests. In addition, physical activity (e.g., playing catch, walks, or going to the park) are never withheld because fitness and endurance are essential to physical health. Extra parent-child activities, however, can be offered as incentives.

ENCOPRESIS FROM STOOL-HOLDING

Definition

About 5 percent of children refuse to be toilet-trained. They get into a tug of war with their parents around using the toilet. Some of these children decide to hold back bowel movements. Other children start holding back after they pass a painful BM and then decide to never experience that again (pain avoidance). Stool-holding can lead to constipation, painful BMs, and even complete blockage (stool impaction). Impacted children constantly leak stool in small amounts. This is called encopresis or soiling. If the impaction persists for very long, the rectum and colon become stretched out of shape and are no longer able to squeeze out stool. Unblocking the child may require enemas. Keeping the child unblocked requires 3 to 6 months of laxatives or stool softeners. Stool-holding is an important problem to recognize early and treat vigorously.

Helping Children with Stool Holding and Encopresis

Clarify the Goal—Review with your child that her job is to make a poop come out every day. Tell her, "Your body makes poop every day" and "The poop wants to come out every day." Emphasize poop production and release. Older children who don't like stool leakage can be told, "If you poop every day and keep your body empty, then nothing will leak out."

Give Laxatives—Most stool-holders need a laxative to keep them empty. Laxatives (bowel stimulants) cause the large intestine to contract, pushing the stool toward the rectum. Most laxatives contain senna, a natural plant extract. Don't worry that your child might become dependent on laxatives (i.e., that the bowels won't move well without them). Children can be gradually withdrawn from laxatives, even after months of using them. The most important goal is keeping the rectum empty. Ask your child's physician to recommend a laxative.

Give Stool Softeners—Stool softeners make the stools softer and easier to pass. Unlike laxatives, they do not cause any bowel contractions or pressure. Some commonly prescribed stool softeners are mineral oil, milk of magnesia, Miralax, and high-fiber products. Increase the dose gradually until your child is passing 1 or 2 soft BMs each day.

Transfer All Responsibility to Your Child—Your child will decide to use the toilet only after she realizes that she has nothing left to resist.

Have one last talk with her about the subject. Tell your child that her body makes poop every day and it belongs to her. Explain that her poop wants to go in the toilet and her job is to help the poop come out. Tell your child you're sorry you forced her to sit on the toilet or reminded her so much. Tell her from now on she doesn't need any help. Then stop all talk about this subject. Pretend you're not worried about this subject. When your child stops receiving pep talks about not going, she will eventually decide to go to the bathroom for the attention.

Stop All Reminders—Let your child decide when she needs to go to the bathroom. She knows what it feels like when she has to poop and where the bathroom is. Reminders are a form of pressure, and pressure keeps the power struggle going. Stop all practice runs and never make her sit on the toilet against her will because this always increases resistance. She needs to gain the feeling of success that comes from doing it her way. Because holding back stool hurts the body, there are some exceptions to not reminding your child:

• If your child is complaining about abdominal pain, clarify how to make it go away. Tell her: "The poop wants to come out," "The poop needs your help," "Holding back causes a tummyache." Offer to help her sit in a basin of warm water to relax the muscles around the anus (anal sphincter). If she refuses, tell her "I can't help you. You have to help yourself." Then ignore your child or put her in time-out. Tell her to come back after the poop is out. Do not give positive attention for holding-back behavior.

• If your child is obviously holding back a BM, initially say nothing in hopes she will do the right thing. If she holds back for more than 5 minutes, give a pleasant verbal reminder. First say "Your body is talking to you. What does it want you to do?" If necessary, add "The poop wants to come out and go in the toilet. The poop needs your help." Tell your child that you want sitting on the potty to be lots of fun. What would she like to do while she's there—maybe read a special book? If she declines your offer to provide a special potty activity, say nothing more and let your child decide how she wishes to respond to the pressure in her rectum.

Put Your Child in "Poop Jail"

• If your child is over age 4 and leaking stool, ground him until he passes a BM. Tell your child: "When poop leaks out, it always means there's a large poop inside trying to get out, and you need time to think about how to help your body get it out." Tell your child he's grounded until he passes a big poop. He can only go to essential events: meals, preschool or school, church, scheduled classes (e.g., music lessons), or team events. Otherwise he's grounded in his bedroom with no TV, videos, computer games, friends over, or playing outside until he completes his assignment. Using the term "poop jail" keeps the intervention humorous and more acceptable for most kids. You can tell your child that this is what the doctor said to do ("doctor's orders") and protect your role as the child's ally. If your child complains, give him a hug and blame the doctor. If this approach doesn't work, consider restricting your child to the bathroom and inform him that he can't come out until he produces a normal-sized poop.

- If your child reaches the end of day 2 (or 3) without passing a BM, again, ground your child until he passes a big poop (at least the size of a banana). Remember that holding it back causes it to become larger and wider. After 4 or 5 days, it will become too wide to pass.

Give Incentives—Your main job is to find the right incentive for going poop in the toilet. Initially err on the side of giving her too much (e.g., several food treats each time). The potency of these incentives is increased by reducing baseline access to them. If you want a breakthrough, make your child an offer she can't refuse (e.g., going somewhere special). See INCENTIVES FOR MOTIVATING CHILDREN, page 293. In addition, give positive feedback, such as praise and hugs every time your child tries to use the toilet. On successful days consider taking 20 extra minutes to play a special game with your child or take her to her favorite playground.

Give Stars—Get a calendar for your child and post it in a conspicuous location. Call it the Good Pooper chart. Have her place a star on it every time she poops in the toilet. Keep this record of progress until your child has gone 1 month without any soiling.

Make the Potty Chair Convenient—Be sure to keep the potty chair in the room she usually plays in. This gives your child a convenient visual reminder about her options whenever she feels the need to pass stool.

Allow Diapers or Pull-Ups—We want your child to look forward to releasing BMs, rather than holding back. If your child refuses to sit on the toilet, having bowel movements in diapers is always better than stool-holding. Therefore, permit access to diapers. However, don't let your child wear diapers all day. Keep your child in loose-fitting underwear so that she has to decide each time she has an urge to pass a BM whether to use the toilet or to come to you for a diaper. To help her make the right choice, offer major incentives (e.g., a trip to a favorite restaurant or toy store) for BMs in the toilet. Offer minor incentives (e.g., candy) for BMs in the diaper. (Note: Staying in underwear also gives her an incentive to maintain bladder control and stay dry.)

Help Your Child Change Her Clothes—Don't ignore soiling. The main role you have in this new program is to enforce the rule "People can't walk around with messy pants." Your child will probably need your help with cleanup, but keep her involved. Make changing pants a neutral, quick interaction. If your child refuses to let you change her, ground her or put her in time-out until she is ready.

Call Your Child's Physician During Office Hours If

- You think your child is blocked up.
- Your child's bowel movements continue to hurt.
- You have other questions or concerns.

ENCOPRESIS AND CONSTIPATION: HOW TO GET BETTER (Note to the School-Age Child)

This information is for children over age 6 who want to get over their constipation and encopresis. Some of these young people are confused about how the body works, and some of them try to prevent stool leakage by holding back BMs rather than releasing them. Ask your youngster to read these instructions (or you read them to him) every morning during breakfast until following them becomes automatic.

Your Wish

- To stay clean and not have poops leak out.
- To not have any pain from big poops.

How to Do It

- Keep your body (rectum) empty of poop.
- Don't let yourself get blocked up ever again.

Your Job

- Go poop every day (don't let it build up inside).
- Sit on the toilet at least 3 times a day. Unless you do this, your medicines won't work.
- Take your medicine every day.
- If your poops aren't coming out like they should, sit on the toilet more often. Also ask your parent for *extra* medicine.
- If only a small poop comes out, sit on the toilet again in 5 minutes.

For Poop That Leaks Out

- The first thing to do is sit on the toilet until a poop comes out.
- Leakage always means there's a big poop inside (in the rectum) trying to get out.
- Clean up *after* you have passed the big poop.

Definitions

- Constipation means no poop for 3 or more days. By 4 or 5 days the poop gets stuck inside.
- *Encopresis* or *soiling* means poop leaks out.

DAYTIME FREQUENCY OF URINATION

Definition

Daytime frequency of urination occurs most often when a child is 4 to 5 years old.

- Your child suddenly starts urinating every 10 to 30 minutes and as often as 30 to 40 times a day.
- Your child passes small amounts of urine each time.
- Your child has no pain with urination.
- Your child does not wet himself during the day.
- Your child does not drink excessive amounts of fluids.
- Your child has been toilet-trained.
- The urinary frequency is not a problem during sleep.

Causes—Frequent urination sometimes reflects emotional tension. It means your child is under pressure. The symptom is involuntary, not deliberate. The urinary frequency may begin within 1 or 2 days of a stressful event or other change in the child's routine. You can make the problem worse by worrying about disease. Punishment, criticism, or teasing also worsens the symptom.

Although physical causes are rare, your child should be examined by a physician. The only test that is usually needed is a check of the urine. No X-rays are needed.

Expected Course—Overall, this is a harmless condition that eventually goes away by itself. If you can identify and deal with whatever is stressing your child, his frequent urination will disappear in 1 to 4 weeks. Without treatment, the symptom usually gets better on its own in 2 or 3 months.

A few children who also have small bladders and problems with bed-wetting may have this symptom more than once.

Helping Children with Daytime Frequency of Urination

Reassure Your Child That He Is Physically Healthy—Tell your child that his body, kidneys, urine, and any other aspect of his health that he is worried about are fine. Because the family (and also possibly physicians) have been concerned about the child's bladder and urine, he may fear there is something wrong with his urinary tract. Reassure him once or twice that he is quite healthy.

Reassure Your Child That He Can Learn to Wait Longer to Urinate—Reassure him that he won't wet himself, which is a common fear. If he has wet himself before, encourage him to talk about his embarrassment and reassure him it happens to many children. Tell him that he will gradually get back to urinating every 2 to 3 hours, or whatever his previous pattern was. If his frequency of urination has gotten worse during shopping trips or travel in general, don't take him with you in public places for a while.

Help Your Child Relax—Frequency of urination can be a barometer of inner tension. Make sure your child has free time and fun time every day. If he is overscheduled with activities, try to lighten the commitments. Relaxation exercises may help your child if he is over 8 years old.

Increasing the happiness and harmony within your home will usually restore your child's sense of security.

Ask the staff at your child's school or day-care center to help reduce any tensions there, such as limits on when a child can use the bathroom.

Try to Figure Out What Is Stressing Your Child—Meet with other family members and try to think of a stressful event that may have occurred 1 or 2 days before the frequency began. Also ask school or day-care staff for ideas. Talk about your ideas with your child and try to help him overcome the stress. Common stressful events are:

• Death in the family
• Accident or other life-threatening event
• Tension in parents' marriage
• A sick parent or sibling
• School entry or a new school
• Too much concern about staying dry at night
• Wetting himself in the presence of peers

Ignore the Symptom of Frequency—When your child is using the toilet frequently, don't comment on it. Comments remind him that the symptom is worrying you. Stop keeping any record of amount or frequency of urination. Do not collect any samples or measure volumes. Don't ask your child about his symptom or watch him urinate. Do not have your child do bladder-stretching exercises. Your child does not need to tell you when he has urinated; you will have a general impression about whether he is getting better or staying the same.

Be sure that none of your child's caretakers or teachers is punishing or criticizing him about this symptom.

Stop all family conversation about the frequency. The less said about it, the less anxious your child will be about it. If your child brings up the topic, reassure him that he will gradually get better.

Avoid Bubble Bath and Other Irritants—Bubble bath can cause frequent urination in children, especially girls. Bubble bath can irritate the opening of the urinary tract. Taking a bath in water that contains shampoo can also cause similar symptoms. In addition, before puberty, be sure your child washes the genital area with water, not soap.

Call Your Child's Physician During Office Hours If

• The frequency of urination is not back to normal after you have followed these recommendations for 1 month.

• Your child begins to have pain or burning when urinating.
• Your child begins to wet himself during the day.
• Your child begins to drink excessive amounts of fluids.
• You have other questions or concerns.

BEDWETTING (Enuresis)

Definition

Enuresis (bedwetting) is the term used for urinating while asleep. It is considered normal until at least age 6.

Causes—Most children who wet the bed have inherited small bladders, which cannot hold all the urine produced in a night. In addition, they are deep sleepers who don't awaken to the signal of a full bladder. The kidneys are normal. Physical causes are very rare, and your physician can easily detect them. Emotional problems do not cause enuresis, but they can occur if it is mishandled.

Measure your child's bladder size to help you understand how important it is for him to get up at night. Do this by having your child hold his urine as long as possible on at least three occasions. Have your child urinate into a container each time. Measure the amount of urine in ounces. The largest of the three measurements can be considered your child's bladder capacity. The normal capacity for children is 1 or more ounces per year of age.

Expected Course—Most children who are bedwetting overcome the problem between ages 6 and 10. Even without treatment, all children eventually get over it. Therefore, treatments that might have harmful complications should not be used. On the other hand, treatments without side effects can be started as soon as your child has had complete bladder control during the daytime for 6 to 12 months.

Helping Children with Bedwetting

Getting Up at Night—This advice is more important than any other. Tell your child at bedtime, "Try to get up when you have to pee."

Access to the Toilet—Put a night-light in the bathroom. If the bathroom is at a distant location, try to put a portable toilet in your child's bedroom. Boys will do fine with a bucket.

Fluid Intake—Encourage your child to drink a lot during the morning and early afternoon. The more your child drinks, the more urine your child will produce, and more urine leads to larger bladders. Discourage your child from drinking a lot during the 2 hours before bedtime. Give gentle reminders about this, but don't worry about normal amounts of drinking. Avoid any drinks containing caffeine.

Empty the Bladder at Bedtime—Sometimes the parent needs to remind the child. Older children may respond better to a sign at their bedside or on the bathroom mirror.

No Diapers or Pull-ups—Although this protective layer makes morning cleanup easier, it can interfere with motivation for getting up at night. Use pull-ups or special absorbent underpants selectively for camping or overnights at other people's homes. Use them only if your child wants to use them. They should rarely be permitted beyond age 8.

Protect the Bed from Urine—Odor becomes a problem if urine soaks into the mattress or blankets. Protect the mattress with a plastic mattress cover.

Include Your Child in Morning Cleanup—Including your child as a helper in stripping the bedclothes and putting them into the washing machine provides a natural disincentive for being wet. Older children can perform this task independently. Also, make sure that your child takes a shower each morning so that he or she does not smell of urine in school.

Respond Positively to Dry Nights—Praise your child on mornings when he wakes up dry. A calendar with gold stars or happy faces for dry nights may also help.

Respond Gently to Wet Nights—Your child does not like being wet. Most bedwetters feel quite guilty and embarrassed about this problem. They need support and encouragement, not blame or punishment. Siblings should not allowed to tease bedwetters. Your home needs to be a safe haven for your child. Punishment or pressure will delay a cure and cause secondary emotional problems.

When Your Child Reaches Age 6

Follow the previous recomendations in addition to the guidelines given below:

Understand the Goal—The key to becoming dry is to learn how to self-awaken every night and find the toilet. Getting up and urinating during the night can keep your child dry regardless of how small the bladder is or how much fluid he drinks. Help your child assume responsibility for doing this. Some children think that enuresis is the parent's problem to solve; they need to be reminded that "only you can solve this."

Bedtime Pep Talk—To help your child remember to awaken himself at night, encourage him to practice the following routine at bedtime:

- Ask him to lie on his bed with his eyes closed.
- Have him pretend it's the middle of the night, and his bladder is full, and he feels the pressure. Have him pretend his bladder is trying to wake him before it's too late. Then tell him to run to the bathroom and empty his bladder.
- Remind him to get up like this during the night.

Daytime Practice of Self-Awakening—Whenever your child has an urge to urinate and you're home, he should go to his bedroom rather than the bathroom. Have him lie down and pretend he's sleeping. Have him tell himself this is how his bladder feels during the night when it tries to awaken him. After a few minutes, have him go to the bathroom and urinate (just as he should at night).

Parent Awakening—If self-awakening fails, use parent awakening to teach your child the correct goal: urinating into the toilet during the night. It makes much more sense than putting your child back into Pull-Ups and having him urinate in bed every night (the wrong goal). Your job is to wake your child up; his job is to locate the bathroom and use the toilet. You can awaken him at your bedtime. Try a hierarchy of prompts (the minimal one being the best), ranging from turning on a light to saying his name, touching him, shaking him, or turning on an alarm clock. If your child is confused and very hard to awaken, try again in 20 minutes. Once he's awake he needs to find the bathroom without any direction or guidance. When he awakens quickly to sound or touch for 7 consecutive nights, he's either cured or ready for an enuresis alarm.

Changing Wet Clothes—If your child wets at night, he should try to get up and change clothes. First, if your child feels any urine leaking out, he should try to stop the flow of urine. Second, he should hurry to the toilet to see if he has any urine left in his bladder. Third, he should change himself and put a dry towel over the wet part of the bed. (This step can be made easier if you always keep dry pajamas and towels on the chair near the bed.)

The child who shows the motivation to carry out these steps is close to being able to awaken from the sensation of a full bladder.

When Your Child Reaches Age 8

Follow the previous recommendations. Talk with your physician about possibly using enuresis alarms or drugs as well, as described below.

Bedwetting Alarms—Alarms are used to teach a child to awaken when he needs to urinate during the night. They go off when they become wet. One type awakens you with a loud noise (buzzer), and the other type uses an annoying vibration. They have the highest cure rate (about 70 percent) of any available approach. They are the treatment of choice for any bedwetter with a small bladder who can't otherwise train himself to awaken at night. The new transistorized alarms are small, lightweight, sensitive to a few drops of urine, not too expensive (about $50), and easy for a child to set up by himself. Some children as young as 5 years want to use them. Children using alarms still need to work on the self-awakening program. (See BEDWETTING ALARMS, page 306.)

Alarm Clock—If your child is unable to awaken himself at night and you can't afford a bedwetting alarm, teach him to use an alarm clock or clock radio. Set it for 3 or 4 hours after your child goes to bed. Put it beyond arm's reach. Encourage your child to practice responding to the alarm during the day while lying on the bed with eyes closed. Have your child set the alarm each night. Praise your child for getting up at night, even if he isn't dry in the morning.

Medication—Most bedwetters need extra help with staying dry during slumber parties, camping trips, vacations, or other overnights. Some take an alarm clock with them and stay dry by awakening once at night. Some are helped by temporarily taking a drug at bedtime. One drug (given by pill or nasal spray) decreases urine production at night and is quite safe. Another drug (taken as a pill) temporarily increases bladder capacity. It is safe at the correct dosage but very dangerous if too much is taken or a younger sibling gets into it.

If you do use a medication, be careful about the amount you use and where you store the drug, and be sure to keep the safety cap on the bottle. The drawback of these medicines is that when they are stopped, the bedwetting usually returns. Therefore, children taking drugs for enuresis should also be using an alarm and learning to get up at night.

Call Your Child's Physician During Office Hours If

- Urination causes pain or burning.
- The stream of urine is weak or dribbly.
- Your child also wets during the daytime.
- Your child also drinks excessive fluids.
- Bedwetting is a new problem (your child used to stay dry).
- Your child is over 12 years old.
- Your child is over 6 years old and is not better after 3 months of following this treatment program.

BEDWETTING ALARMS

Definition

Almost all children and teens who wet the bed need to get up during the night to urinate. A bedwetting (enuresis) alarm, which is activated by moisture, can help your child learn to awaken in time to go to the bathroom. The new models are lightweight and easy for the child to operate. Enuresis alarms can be used on any child age 5 and up who wants to try one. On the other hand, they should never be imposed on children at any age, even teenagers, if they don't want to use one.

How to Use an Enuresis Alarm: Instructions for the Young Person

When you buy an alarm, give your child the following instructions:

1. This is your alarm. It can help you cure your bedwetting if you use it correctly. Remember that the main purpose of the alarm is to help you get up during the night and use the toilet. The alarm won't work unless you listen for it carefully and get up as soon as you hear it. Better yet, get up before the alarm goes off.

2. Hook up the alarm system by yourself. Trigger the buzzer a few times by touching the moisture sensor with a wet finger and practice going to the bathroom as you will do if it goes off during the night.

3. Have a night-light or flashlight near your bed so it will be easy to see what you are doing when the alarm sounds. Turn on the night-light when you go to bed.

4. Give yourself a pep talk at bedtime. Remind yourself that you want to try to "beat the buzzer." You want to wake up when your bladder feels full but before any urine leaks out. If the buzzer does go off, you are going to try to wake up and stop urinating as soon as you think you hear the alarm, even if you think you are hearing it in a dream.

5. As soon as you hear the alarm when you are sleeping, wake yourself up and close the valve to your bladder to stop urinating. Then jump out of bed and run to the bathroom.

6. In the bathroom empty your bladder to see how much urine you were able to hold back. Then work on turning off the buzzer by disconnecting and removing the sensor from the wet underwear.

7. Put on dry underwear and pajamas and reconnect the alarm. Put a dry towel over the wet spot on your bed. Remind yourself to get up before the alarm buzzes the next time.

8. In the morning, write on your calendar for that day "Dry" (meaning no alarm), "Wet Spot" (you got up after the alarm went off), or "Wet" (you didn't get up).

9. Use the alarm every night until you go 3 or 4 weeks without wetting the bed. It usually takes 2 to 3 months before you can go 3 or 4 weeks without wetting, so keep working at it.

A Self-Awakening Program for Your Youngster

While your child is using the alarm, it's very important that he also practice the following self-awakening program at bedtime. Your child is trying to teach himself to awaken during the night and use the toilet when the bladder feels full. Until he learns how to do this, he won't stay dry.

Have your child practice waking up. Tell your child to:

• Lie on your bed with your eyes closed.

• Pretend it's the middle of the night.

• Pretend your bladder is full.

• Pretend you feel the pressure.

- Pretend your bladder is trying to wake you up.
- Pretend it's saying, "Get up before it's too late."
- Run to the bathroom and empty your bladder.
- Remind yourself to get up like this during the night.

Parent's Role

If your child doesn't awaken immediately to the sound of the buzzer, he needs your help. You may need to help your child every night for the first 2 to 3 weeks.

1. When you hear the alarm go to your child's room as quickly as you can. Turn on the light and say loudly, "Get out of bed and stand up."

2. If that doesn't work, help your child sit up. Wipe his face with a cold washcloth to bring him out of his deep sleep.

3. Only after your child is standing, remind him to turn off the alarm. By all means, do not turn off the buzzer for him. Your child has to learn to carry out this step for himself.

4. Make sure your child is wide-awake and walks into the bathroom before you leave him. If necessary, ask him questions to help awaken him.

5. Your goal is to help your child awaken immediately and get out of bed when the buzzer sounds. Stop helping him as soon as he appears to be able to wake up and get up without your help. Going to bed with the radio off, going to bed at a reasonable hour, and using a night-light can help your child respond faster to the alarm.

How to Order an Enuresis Alarm

Order alarms and information from:

- Nytone Alarm: Nytone Medical Products, 2424 South 900 West, Salt Lake City, UT 84119; 1-801-973-4090.
- Wet-Stop Alarm: Palco Laboratories, 8030 Soquel Avenue, Suite 104, Santa Cruz, CA 95062; 1-800-346-4488.
- Potty Pager (silent alarm): Ideas for Living, 1285 North Cedarbrook, Boulder, CO 80304; 1-800-497-6573.

An alarm may be covered by health insurance if your physician writes an order for it.

DISCIPLINE PROBLEMS

DISCIPLINE BASICS

Goals of Discipline

The first goal of discipline is to protect your child from danger. Another very important goal is to teach your child an understanding of right and wrong. Good discipline gradually changes a self-centered child into a mature teen who is responsible, thoughtful, and respectful of others, assertive without being hostile, and in control of his or her impulses. Reasonable limit-setting keeps us from raising a spoiled child (see pages 327–31). Discipline means to teach, not to punish. To teach respect for the rights of others, first teach your child to respect your rights. Children need a parent who is "in charge." Begin external controls by 4 months of age when you gradually change from a demand schedule of feeding to fitting your child into your schedule. Children don't start to develop internal controls (self-control) until 3 or 4 years of age. They continue to need external controls (in gradually decreasing amounts) through adolescence.

How to Begin a Discipline Program

If your child has several discipline problems or is out of control, start here. If you are reading to learn more about normal discipline, go directly to RULES FOR STOPPING MISBEHAVIOR, page 311.

List Problem Behaviors—What do you want to change? Take 3 or 4 days to note and write down your child's inappropriate or annoying behavior traits.

Set Priorities—Some modes of behavior need immediate attention—for instance, those that might cause harm to your child or others. Some are too annoying or obnoxious to be ignored (such as not going to bed). Some instances of unpleasant behavior (such as negativism) are normal and must be tolerated (see THE TERRIBLE TWOS AND STUBBORN TODDLERS, page 331). Some families who have an out-of-control child have too many rules and need to rethink what can be overlooked.

Write House Rules—Decide which are the most important kinds of misbehavior. (See RULES FOR STOPPING MISBEHAVIOR, page 311).

Devise a Discipline Response—(See DISCIPLINE TECHNIQUES AND CONSEQUENCES FOR STOPPING MISBEHAVIOR, page 312). All behavior, regardless of cause, can be changed. Behavior is predominantly shaped by consequences. If the consequence is pleasant (a reward or praise), behavior is more likely to be repeated. If the consequence is unpleasant (a punishment), behavior is less likely to be repeated. Young children usually do not respond to lectures or reminders. The best way to get your child to stop doing something is to take action. The most helpful actions are ignoring the misbehavior, redirecting to appropriate behavior, or putting your child into time-out.

Discontinue Physical Punishment—(See PHYSICAL PUNISHMENT AND SPANKING, page 318). Most out-of-control children are already too aggressive. Physical punishment teaches them that aggression is acceptable for solving problems.

Discontinue Yelling—Yelling and screaming teach your child to yell back, thereby legitimizing shouting matches. They also convey that you are not in charge. Yelling often escalates the disagreement and turns it into a win-lose battle. Your child will respond better in the long run to a pleasant tone of voice and words of diplomacy.

Limit Going Out in Public—Don't take your child to public places until his or her behavior is under control at home. Misbehaving children are usually more difficult to control in a shopping mall or supermarket. Leave your child with a baby-sitter or spouse when you need to go to these places.

Take Daily Breaks from Your Child—Ask your spouse to spell you from supervising your young child, to take over all the discipline for a few hours. If this is impossible, hire a teenager a few times a week to look after your child while you go out. Also make a "date" for a weekly night out with your spouse.

Give More Positive Feedback—(See POSITIVE REINFORCEMENT OF DESIRED BEHAVIOR, page 317). Children respond to discipline from people they feel loved by and want to please. Every child needs daily praise, smiles, and hugs (time-ins). Give your child this increased attention when he is not demanding it, especially if he is behaving in an adaptive way. When all is quiet in your house, make the rounds and catch your child being good. If your child receives more negative comments and criticisms each day than positive responses, you need to restore an emotionally healthy balance by reducing the rules, reducing the criticism, and increasing the positive contacts. Many experts feel that it takes several positive contacts to counter one negative one.

Protect Your Child's Self-Esteem—Your child's self-esteem is as important as how well disciplined he or she is. Don't discuss his discipline problems and your concerns about him when he is around. Correct your child in a kindly way. Sometimes begin your correction with "I'm sorry I can't let you ———." Don't label your child a "bad girl" or "bad boy." After punishment is over, accept your child back into the family circle, convey that all is forgiven, and give him a clean slate.

Rules for Stopping Misbehavior

Begin Discipline After 4 Months of Age—Prior to 4 months of age, infants don't need any discipline. Starting at this age, however, parents can begin to clarify their own rights. If your child kicks and wiggles during a diaper change, making the process difficult, you can say firmly, "No, help Mommy change your diaper." By the time they start to crawl (8 months of age), all children need rules for their safety.

Set Clear Rules—Express each example of misbehavior as a clear and concrete rule. Vague descriptions of misbehavior (such as "hyperactive," "irresponsible," or "mean") are not helpful. The younger the child, the more concrete the rule must be. Examples of clear rules are "Don't push your brother" and "Don't interrupt me while I'm on the telephone."

Outline Desired Behaviors—Also state the acceptable, desired, adaptive, or appropriate behavior. Your child needs to know what is expected of him or her. Examples are: "Play with your brother," "Look at books when I'm on the telephone," or "Walk, don't run." Praise your child at these times. Make your praise specific (e.g., "Thank you for being quiet").

Ignore Unimportant or Irrelevant Misbehavior—The more rules you have, the less likely your child is to listen. Constant criticism is usually ineffective. Behaviors such as swinging the legs, poor table manners, or normal negativism are unimportant during the early years.

Use Rules That Are Fair and Attainable—Rules must be age-appropriate. A child should not be punished for clumsiness when he or she is learning to walk, nor for poor pronunciation when learning to speak. In addition, a child should not be punished for behavior that is part of normal emotional development, such as thumbsucking, separation fears, and toilet-training confusion.

Concentrate on Two or Three Rules—The highest priority is given to issues of safety, such as not running into the street. Of equal importance is the prevention of harm to others—parents, other children and adults, or animals. Destructive behavior toward property is of the next importance. Then come all the annoying behaviors that wear you down.

Avoid Power Struggles—This type of misbehavior usually involves a body part. Examples are wetting, soiling, hair-pulling, thumbsucking, body rocking, masturbation, not eating enough, not going to sleep, and refusing to complete schoolwork. No-win behavior is usually uncontrollable by the parent if the child decides to continue it. The first step in resolving a power struggle is to withdraw from the conflict. Then apply positive approaches (see POSITIVE REINFORCEMENT OF DESIRED BEHAVIOR, page 317).

Apply the Rules Consistently—After the parents agree on the rules, it may be helpful to print them out and post them in a conspicuous place in the home.

Discipline Techniques and Consequences for Stopping Misbehavior

Discipline Techniques to Use for Different Ages—The techniques mentioned here are further described after this list.

- From birth to 4 months: no discipline necessary
- From 4 to 8 months: mild verbal disapproval
- From 8 to 18 months: structuring the environment, distracting, ignoring, verbal and nonverbal disapproval, physically moving or escorting, and temporary time-out in a playpen
- From 18 months to 3 years: the preceding techniques plus temporary time-out in a chair
- From 3 years to 5 years: the preceding techniques plus temporary time-out in a room, natural consequences, logical consequences, restricting places where the child can misbehave

- From 5 years to adolescence: the preceding techniques plus delay of a privilege, negotiation and family conferences, and "I" messages
- Adolescence: mainly logical consequences and family conferences about house rules. We can't discipline adolescents the way we discipline preschoolers (and vice versa). By the time your child is an adolescent you should discontinue manual guidance and time-out techniques (see ADOLESCENTS: DEALING WITH NORMAL REBELLION, page 419).

Structuring the Home Environment—The surroundings can be modified so that an object or situation that could potentially cause a problem is eliminated. Examples are putting breakables out of reach, fencing in a yard, setting up gates, putting locks on a special desk, or locking certain rooms.

Distracting, Redirecting, or Diverting Your Child from Misbehavior—Distracting a child counteracts an unacceptable activity with a parent-approved one. Distraction is especially helpful with young children when they are in someone else's house, a physician's office, or a store where other options for discipline (such as time-out) would be difficult to employ. It also can be used preventively if you're going to be busy at home with guests, the telephone, or feeding a baby. Most children can be distracted with toys or food. School-age children may need books, games, or other activities to keep their attention.

Ignoring the Misbehavior—Ignoring, or extinction, is a technique that is helpful for eliminating unacceptable behavior that is harmless, such as tantrums, sulking, whining, quarreling, or interrupting. The proper way to ignore is to move away from your child, turn your back, avoid eye contact, and stop any conversation with your child. Ignore any protests or excuses. At times, you may need to leave the area where your child is misbehaving.

Verbal and Nonverbal Disapproval—Mild disapproval is often all that is required to stop a young child's misbehavior. The proper technique is to move close to your child, make eye contact, assume a stern facial expression, and give a brief, direct instruction such as "no" or "stop." Your comments can be made in a soft but disapproving tone, since you are close to your child. Also show your child what you want him to do (the adaptive behavior). You may want to underscore your serious intent by pointing or shaking your finger. The most common mistake in using this technique is smiling or laughing.

Physically Move or Escort (Manual Guidance)—Manual guidance is the process of moving a child from one place to another against his or her will. Sometimes children must be physically removed from a place where they are causing trouble to a time-out chair. Other children must be physically taken to the bed, bath, or car when they refuse to go. The correct technique is guiding your child by the hand or forearm. If he refuses to be led, pick him up from behind and carry him.

Temporary Time-out or Social Isolation—Temporary time-out is the most effective discipline technique available to parents for dealing with misbehaving infants and young children. See TIME-OUT TECHNIQUE FOR DISCIPLINE (page 320) for details. Time-out should be applied briefly, on the order of 1 minute per year of age.

Natural Consequences—Natural consequences are the negative results of your child's own actions. They permit your child to learn from the natural laws of the physical world. For example, coming to dinner late means the food will be cold; not dressing properly for the weather means your child will be cold or wet; not wearing mittens while playing in the snow will lead to cold hands; running on ice will usually lead to falling down; putting sand in the mouth leads to an unpleasant taste; breaking a toy means it's no longer playworthy; and going to bed late means being sleepy in the morning. Although it is very helpful for children to learn from their mistakes, it is important that they not be allowed to engage in behavior that could be harmful, such as playing with matches or running into the street.

Restricting Places Where a Child Can Misbehave—This technique is especially helpful for behavior problems that can't be eliminated. For thumbsucking, nose picking, and masturbation, allowing the misbehavior in your child's room prevents an unnecessary power struggle. Roughhousing can be restricted to outdoors. The child's tricycle can be restricted to the basement in the wintertime.

Delay of a Privilege—This technique requires that a less preferable activity be completed before a more preferable one is allowed (work before play). Examples are: "After you clean your room, you can go out and play"; "When you finish your homework, you can watch TV"; "When you have tasted all your foods, you can have your dessert."

Temporary Removal of a Privilege or Possession (Logical Consequences)—Logical consequences permit children to learn from the reality of the social order. These consequences should be logically related to the unacceptable behavior. Many logical consequences are simply the temporary removal of a possession or privilege. Examples are removal of toys or crayons that are mishandled, not replacing a lost toy, not repairing a broken toy, sending your child to school partially dressed if she won't dress herself, having your child clean up milk he has spilled or a floor he has tracked mud on, having your child clean up underwear if she has soiled it, and turning off the TV if siblings are quarreling about it. In addition, TV, telephone, shopping, bicycle, and car privileges can all be temporarily suspended if they are misused. The schoolteacher will provide appropriate logical consequences if your child does not complete homework assignments.

Some mistakes made by parents in the area of providing consequences are depriving children of basic essentials, such as a meal; activities with an organized peer group, like a team or Scout troop; or greatly anticipated events, such as going to the circus. The main thrust of logical consequences is to make your child accountable for his or her problems and decisions. It is important for children to learn from experience and not be sheltered from realities.

"I" Messages—When your child misbehaves, preface your correction by telling your child how you feel. Say "I am angry" or "I am upset when you do such and such." Your child is more likely to listen to this than a message that starts with "you." "You" messages usually trigger a defensive reaction. (For details see ADOLESCENTS: DEALING WITH NORMAL REBELLION, page 419.)

Negotiation and Family Conferences—As children become older they need more communication and discussion with their parents. A parent can initiate such a conversation by stating: "We need to change these things. Where do you want to start?" Discussions involving the whole family (family conferences) also become helpful (see ADOLESCENTS: DEALING WITH NORMAL REBELLION, page 419). Don't forget to reward acceptable (desired) behavior (see page 317).

Consequences: How to Deliver

- *Be unambivalent.* Mean what you say and follow through. Be stern and tough. You know the rules, so take charge.
- *Correct with love.* Talk to your child the way you would want to be talked to. Avoid yelling or using a disrespectful tone of voice. For example, say, "I'm sorry you left the yard, but now you must stay in the house."

- *Precede the consequence by one warning or reminder.* After the rule is clearly understood, this warning is unnecessary and you can punish your child without a warning. Avoid repeated threats of consequences if your child doesn't stop what he is doing.

- *With aggressive behavior, punish your child for clear intent.* Try to interrupt your child before someone is hurt or damage is done. An example would be that you see your child raising a toy to hit a playmate. Intervene before the friend is injured.

- *Apply the consequence immediately.* Delayed consequences are less effective, because young children forget why they are being punished. Punishment should occur close in time to the misdeed and be administered by the adult who witnessed the misbehavior. An exception for children older than 4 or 5 years of age is: when they misbehave outside the home and you don't want to improvise a time-out, you may put check marks on your child's hand with a felt-tip pen to indicate the number of punishments to be meted out when you get home. Punishment might be 30 minutes of lost TV time for each check mark.

- *Make a one-sentence comment about the rule during correction.* Avoid making a long speech.

- *Ignore your child's arguments during correction.* This is the child's way of delaying punishment. Especially under 3 years of age, children mainly understand action, not words.

- *Make the punishment brief.* Toys can be taken out of circulation for no more than 1 or 2 days. Time-out should be on the order of 1 minute per year of age.

- *Keep the consequence in proportion to the misbehavior.* Also try to make the consequence relate to the misbehavior (see LOGICAL CONSEQUENCES, pages 314–15).

- *Follow the consequence with love and trust.* Welcome your child back into the family circle and do not comment upon the previous misbehavior or require an apology for it.

- *Direct the punishment against the misbehavior, not the person.* Avoid degrading comments such as "You never do anything right."

- *Expect the behavior to get worse before it gets better.* Don't be surprised if your child temporarily shows an increased frequency of bad behavior once you start disciplining him more consistently. Children who are out of control initially go through a phase of testing their parents before they comply with the new system. This testing usually lasts 2 or 3 days.

Positive Reinforcement of Desired Behavior

Most parents don't give enough positive reinforcement—especially touching and hugs. Dr. Edward Christophersen, an eminent pediatric psychologist, calls these brief, nonverbal physical contracts "time-in" (in contrast to time-out). When you give positive social reinforcement (positive strokes), move close to your child, look at him or her, smile, and be physically affectionate. Although it takes little time or energy, a parent's affection and attention are the favorite rewards of most children.

Social reinforcement should principally be used when your child behaves in an adaptive or desired way. Don't take good behavior for granted. Watch for behavior you like, then praise your child by saying such things as "I like the way you ———," or "I appreciate ———." Praise the behavior, not the person. Examples are sharing toys, demonstrating good manners, doing chores, playing cooperatively, treating the baby gently, petting the dog, being a good sport, cleaning the room, or reading a book. Your child can also be praised for trying, such as trying to use the potty or attempting something difficult, like a puzzle. Positive reinforcement will increase the frequency of desired behavior.

You should try to catch your child being good, and comment on it three or more times for every one time you discipline or criticize your child. Although difficult, this can be achieved. Some families with teenagers have increased everybody's ability to pay attention to positives by providing each member with ten thank-you cards, one of which is given to a family member whenever one is helpful to another. This increases everybody's awareness of working cooperatively. Social reinforcers are especially helpful when a child is having a bad day.

Special material reinforcers or incentives are things such as favorite foods, money, or video time. While these tangible reinforcers tend to be overused by many parents, other parents are completely opposed to them. They consider them to be bribes. To my way of thinking, a bribe is when something like candy is given to a child for not doing something bad. This type of misbehavior could be dealt with by isolation or some other form of punishment. When I suggest material reinforcers, they are as incentives rather than bribes. As incentives, they are used for increasing the frequency of more responsible behavior. Incentives may be helpful in overcoming inertia when children need to engage in an unpleasant behavior, such as eating less for weight loss. They may be useful in overcoming resistance when children are entrenched in power struggles around no-win behaviors (e.g., soiling). (See INCENTIVES FOR

MOTIVATING CHILDREN, page 293.) These reinforcers should be used for only one problem behavior at a time and when praise alone hasn't worked. They should be phased out and replaced by natural (social) reinforcers as soon as possible.

Call Your Child's Physician During Office Hours If

- The misbehavior is dangerous.
- The instances of misbehavior seem too numerous to count.
- Your child is also having behavior problems at school.
- Your child doesn't seem to have many good points.
- Your child seems depressed.
- The parents can't agree on discipline.
- You can't give up physical punishment. (Note: Call immediately if you are afraid you might hurt your child.)
- The misbehavior does not improve in one month using this approach.

PHYSICAL PUNISHMENT AND SPANKING

The American Academy of Pediatrics, the National Education Association, and many other national organizations are strongly opposed to spanking. All children need discipline on occasion, but there are alternatives to spanking. Redirecting (distracting) the child, taking away a privilege, or sending a child to his or her room are some of the other ways to discipline. We can raise children to be agreeable, responsible, productive adults without ever spanking them.

There are several good arguments for not spanking. Spanking carries the risk of triggering an angry chain reaction that sometimes ends in child abuse. Also, spanking makes aggressive behavior worse because it teaches a child to lash out when he or she is angry. Other forms of discipline can be more constructive, leaving a child with some sense of guilt and helping her to form a conscience. Finally, parents who turn to spanking in order to "break the child's will" usually find that they have underestimated their child's will.

Also consider the legal argument. If physical punishment were directed against another adult, it would be called assault and battery, and that's illegal. Also consider the following facts from societies more protective of children than our own: Physical punishment was first banned by law in Sweden, Norway, Finland, and Denmark over 20 years ago. Currently all European countries (except England), Israel, Japan, and many others prohibit physical punishment of children by law. Physical punishment by school staff is illegal in all countries except the United States and South Africa. On the brighter side, it is currently prohibited by state boards of education in 37 out of 50 states.

Safe Physical Punishment

We would prefer that you not use spanking to discipline your child. At this time, less than 50 percent of American parents still use some physical punishment in child-rearing. It's gradually becoming socially unacceptable. So if you have not changed your mind after reading these facts, please follow guidelines for safe physical punishment:

- Always use other techniques (such as time-out) first. Only use spanking for behaviors that are dangerous or deliberately defiant of your instructions.
- Hit only with an open hand. It is difficult to judge how hard you are hitting your child if you hit him or her with an object other than your hand. Paddles and belts may cause bruises. Spanking should never leave more than temporary redness of the skin.
- Hit only on the buttocks, legs, or hands. Hitting a child on the face is demeaning as well as dangerous. In fact, slapping the face is inappropriate at any age. Your child could suddenly turn his head and the slap could damage his vision or hearing.
- Give only one swat. That's enough to change behavior. Spanking your child more than once may relieve your anger but will probably not teach your child anything else.
- Don't spank children less than 18 months old. Spanking is absolutely inappropriate before your child has learned to walk. Spanking should be unnecessary after the age of 6 years. After that you should be able to discuss problems with your child.
- Because of the serious risk of causing bleeding in the brain, never shake a young child.
- Use spanking no more than once a day. The more your child is spanked, the less effect it will have.
- Learn alternatives to spanking. Isolating a child in a corner or bedroom for a time-out is much more civilized and effective. Learn how to use

other forms of discipline. Spanking should never be the main form of discipline a child receives.

- Never spank your child when you are out of control, scared, or drinking. A few parents can't stop hitting their child once they start. They can't control their rage and things always escalate. They must learn to walk away from their children and never use physical punishment. They should seek help for themselves from Parents Anonymous or other self-help groups.
- Do not spank your child for aggressive misbehavior, such as biting, hitting, or kicking. This teaches a child that it is all right for a bigger person to hit a smaller person. Aggressive children need to be taught restraint and self-control. They respond best to time-outs, which give them an opportunity to think about the pain they have caused. If you are not using time-outs, read more on how to make them work for you.
- Do not allow baby-sitters, child-care staff, and teachers to spank your children.

TIME-OUT TECHNIQUE FOR DISCIPLINE

Time-out consists of immediately isolating a child in a boring place for a few minutes whenever she or he misbehaves. Time-out is also called quiet time, thinking time, or cooling-off time. Time-out has the advantage of providing a cooling-off period to allow both child and parent to calm down and regain control of their emotions.

Used repeatedly and correctly, the time-out technique can change almost any childhood behavior. Time-out is the most effective consequence for toddlers and preschoolers who misbehave—much better than threatening, shouting, or spanking. Every parent needs to know how to give time-out.

Time-out is most useful for aggressive, harmful, or disruptive behavior that cannot be ignored. Time-out is unnecessary for most temper tantrums. Time-out is not needed until a child is at least 8 months old and beginning to crawl. Time-out is rarely needed for children younger than 18 months because they usually respond to verbal disapproval. The peak age for using time-out is 2 to 4 years. During these years children respond to action much better than to words.

Choosing a Place for Time-out

Time-out Chair—When a chair is designated for time-out, it gives time-out a destination. The chair should be in a boring location, facing a blank wall or a corner. Don't allow your child to take anything with him to time-out, such as a toy, pacifier, security blanket, or pet. The child shouldn't be able to see TV or other people from the location. A good chair is a heavy one with side arms. Placed in a corner, such a chair surrounds the child with boundaries, leaves a small space for the legs, and reduces thoughts of escape. Alternatives to chairs are standing in a particular corner, sitting on a particular spot on the floor, or being in a playpen (if the child is not old enough to climb out of it).

Usually the chair is placed in an adjacent hallway or room. Some children less than 2 years old have separation fears and need the time-out chair (or playpen) to be in the same room as the parent. When you are in the same room as your child, carefully avoid making eye contact with the child.

Time-out Room—Children who refuse to stay in a time-out chair need to be sent to a time-out room. Confinement to a room is easier to enforce. The room should be one that is safe for the child and contains no valuables. The child's bedroom is often the most convenient and safe place for time-out. Although toys are available in the bedroom, the child does not initially play with them because she is upset about being excluded from mainstream activities. Forbid turning on the radio, stereo, or video games during time-out in the bedroom. Avoid any room that is dark or scary (such as some basements), contains hot water (bathrooms), or has filing cabinets or bookshelves that could be pulled down on the child.

Time-out Away from Home—Time-out can be effectively used in any setting. In a supermarket, younger children can be put back in the grocery cart and older children may need to stand in a corner. In shopping malls, children can take their time-out sitting on a bench or in a restroom. Sometimes a child needs to be taken to the car and made to sit on the floor of the backseat for the required minutes. If the child is outdoors and misbehaves, you can ask him to stand facing a tree.

How to Administer Time-out

Deciding the Length of Time-out—Time-out should be short enough to allow your child to have many chances to go back to the original situation and learn the acceptable behavior. A good rule of thumb is 1 minute per year of age (with a maximum of 10 minutes). After age 6, most children can be told they are in time-out "until you can behave," allowing them to choose how long they stay there. If the problem behavior recurs, the next time-out should last the recommended time for their age.

Setting a portable kitchen timer for the required number of minutes is helpful. The best type ticks continuously and rings when the time is up. A timer can stop a child from asking the parents when he can come out.

Sending Your Child to Time-out—Older children will usually go to time-out on their own. Younger children often need to be led there by the wrist, or in some cases carried there protesting. If your child doesn't go to time-out within 5 seconds, take her there. Tell your child what she did wrong in once sentence (such as "No hitting"). If possible, also clarify the preferred behavior (such as "Be kind to George"). These brief comments give your child something to think about during the time-out.

Requiring Quiet Behavior in Time-out—The minimum requirement for time-out completion is that your child does not leave the chair or time-out place until the time-out is over. If your child leaves ahead of time, reset the timer.

Some parents do not consider a time-out to be completed until the child has been quiet for the entire time. However, until 4 years of age, many children are unwilling or unable to stay quiet. Ignore tantrums in time-out, just as you should ignore tantrums outside of time-out. After age 4, quiet time is preferred but not required. You can tell your child, "Time-out is supposed to be for thinking, and to think you've got to be quiet. If you yell or fuss, the time will start over."

Dealing with Room Damage—If your child makes a mess in his room (for example, empties clothing out of drawers or takes the bed apart), he must clean it up before he is released from time-out. Toys that were misused can be packed away. Some damage can be prevented by removing any scissors or crayons from the room before the time-out begins.

Releasing Your Child from Time-out—To be released, your child must have performed a successful time-out. This means she stayed in time-out for the required number of minutes. Your child can leave time-out when the timer rings. If you don't have a timer, she can leave when you tell her, "Time-out is over. You can get up now." Many parents of children over 4 years old require their children to be quiet at the end of time-out. If a child is still noisy when the timer rings, it can be reset for 1 minute.

Keeping Your Child in Time-out

The Younger Child Who Refuses to Stay in Time-out—In general, if a child escapes from time-out (gets up from the chair or spot), you should quickly take the child back to time-out and reset the timer. This approach works for most children. If a child refuses to stay in time-out, the parent should take action rather than arguing with or scolding the child. You may temporarily need to hold a strong-willed, 2- or 3-year-old child in time-out. Holding your child in time-out teaches your child that you mean what you say and that he must obey you. Place your child in the time-out chair and hold him by the shoulders from behind. Tell your child that you will stop holding him when he stops trying to escape. Then avoid eye contact and any more talking. Pretend that you don't mind doing this and are thinking of something else or listening to music. Your child will probably stop trying to escape after a week of this approach.

A last resort for young children who continue to resist sitting in a chair is putting them in the bedroom with a gate blocking the door. Occasionally a parent with carpentry skills can install a half-door. If you cannot devise a barricade, then you can close the door. You can hold the door closed for the 3 to 5 minutes it takes to complete the time-out period. If you don't want to hold the door, you can put a latch on the door that allows it to be temporarily locked. Most children need their door closed only two or three times.

The Older Child Who Refuses to Stay in Time-out—An older child can be defined in this context as one who is too strong for the parent to hold in a time-out chair. In general, any child older than 5 years who does not take time-out quickly should be considered a refuser. In such cases the discipline should escalate to a consequence that matters to the child. First, you can make the time-out longer, adding one extra minute for each minute of delay. Second, if 5 minutes pass without your child going to time-out, your child can be grounded. "Grounded" is defined as no TV, radio, stereo, video games, toys, telephone access, outside play, snacks, or visits with friends. After grounding your child, walk away and no longer talk to her. Your child becomes "ungrounded" only after she takes her regular time-out plus the 5 minutes of penalty time. Until then, her day is very boring. If your child refuses the conditions of grounding, she can be sent to bed 15 minutes earlier for each time she breaks the grounding requirements. The child whose behavior doesn't improve with this approach usually needs to be evaluated by a mental health professional.

Practicing Time-out with Your Child

If you have not used time-out before, go over it with your child before you start using it. Tell your child it will replace spanking, yelling, and other forms of discipline. Review the kinds of negative behavior that will lead to placement in time-out. Also review the positive behavior that you would prefer. Then pretend with your child that he has broken one of the rules. Take him through the steps of time-out so he will understand your directions when you send him to time-out in the future. Also teach this technique to your baby-sitter.

TIME-OUT: WHEN IT DOESN'T SEEM TO BE WORKING

Some parents become discouraged with time-out because their child repeats misbehavior immediately after release from time-out. Other children seem to improve temporarily but by the next day are repeating the behavior the parent is trying to stop. Some children refuse to go to time-out or won't stay there. None of these examples means that time-out should be abandoned. It remains the best discipline technique for 2- to 5-year-old children. If you use time-out repeatedly, consistently, and correctly, your child will eventually improve. The following recommendations may help you fine-tune how you are using time-out.

Helping Time-out Succeed

Give Your Child More Physical Affection—Be sure your child receives two time-ins for every time-out each day. A time-in is a positive, close, brief human interaction. Try to restore the positive side of your relationship with your child. Catch him being good. Try to hold your child for 1 or 2 minutes every 15 minutes when he's not in time-out or misbehaving. Play with your child more. Children who feel neglected or overly criticized don't want to please their parents.

Use Time-out Consistently—Employ time out every time your child engages in the behavior you are trying to change (target behavior). For the first 2 or 3 days you may need to use time-outs 20 or more times a day to gain a defiant toddler's attention. Brief time-outs are harmless and there is no upper limit on how many times you can use them as long as you offset them with positive interactions.

Don't Just Threaten—For aggressive behaviors, give no warnings; just put your child in time-out. Better yet, intercept your child when you see her starting to raise her arm or clench her fist and before she makes others cry. For other behaviors, remind your child of the rule, count to three, and if she doesn't stop immediately, put her in time-out.

Use It Early—Put your child in time-out before his behavior worsens. Your child is more likely to accept a time-out calmly if he's put in early rather than if he's put in late (and screaming). Also, putting him in early means you will be more in control of your emotions. Try to put your child in time-out before you become angry. If you are still yelling when you put your child in time-out, it will not work.

Use It Quickly—Don't talk about it first. When your child breaks a rule, have her in time-out within 10 seconds.

No Talking—Don't talk to your child during time-out. Don't answer his questions or complaints. Don't try to lecture your child.

Ignore Tantrums—Don't insist on quietness during time-out because it makes it harder to finish the time-out.

Handling Escapes—Return your child to time-out if he escapes. Have a backup plan for further discipline—for example, holding a young child in the time-out chair or grounding an older child.

Consider Increasing the Length—If your child is over 3 years old and needs to be placed in time-out more than 10 times each day, a longer time-out may be needed to get her attention. A preschooler with a strong-willed temperament may temporarily need a time-out that lasts 2 or 3 minutes per year of her age. Children younger than 3 years should receive only brief time-outs (1 minute per year of age) because it is difficult for them to stay in time-out any longer.

Make It Boring—If your child doesn't seem to mind the time-outs, eliminate sources of entertainment. Move the time-out chair to a more boring location. If you use your child's bedroom, close the blinds or shades. Make sure that siblings or pets aren't visiting. Temporarily remove all toys and games from the bedroom and store them elsewhere.

Time It—Use a portable timer for keeping track of the time. Your child is more likely to obey a timer than to obey you.

Be Kind—Try to be kinder in your delivery of time-out. This will help reduce your child's anger. Say you're sorry he needs a time-out, but be firm about it. Try to handle your child gently when you take him to time-out.

Praise—Praise your child for taking a good time-out. Forgive your child completely when you release her from time-out. Don't give lectures or ask for an apology. Give your child a clean slate and don't tell her other parent or relatives how many time-outs she needed that day.

Allow Normal Anger—Don't punish your child for the normal expression of anger, such as saying angry things or looking angry. Don't try to control your child too much.

Provide Choices—Give your child choices about how he takes his time-out. Ask, "Do you want to take a time-out by yourself or do you want me to hold you in your chair? It doesn't matter to me." For older children, the choice can be, "Do you want to do it by yourself or do you want to be grounded?"

Coming Out Early—Give your child the option of coming out of time-out as soon as she is under control rather than taking the specified number of minutes.

Use a Variety of Consequences—Ignore harmless behaviors. Also, use distraction for bad habits. Use logical consequences—such as removal of toys, other possessions, or privileges—for some misbehavior.

Clarify—Make sure your child knows what you want him to do. Also clarify the house rules. Review this at a time when your child is in a good mood. This will help him be more successful.

Use Time-out with Siblings When Appropriate—Be sure that one sibling isn't being treated preferentially. If siblings touch the timer or tease the child in time-out, they should also be placed in time-out.

Time-out by Others—Teach all caretakers to use time-out correctly and consistently.

Call Your Child's Physician During Office Hours If

- Your child hurts himself during time-out.
- Your child runs out of the house to avoid time-out.

- Your child needs to be kept in her room with the gate up for time-outs for more than 1 week.
- Your child refuses to take time-outs despite being grounded for 3 days.
- Your child refuses to cooperate with time-outs after using this approach for 1 month.
- Your child has many other behavioral problems.

SPOILED CHILDREN, PREVENTION OF

Definition

A spoiled child is undisciplined, manipulative, and unpleasant to be with. He has many of the following behaviors:

- Doesn't follow rules or cooperate with suggestions
- Doesn't respond to "no," "stop," or other commands
- Protests everything
- Doesn't know the difference between his needs and his wants
- Insists on having his own way
- Makes unfair or excessive demands on others
- Doesn't respect other people's rights
- Tries to control other people
- Has a low frustration tolerance
- Frequently whines or throws tantrums
- Constantly complains about being bored

Causes—The main cause of spoiled children is a lenient, permissive parent who doesn't set limits and gives in to tantrums and whining. If the parent gives the child too much power, he will become more self-centered. Such parents also rescue the child from normal frustrations. Occasionally the child of working parents is left with a nanny or baby-sitter who spoils the child by providing constant entertainment and giving in to unrealistic demands.

The reason some parents are overly lenient is that they confuse the child's needs (e.g., for demand feeding) with the child's wants or whims (e.g., for demand play). They do not want to hurt their child's feelings or to cause any crying. In the process, they may take the short-term solution of doing whatever prevents crying, which, in the long run, causes more crying. The child's ability to cry and fuss deliberately to get something usually doesn't begin before five or six months of age. There may be a small epidemic of spoiling in our country because some working parents come home feeling guilty about not having enough total time for their children and so spend their free time together trying to avoid any friction or limit-setting.

Confusion exists about the differences between giving attention to children and spoiling children. In general, attention is good for children. Attention can become harmful if it is excessive, given at the wrong time, or always given immediately. Attention from you is excessive if it interferes with your child's learning to play by himself or with other children. An example of giving attention at the wrong time is when you are busy and your child is demanding attention. Another wrong time is when a child has just misbehaved and needs to be ignored. If attention is always given immediately, your child won't learn to wait.

Holding is a form of attention that some parents unnecessarily worry about. Holding babies is equivalent to loving them. Most cultures hold their babies much more than we do. Lots of holding by the mother and father does not cause a spoiled infant or child.

Expected Outcome—Without intervention, spoiled children run into trouble by school age. Other children do not like them because they are too bossy and selfish. Adults do not like them because they are rude and make excessive demands on them. Eventually they become hard for even the parent to love because of their behaviors. As a reaction to not getting along well with other children and adults, spoiled children eventually become unhappy. Spoiled children may show reduced motivation and reduced perseverance in schoolwork. There is also an association with risk-taking behaviors, such as drug abuse. Overall, spoiling a child prepares him poorly for life in the real world.

How to Avoid Spoiling a Child

Provide Age-Appropriate Limits or Rules—Parents have the right and the responsibility to take charge and make rules. Adults must keep their child's environment safe. Age-appropriate discipline must begin by the age of crawling. Saying "no" occasionally is good for children. Children need external controls until they develop self-control and self-discipline. Your child will still love you after you say "no" to him.

Require Cooperation with Important Rules—It is important that your child be in the habit of responding properly to your demands long before he enters school. Important rules include staying in the car seat, not hitting other children, being ready to leave on time in the morning, going to bed, and so forth. These adult decisions are not open to negotiation. Do not give your child a choice when there is none.

Child decisions, however, involve such things as which cereal to eat, book to read, toys to take into the tub, clothes to wear, etc. Make sure your child understands the difference between areas in which he has choices (options) and your rules (commands). Try to keep your important rules to no more than 10 or 20 items, and be willing to go to the mat about these. Also, be sure that all adult caretakers consistently enforce these rules.

Expect Crying—Distinguish between crying for needs and crying for wants. Needs include pain, hunger, or fear. In these cases, respond immediately. Other crying usually relates to your child's wants or whims. Crying is a normal response to change or frustration. When the crying is part of a tantrum, ignore it. There are times when it is necessary to withhold overt affection temporarily to help your child learn something important. Don't punish him for crying, tell him he's a crybaby, or tell him he shouldn't cry. While not denying him his feelings, don't be moved by his crying. To compensate for the extra crying your child does during a time when you are tightening up on the rules, provide extra cuddling (time-ins) and enjoyable activities when he is not crying or having a tantrum.

Do Not Allow Tantrums to Work—Children throw temper tantrums to get your attention, to wear you down, to change your mind, and to get their way. The crying is to change your no vote to a yes vote. Tantrums may include whining, complaining, crying, breath-holding, pounding the floor, shouting, or slamming a door. As long as your child stays in one place and is not too disruptive, you can leave him alone at these times. By all means don't give in to tantrums.

Include Discipline During Quality Time—If you are working parents, you will want to spend part of each evening with your child. This special time needs to be enjoyable but also reality-based. Don't ease up on the rules. If your child misbehaves, remind him of the existing limits. Even during fun activities, you occasionally need to be the parent.

Don't Try to Negotiate with Young Children—Don't give away your power as a parent. At age 2 and 3, be careful not to talk too much with your toddler about the rules. Toddlers don't play by the rules. A young child mainly understands actions, not words. By age 4 or 5, you can begin to reason with your child about discipline issues, but he still lacks the judgment necessary to make the rules. By ages 14 to 16, an adolescent can be negotiated with as an adult. At that time you can ask for his input about what rules or consequences would be fair.

The more democratic the parents are during the early years, the more demanding the children tend to become. Generally, young children do not know what to do with power. Left to their own devices, they usually spoil themselves. If you have given away your power, take it back. You don't have to explain the reason for every rule. Sometimes it is just because "I said so."

Teach Your Child to Get Himself Unbored—Your job is to provide toys, books, and art supplies. Your child's job is to play with them. Assuming you talk and play with your child several hours a day, you do not need to become his constant playmate. Nor do you need to provide him with an outside friend constantly. When you're busy, expect your child to amuse himself. Even 1-year-olds can keep themselves occupied for 15-minute blocks of time. By 3 years, most children can entertain themselves half the time. Sending your child outside to "find something to do" is doing him a favor. Much good creative play, thinking, and daydreaming come out of solving boredom. If you can't seem to resign as social director, enroll your child in a playschool or preschool.

Teach Your Child to Wait—Waiting helps children deal better with frustration. All jobs in the adult world carry some degree of frustration. Delaying immediate gratification is a trait your child must gradually learn, and it takes practice. Don't feel guilty if you have to make your child wait a few minutes now and then (e.g., don't allow your child to interrupt your conversations with others in person or on the telephone). Waiting doesn't hurt him as long as he doesn't become overwhelmed or unglued by waiting. His perseverance and emotional fitness will be enhanced.

Don't Rescue Your Child from Normal Life Challenges—Changes such as moving and starting school are normal life stressors. These are opportunities for learning and problem-solving. Always be available and supportive, but don't help your child if he can handle it himself. Overall, make your child's life as realistic as he can tolerate for his age, rather than going out of your way to make it as pleasant as possible. His coping skills and self-confidence will benefit from this practice.

Don't Overpraise—Children need praise, but it can be overdone. Praise your child for good behavior and following the rules. Encourage him to try new things and work on difficult tasks. But teach him to do things for his own reasons, too. Self-confidence and a sense of accomplishment come from doing and completing things he is proud of. Praising your child while he is in the process of doing something may make him stop at each step and want more praise. Giving your child constant attention can make him "praise-dependent" and demanding. Avoid the tendency (so common with the firstborn) to overpraise your child's normal development.

Teach Your Child to Respect Parents' Rights—The needs of your children for love, food, clothing, safety, and security obviously come first. However, your needs should come next. Your children's wants (e.g., for play) and whims (e.g., for an extra bedtime story) should come after your needs are met and as time is available on that day. This is especially important for working parents where family time is limited. It is both the quality and quantity of time that you spend with your children that is important. Quality time is time that is enjoyable, interactive, and focused on your child. Children need some quality time with their parents every day. Spending every free moment of every evening and weekend with your child is not good for your child or your marriage. You need a balance to preserve your mental health. Scheduled nights out with your mate will not only nurture your marriage but also help you to return to parenting with more to give. Your child needs to learn to trust other adults and that he can survive separations from you. If your child isn't taught to respect your rights, he may not respect the rights of other adults.

THE TERRIBLE TWOS AND STUBBORN TODDLERS

From 18 months to 3 years of age many children are in the "Terrible Twos." Stubbornness, opposition, or outright defiance may principally characterize their behavior. They normally are noisy (not quiet), busy (not still), distractible (not focused), impulsive (not cautious), and negative (not cooperative). No matter how calm and gentle a parent you are, your child will throw some temper tantrums. Your child will say no to many of your reasonable requests. You may feel helpless and at your child's mercy. Not until adolescence will you again be put through such an ordeal.

The Terrible Twos are a normal phase in child development. Your child is not deliberately trying to irritate you. Negativism is a normal step in becoming independent. Temper tantrums are a normal step in becoming more verbal. The children who have the most severe form of the Terrible Twos usually are "difficult" children by temperament. From birth they stand out as infants who resist anything new, react intensely, and are unpredictable in their behavior. Occasionally a parent makes the Terrible Twos worse by being excessively strict or having unreasonable expectations. Fortunately all children pass through this phase into a more cooperative one.

Dealing with Stubborn Toddlers

Negativism is a normal phase seen in most children between 18 months and 3 years of age. It begins when children discover they have the power to refuse other people's requests. Once the Terrible Twos are in full swing, children become more stubborn and less cooperative. They respond negatively to many requests (including pleasant ones). They delight in refusing a suggestion, be it to get dressed or take off their clothes, take a bath or get out of the bathtub, go to bed or get up. Unless understood, this behavior can become extremely frustrating for parents. Handled appropriately, it lasts about a year. As a bonus, the better you handle this phase, the fewer temper tantrums your child will have. Consider the following guidelines for helping your child through this phase.

Don't Take This Normal Phase Too Personally—To your child, "No" means "Do I have to?" or "Do you mean it?" A negative response should not be confused with disrespect. Also, it is not meant to annoy you. This phase is critical to the development of independence and identity. Try to look at it with a sense of humor and amazement.

Don't Punish for Saying "No"—Punishment should be for what your child does, not what he or she says. Since saying "no" is not something you can control, ignore it. If you argue with your child about saying "no," you will probably prolong this behavior.

Give Your Child Plenty of Choices—This is the best way to increase your child's sense of freedom and control, so that he or she will become more cooperative. Examples of choices are letting your child choose between a shower or a bath, choose which book is read, which toys go in the tub, which fruit is eaten for a snack, which clothes or shoes will be worn, which breakfast cereal is eaten, which game is played, whether inside or outside, in the park or in the yard, and so forth. Even for a task your child doesn't like, he can be given a say in the matter by asking him, "Do you want to do it slow or fast?" or "Do you want me to do it, or you?" The more quickly your child gains a feeling that he is a decision-maker, the sooner he will become cooperative.

Don't Provide a Choice When There Is None—Safety rules are not open to discussion. Taking a bath, going to bed, or going to day care also are not things that can be negotiated. Don't ask a question when there's only one answer. When a request such as this must be made, it can be presented in as kind a way as possible (e.g., "I'm sorry, but now you have to put away your airplanes and go to bed."). Directives ("Do this or else") should be avoided.

Give Transition Time When Changing Activities—If your child is having fun and must change to another activity, he or she probably needs a transition time. For example, when playing with trucks as dinnertime approaches, your child needs a 5-minute warning. A kitchen timer sometimes helps a child accept the change better. Set the timer and say, "In five minutes, it will be time to stop playing and come to eat dinner."

Eliminate Excessive Rules—The more rules you have, the less likely it is that your child will be agreeable about them. Eliminate unnecessary expectations and arguing about wearing socks, cleaning her plate, or sleeping in bed. Help your child feel less controlled by making your positive contacts greater than your negative contacts each day.

Try to Respond Positively to Your Child's Requests—Avoid excessive nos. Be a model of agreeableness. When your child requests something and you're unsure, try to say yes, or postpone your decision by saying, "Let me think about it." If you're going to grant a request, do it right away, before your child whines or begs for it. When you must say no, say you're sorry and give your child a reason.

TEMPER TANTRUMS

Temper tantrums are immature ways of expressing anger. There are several types of temper tantrums. Some are to get something, others are to avoid doing something. Try to teach your child that temper tantrums don't work, that you don't change your mind or give in because of them. By 3 years of age, you can begin to teach your child to verbalize his feelings ("You feel angry because ———"). We need to teach children that anger is normal but that it must be channeled appropriately. By school age, temper tantrums should be rare. During adolescence, tantrums reappear, but your teenager can be reminded that blowing up creates a bad impression. Teach your teenager how to keep temper tantrums in check by counting to 10 and pausing long enough to regain control.

Temper Tantrums of Younger Children

Overall, praise your child when he controls his temper, verbally expresses his anger, and is cooperative. Be a good model by staying calm and not screaming or having adult tantrums. Avoid spanking for tantrums because it conveys to your child that you are out of control. Try using the following responses to the different types of temper tantrums.

Support and Help Children Having Frustration- or Fatigue-Related Tantrums—Children normally have temper tantrums when they are frustrated with themselves. They may be frustrated because they can't put something back together. Young children may be frustrated because their parents cannot understand their speech. Older children may be frustrated with their inability to do their homework.

At these times your child needs encouragement and a parent who listens. Put an arm around him and say something brief that shows understanding, such as "I know it's hard, but you'll get better at it. Is there something I can do to help you?" Also give praise for not giving up. Some of these tantrums can be prevented by steering your child away from tasks he can't do well.

Temper tantrums also normally increase when children are tired (for instance when they've missed a nap) or exhausted (as during a party), because they are less able to cope with frustrating situations. At these times put your child to bed. Hunger can also contribute to temper tantrums. If you suspect this, give your child a snack. Temper tantrums also increase during sickness. Mood is clearly affected by a child's physical state.

Ignore Attention-Seeking or Demanding-Type Tantrums—Young children commonly throw temper tantrums to get their way. They may want something to eat right before dinner, want to go with you rather than be left with the baby-sitter, want candy, want to empty a desk drawer, or want to go outside in bad weather. They don't accept rules for their safety.

As long as your child stays in one place during the tantrum and is not too disruptive, you can leave him alone. Harmless behavior can be ignored.

If you recognize that a certain event is going to push your child over the edge, try to shift his attention to something else. However, don't give in to your child's demands. During the temper tantrum, ignore it completely. Once a tantrum has started, it rarely can be stopped.

Move away, even to a different room; you are thereby removing the child's audience. Don't talk to or try to reason with your child; it will only make the tantrum worse. Simply state, "I can see you're very angry. I'll leave you alone until you cool off. Let me know if you want to talk." Don't hold your child during the temper tantrum. And by all means, don't give in to your child's demands. Let your child regain control. After the tantrum, be friendly and try to return things to normal. You can prevent some of these tantrums by saying "no" less often.

The following types of temper tantrum can be ignored:

- Crying and screaming to get attention.
- Whining to get attention (see WHINING, page 337).
- Minor displays of anger such as slamming a door, sticking out the tongue, or making a face. These harmless releases of anger when your child is overruled should be permitted.
- Temper tantrum with pounding and kicking the floor, wall, or door. The only limitation is if your child is damaging property.
- A temper tantrum with head banging. You can assume your child won't hurt herself, since children don't like pain. If she has such a complete loss of control that she throws herself backward and has caused a bump on the back of her head, as a last resort you can throw a glass of water on her when she starts to have a temper tantrum, and then leave the room. Don't rush to her to try to prevent her falls, since this will lead to more frequent tantrums.
- Temper tantrums with breath-holding. While your child will turn blue and pass out for 30 to 60 seconds, he won't hurt himself (see BREATH-HOLDING SPELLS, page 370).

Physically Move Children Having Refusal-Type or Avoidance-Type Tantrums—If your child refuses something unimportant (such as a snack or lying down in bed), let it go before a tantrum begins. However, if your child must do something important, such as going to bed or to day care, he should not be able to avoid it by having a tantrum.

Some of these tantrums can be prevented by giving your child a 5-minute warning instead of asking him suddenly to stop what he is doing. Once a tantrum has begun, let your child have the tantrum for 2 or 3 minutes. Try to put his displeasure into words: "You want to play some more, but it's bedtime." Then take him to the intended destination (e.g., the bed), helping him as much as is needed (including carrying). And change the bedtime ritual to a brief, no-frills type.

Use Time-outs for Disruptive Tantrums—Some temper tantrums are too disruptive or aggressive for the parents to ignore. On such occasions, children need to be sent or taken to their rooms for 2 to 5 minutes (see TIME-OUT TECHNIQUE FOR DISCIPLINE, page 320). Examples are:

- Clinging to you or following you around during the tantrum. This type of interruption should not be tolerated.
- Hitting you during the temper tantrum. This is no longer a temper tantrum but has become aggressive behavior and should be treated as such.
- Throwing something or damaging property during a temper tantrum.
- Prolonged screaming or yelling that gets on your nerves. (See SCREAMING AND SHOUTING, page 338.)
- Having a temper tantrum in a public place such as a restaurant or church. Move your child to another place for his time-out. The rights of other people need to be protected.

Hold Children Having Harmful or Rage-Type Tantrums—If your child is totally out of control and screaming wildly, consider holding him. His loss of control probably scares him. Also hold your child when he is having tantrums that carry a danger of self-injury (such as if he is violently throwing himself backward).

Take your child in your arms, tell him you know he is angry, and offer him your sense of control. Hold him until you feel his body start to relax. This usually takes 1 to 3 minutes. Then let him go. This comforting response is rarely needed after 3 years of age, unless your child has a developmental disability.

Some children won't want you to comfort them. Hold your child only if it helps. If your child says "Go away," do so. After the tantrum subsides, your child will often want to be held briefly. This is a good way to get him back into family activities.

Call Your Child's Physician During Office Hours If

- Your child has hurt himself or others during tantrums.
- The tantrums occur 5 or more times per day.
- The tantrums also occur in school.
- Your child has several other behavior problems.
- One of the parents has tantrums or screaming bouts and can't give them up.
- This approach does not bring improvement within 2 weeks.
- You have other questions or concerns.

Verbal Temper Tantrums of Older Children

Verbal disagreement (normal arguing) is healthy; so is the expression of feelings. We want children to express their anger through talking. Some talking back to parents is also normal. When a school-age child challenges our decisions in a logical way, we need to listen. As long as your child is reasonable, he or she needs to be heard. However, if a rule is important to the parent (for instance, not paying to see the same movie twice), the parent can cut off the discussion in 3 to 5 minutes by saying something like: "I've heard your side of it, but the rule stands. Now let me get back to my work." Try to teach your child to argue without whining, screaming, exaggerating, being rude, or swearing.

Whining—The whining child keeps asking and pestering us to do something he's been told he can't do. He may want an extra snack or to go outside after dark. His requests are unremitting and irritating. There's nothing mysterious about what causes whining. Whining is a low-grade, minor-league type of temper tantrum. It's the opposite of a screaming tantrum. You must teach your child that whining never works. Dealing with whining now is important to prevent complaining behavior in adults. Here's how to eliminate whining:

- Tell your child what you expect: "I can't understand you when you're whining. Come back to me when you can talk in your normal voice."
- If whining continues, ignore your child completely. No eye contact and no conversation. Don't try to reason with your child. If necessary, go to a different room.
- If the whining is loud or nerve-wracking, tell your child to take a

3-minute time-out in the "whining chair." That should be somewhere boring and at the other end of the house.

- Give your child lots of positive attention when he's not whining.

Screaming and Shouting—Screaming is a super-duper temper tantrum, unleashed by a youngster with exceptional vocal cords and lungs. Screaming tends to recur because it usually works. It either gets the parent to hand over an unconditional surrender or it causes the parent to scream back. Try this instead:

- Clarify the house rule for your child: "We don't scream in this house. Either talk in a calm voice or go to your room."
- If the screaming continues, take your child to her bedroom for a brief time-out. Don't try to ignore this disruptive tantrum. Close the door to the "screaming room" to preserve your sanity.
- Every 4 or 5 minutes, open the door and tell your child, "I hope you feel good enough to come out now." Give her lots of chances to rejoin the family. But if she comes out screaming, return her.
- Be sure none of the adults who care for your child yells or screams. Kids are marvelous copycats.

Giving Excuses—Without being verbally abusive, your child may present outlandish comments in order to postpone his punishment. In young children less than 3 years of age, these stalling tactics can be ended by saying: "For the last time, go to your room." If they don't go, they can be taken there. Other children may try to put their parents on a guilt trip by saying: "Everyone else does it," "You never listen to me," or "You don't love me." Your response can be: "Of course I love you, but that has nothing to do with this," and then stick to your guns about the consequence.

Making Threats or Hurtful Comments—When young children are angry, they scream or throw a tantrum. As they become older, they say hurtful things, like "I hate you." When they're mad, they go right for the jugular. Such remarks are called "show-stoppers." How should you respond?

- Respect your child's need to express angry feelings. Don't take these exaggerated comments personally. You can reply: "Well, I love you anyway, but you still need to take that time-out." Don't allow her comment to change the rule.
- At a later time, discuss anger with your child. Explain how people who live together normally have both positive and negative feelings about

each other. You can add, "Sometimes I get angry with you, but I always care about you."

- If your youngster threatens to run away, you can calmly state, "That would make me very sad." Most children then drop the subject. An adolescent who threatens to run away needs to be taken more seriously.
- Do children try to play psychological games on us? What do you think?

Rudeness and Insults—Verbal abuse can be defined as making derogatory comments about the parent. These include calling the parent stupid, a liar, or a jerk. The parent should not tolerate such comments. If the young person is allowed to continue this type of behavior, he or she will have difficulty keeping friends or pleasing other adults. You can give an "I" message, such as "I feel very hurt when you say rude things like that," in a nonangry voice. You can then send your child to his or her room, or outside. It's very important that you not retaliate with a similar verbal attack. Try to present a model of objective, constructive disagreement. Don't forget to praise your child when she uses politeness and diplomacy in stating her case.

Swearing—Swearing has become commonplace in our society—largely due to TV and the movies, not to mention bumper stickers and T-shirts. Children today hear in grade school bad language that used to start in high school. But that doesn't mean you have to listen to it. Here are some suggestions:

- Have a rule that swearing is not allowed in the house. You can enforce that, but define in advance any words you allow (e.g., *damn*). And tell him not to swear around teachers or other adults. Enforcing this is more complicated, but back up the school. Then accept the fact that how your youngster talks with his friends in private is something you can't control.
- If your youngster swears around you or other adults, send him to his room for a time-out. If he does it repeatedly, ground him for a day. But don't wash his mouth out with soap; that's too barbaric and it doesn't work.
- When your child is angry at someone, suggest he tell you about it without swearing. If he can't, suggest he swear in his room or hit a pillow.
- Praise your child for not swearing when he gets mad.
- Clean up your act. You won't be able to get your youngster to give up any four-letter words that you continue to use. Have you tried *darn it* lately? How about *rats*?

BITING

Biting another child is one of the more unacceptable aggressive behaviors in our society. The parent of the child who has been bitten is usually very upset and worried about the risk of infection. If it happens in a child-care setting, the other parents may want the biter to be expelled. If it happens in another's home, the child is often told never to return. Adults tend to forget that some biting behavior in a group of toddlers is to be expected. Most children first learn to bite by doing it to their parents playfully. It is important to try to interrupt this primitive behavior at this early stage.

Causes—Biting is usually a chance discovery around 1 year of age, at a time when teething and mouthing are normal behaviors. It often continues because the parents initially think it is cute and the child considers it a type of game to get attention. Later, children may use it when they are frustrated and want something from another child. At this age, for children with minimal verbal skills, biting becomes a primitive form of communication. Only after age 2 or 3 can it become a deliberate way to express anger and intimidate others.

Recommendations

Establish a Rule—Give your child a reason for the rule "We never bite people"—that biting hurts. Other reasons (that won't interest him at his age) are that bites can lead to infection or scarring.

Suggest a Safe Alternative Behavior—Tell your child that if he wants something he should come to you and ask for help or point to it, rather than biting the person who has it. If he bites when he is angry, tell him "If you are mad, come to me and tell me." If your child is at the chewing-everything stage (usually less than 18 months), help him choose a toy he can bite rather than telling him he cannot bite anything. A firm toy or teething ring will do. Encourage him to carry his "chewy" with him for a few days.

Interrupt Biting with a Sharp "No"—Be sure to use an unfriendly voice, and look him straight in the eye. Try to interrupt him when he looks like he might bite somebody but before he actually does it, leaving the victim hurt and screaming. Extra-close supervision may be necessary until the biting has stopped.

Give Your Child a Time-out If He Bites Others—Send him to a boring place for approximately 1 minute per year of age. If he attempts to bite you while you are holding him, say "No," put him down immediately, and walk away (a form of time-out). If time-out does not work, take away a favorite toy for the remainder of the day.

Never Bite Your Child for Biting Someone Else—Biting back will make your child upset that you hurt him and may teach him that it is okay to bite if you are bigger. Also do not wash the mouth out with soap, pinch the cheek, or slap the mouth. In fact, if your child tends to be aggressive, avoid physical punishment in general (e.g., spanking). Also eliminate "love bites," since your child will be unable to distinguish them from painful biting.

Praise Your Child for Not Biting—The most important times to praise him are when he is in situations where or with particular children whom he used to bite frequently. Give him a kind reminder just prior to these high-risk visits. Then praise him afterward for good behavior.

Biting in Child-Care Settings—Biting behavior is common in child-care settings. The preceding approach should be used by day-care staff to eliminate the behavior in their setting. Provide careful supervision and quickly place the biting child in time-out, even when he acts like he might bite someone. In general, biting is harmless since most bites by younger children don't puncture the skin. Calling the parent at work is pointless since the problem should be dealt with immediately by whoever witnesses it.

Prevention—The best time to stop a biting behavior from becoming a habit is when it first starts. Be sure that no one laughs when he bites and that no one treats it like a game (this includes older siblings). Also never "give in" to your child's demands because of biting. Since biting not uncommonly occurs in child-care settings, be sure the providers understand your approach and are willing to apply it.

Call Your Child's Physician

Immediately If
- Biting causes a puncture or a cut that completely breaks the skin.

During Office Hours If
- Biting behavior lasts for more than 4 weeks with this approach.
- Your child bites or hurts himself.
- Your child has several other behavior problems.
- You have other questions or concerns.

HURTING ANOTHER CHILD

Some aggressive behaviors that children experiment with are hitting, slapping, pinching, scratching, poking, hair-pulling, biting, kicking, shoving, and knocking down. Since these behaviors are unacceptable in the adult world and potentially harmful, they should not be allowed between children.

Causes—Many children fight when they are angry. They do not like something another child did, and they retaliate. They want something another child has and see force as the easiest way to get it. Most children try aggressive behaviors because they see this behavior in playmates or on TV. If children get their way through hitting, it will only become more frequent. Occasionally children become excessively aggressive because they receive lots of spankings at home or witness spouse or sibling abuse.

Recommendations

Establish a Rule—Explain the rule to your child: "Do not hit, because it hurts. We do not hurt people."

Use Brief Time-outs—Being in a time-out helps a child learn to cool down (rather than blow up) when he is angry. When it looks as if your child might hurt someone, intervene immediately. Stop the behavior at the early threatening or shoving stage. Do not wait until the victim is hurt or screams. If a time-out does not seem to be effective, also take away your child's favorite toy or television time for the remainder of the day.

Suggest Acceptable Ways to Express Anger—In the long run you want your child to be able to verbalize his anger in a calm but assertive way. Encourage your child to come to you when he's angry and talk about it until he feels better. A second option is to teach your child to stop and count to 10 before doing anything about his anger. A third option is to help him learn to walk away from a bad situation. Giving your child a time-out is one way of teaching him to walk away from anger.

Younger children with limited expressive language (less than 3 or 4 years old) need time to develop these skills. When they are in a time-out, don't be surprised if they pout, mutter to themselves, yell in their room, or pound on their door. If these physical outlets for anger are blocked, a more aggressive outburst may occur. As long as the behavior is not destructive, ignore it. Teaching your child how to control anger provides him with a valuable resource.

Verbalize Your Child's Feelings for Him—If your child can't talk about his anger, put it into words for him: "I know that you feel angry." It is unrealistic to expect your child not to feel anger. You may need to make an understanding statement such as "You wish you could punch your brother, but we cannot hurt other people."

Teach Your Child Acceptable Ways to Get What He Wants—Teach him how to negotiate (ask for) what he wants, rather than taking it. Teach him how to take turns or how to trade one of his toys to gain use of another child's toy.

Give Special Attention to the Victim—After putting your child in a time-out, pick up the child who has been injured and give him extra sympathy and attention. It is especially helpful if you can rescue the victim before he is hurt. In your child's mind the attention he wanted is now being given to the other person, and that should give him some food for thought. If fighting is a pattern with certain playmates or siblings, be sure the "victim" isn't setting up the "perpetrator" to gain attention.

Never Hit Your Child for Hitting Someone Else—Hitting your child only teaches that it is fine to hit if you are bigger. If your child tends to be aggressive, it's critical to eliminate all physical punishment (such as spanking). You can use many other consequences (such as a time-out) to teach your child right from wrong.

Praise Your Child for Friendly Behavior—Praise him for being nice to people, playing with agemates in a friendly way, sharing things, and helping other children. Remind your child that people like to be treated kindly, not hurt. Some children respond to a system of receiving a treat or star chart for each day they go without any "hitting"-type behavior.

Prevention—Set a good example. Show self-control and verbal problem-solving. Avoid playmates who often tease or other situations where your child frequently gets into fights. And when your child becomes tired or hungry, leave the play setting until these needs are met.

Call Your Child's Physician During Office Hours If

- The aggressive behavior is very frequent.
- Your child has seriously hurt another child.
- Your child can't keep friends.
- Your child seems very angry.
- The misbehavior lasts more than 4 weeks with this approach.
- You have other questions or concerns.

SIBLING ARGUING AND QUARRELING

Most siblings argue and bicker occasionally. They fight over possessions, space on the sofa, time in the bathroom, the last doughnut, etc. Quarreling is an inevitable part of sibling relationships. On some days, brothers and sisters are rivals and competitors. But on most days, they are friends and companions. This ambivalence between love and hate is part of all close relationships, and it becomes more intense in siblings because both want to gain their parents' attention and be their parents' favorite. The positive side of this sibling rivalry is that it gives children a chance to learn to give and take, share, and stand up for their rights.

Recommendations

Encourage Children to Settle Their Own Disagreements—Have a rule: "Settle your own arguments, but no hitting, property damage, or name-calling." The more you intervene, the more you will be called upon to intervene. When possible, stay out of disagreements as long as they remain verbal. Children can't go through life having a referee to resolve their differences. They need to learn how to negotiate with people and find common ground. Arguing with siblings and peers provides this experience. The only exception is if they are both under age 2 or 3 and one of them is aggressive. At this age they do not understand the potential dangers of fighting and need to be supervised more closely.

Stay Out of the Middle—Try to keep your children from bringing their argument to you for an opinion. Remind them again to settle it themselves. If you do become involved, help them clarify what they are arguing about. To achieve this, try to teach them to listen better. Encourage each child to describe the problem for a minute or so without being interrupted by the other. If they still don't understand the issue, reframe it for them. Unless there's an obvious culprit, do not try to decide who is to blame, who started it, or who is right. Interrogation in this area can be counterproductive because it may cause them to exaggerate or lie. Also do not impose a solution. Since it's their problem, let them find their own solution whenever possible.

If an Argument Becomes Too Loud, Do Something About It—If the arguing becomes annoying or interferes with your ability to think, go to your children and tell them "I do not want to hear your arguing. Please settle your differences quietly or find another place to argue." If they do not change at that point, send them to the basement, outdoors, or to time-out in separate rooms. If they are arguing over an object such as the TV, take it away. If they are arguing over who gets to sit in the front seat of the car, have them both sit in the backseat. If they are arguing about going somewhere, cancel the trip for both.

Do Not Permit Hitting, Breaking Things, or Name-Calling—Under these circumstances, punish both of your children. If they are hurting each other, send them both to time-out in separate places no matter who you see doing the hitting when you come on the scene. That may not be the person who took the first swing or provoked it. Name-calling or teasing hurts people's feelings and should never be allowed (e.g., calling a child who is not good in school "dummy," one who is not athletic "clumsy," or one who has a bedwetting problem "smelly"). Derogatory comments such as these can be harmful to self-esteem and should not be permitted.

Stop Any Arguing That Occurs in Public Places—If you are in a shopping mall, restaurant, or movie theater and your children begin arguing, you need to stop them because it is annoying to other people. If the arguing continues after a warning, separate them (e.g., by sitting between them). If that doesn't work, give them a brief (2 to 5 minutes) time-out outside or at an out-of-the-way spot. If they are over age 4 or 5, you can sometimes tell them to stop or they'll get a 30-minute time-out (or a 30-minute loss of TV time) upon arrival at home. Sometimes you will have to leave the public setting and take them home.

Protect Each Child's Personal Possessions, Privacy, and Friendships—When children argue over toys, if the toy belongs to one of the children, return it to that child. Although children don't have to share their possessions, warn them that sharing works both ways. For family "toys" (such as video games or board games), teach taking turns. Also teach sharing toys when friends come over. Sharing is a skill they will need in order to have friends and to get along in school. Younger siblings often intrude on older siblings' friendships and play. It is helpful if the younger sibling is provided with a playmate or special activity when your older child has a friend over. Your child's study time also deserves protection from interruption. Designating a study room often helps.

Avoid Showing Favoritism—It is critical that all punishments for arguing or fighting be "group punishments." Parents must avoid the myth that fighting is always started by the brother rather than the sister, by the older child rather than the younger one, or by one child who is the "troublemaker." Rivalry will be intense if the parent shows favoritism. Try to treat your children as unique and special individuals. Do not take sides. Do not compare them, and do not polarize them into good ones and bad ones. Do not listen to tattling. And if one of your children complains about you not being fair, either ignore this comment or restate the rule that has been broken. If you're feeling guilty, remind yourself that "it all balances out."

Praise Cooperative Behavior—Catch your children "being good"— namely, playing together in a friendly way. Give "group praise" whenever possible. Compliment them for helping each other and settling disagreements politely.

Prevent Fighting or Name-Calling—First, help your children acknowledge their feelings. Let them know it is all right to be angry toward a sibling but that they should not vent their anger by fighting or name-calling. Give them useful alternatives to hurtful arguing, such as talking to you about it. Second, provide access to outside friends and different settings, rather than expecting your children to play constantly with each other. Third, avoid showing favoritism toward one child over another. Try to talk with each child every day and to schedule a special individualized activity once or twice a week. Most importantly, show your child how to settle disagreements peacefully and in a calm voice. Try not to act disrespectful, disagreeable, or ill-tempered to your children or to other people.

Call Your Child's Physician During Office Hours If

• Sibling interactions have not improved after using this approach for 6 weeks.
• Your children constantly fight with each other.
• Your children have several other behavior problems.
• One of your children constantly teases the other.
• One of your children has physically harmed the other.
• You have other questions or concerns.

DISCIPLINE PROBLEMS: OTHER STRATEGIES

These guidelines cover specific types of misbehavior and how to deal with them. Most of these discipline problems can occur in well-adjusted children with reasonable parents. Each type of misbehavior includes recommendations on how to phrase the rule, the preferred discipline technique, the adaptive behaviors that should be praised, and the parent behaviors that should be modeled to help your child behave better. Refer to DISCIPLINE BASICS (page 309) or TIME-OUT TECHNIQUE FOR DISCIPLINE (page 320) for details on how to implement the different types of consequences or praise recommended in this guideline. The categories of misbehavior are described in the following order: safety, aggression, siblings or peers, pets, destructive behavior toward property, public places, interrupting others, delaying or ignoring others, dressing, sleep, eating, washing and bathing, and miscellaneous. Specific recommendations for dealing with negativism and different types of temper tantrums are reviewed in THE TERRIBLE TWOS AND STUBBORN TODDLERS and TEMPER TANTRUMS (pages 331 and 333).

Safety Misbehavior

Runs Out of the House or Yard

Rule: "Don't go outside" or "Don't leave your yard."

Until age 3 or 4 most children can't be trusted to stay in their yards. They may wander off and may be harmed on a street, railroad track, pond, or swimming pool.

Discipline technique: Structure your child's environment so that you do not have to supervise him or her to prevent this misbehavior. Lock the outside doors to keep children inside. Leave them outside alone only if you have a safe, fenced-in yard.

Runs Away from the Parent When Walking

Rule: "Stay on the sidewalk or path when you're walking with me" and "Hold my hand when we cross the street."

Discipline technique: If your child starts to run off, catch him immediately. Make this a very serious matter and tell him sternly: "Never run off again." Don't let your child tease you about this or allow running off to become a game. Say firmly, "That's not funny."

If your child repeats running off, routinely hold his hand when you go walking.

If this is unsuccessful, take a children's harness with you when you go walking. The harness can be put on if your child breaks the rule and taken off after approximately 5 minutes. If your child breaks the rule a second time, the harness can be put on for 10 minutes. Using a harness occasionally is harmless.

Praise your child: For staying close to you.

Model: Cross streets carefully.

Plays with Electricity or Gas

Rule: "Never touch that, because you can get hurt."

Examples: Chewing on electrical cords, playing with electrical outlets, or turning the knobs on the stove.

Discipline technique: Give your child strong verbal disapproval. Don't let this behavior become something your child can tease you about. Also, put your child in time-out. Some of these hazards can be eliminated by using safety plugs or rerouting electrical cords. Since chewing on an electrical cord can cause severe burns to the mouth, you may wish to underscore your special concern about this behavior by slapping your child once on the hand.

Lights Matches

Rule: "Don't play with matches. They can start fires."

Discipline technique: Remove all matches from your child's reach. Consider teaching your child how to use matches properly after 8 years of age.

Model: The appropriate use of matches.

Climbs Trees or Fences

Rule: "Don't climb trees or fences, because you can fall and be seriously hurt."

You might specify that your child can climb certain trees after reaching an appropriate age, such as 6.

Discipline technique: Time-out. To help your child through this phase, consider designating a safe place to practice climbing, such as on an old sofa or a jungle gym at the playground.

Unfastens Seat Belts in the Car

Rule: "We don't drive unless everyone is buckled up."

Discipline technique: Immediate time-out. Don't start the car until all passengers have buckled their seat belts. As soon as anyone unbuckles, pull your car off the road into a boring place, such as a parking lot. Read a book until your child puts the seat belt on or asks for your help. Children usually want to go somewhere rather than sit in the car.

Praise your child: For keeping the seat belt buckled.

Model: Buckling yourself in.

Rides Bicycle Unsafely

Rule: "Obey the bicycle safety rules."

Discipline technique: Logical consequences: not being able to use the bike for 2 or 3 days.

Praise your child: For riding a bike safely.

Model: Appropriate use of your bicycle and wearing your bike helmet.

Aggression

Hurting Another Child (see page 342)

Two Children Physically Fight with Each Other

Definition: Two children are angry with each other and hitting, kicking, or shoving. This is not wrestling. In wrestling, children are not angry with each other but are practicing their physical skills. Wrestling is fine as long as it's done outside or in a recreation room and the opponents are reasonably well matched.

Rule: "Don't fight with each other, because disagreements can't be settled by hitting."

Discipline technique: Intervene at the early shoving stage and separate the children without interrogation. Send both to time-out in separate rooms or separate corners. Another option is to send one child home. Also see SIBLING ARGUING AND QUARRELING (page 344) for details.

Refuses to Fight

Definition: While you can have a rule against fighting in your home and yard, you can't control what goes on in the neighborhood or school. Some parents teach their children to fight (but fight fairly). Another option is to teach your child to say "I don't believe in fighting" and to walk away from aggressors. Although the chance of being seriously hurt in a fight is slim, it can happen. Sometimes it's better to be smart than to be brave. Most disagreements can be settled by words, and most bullies can be ignored. You don't have to teach your child to defend himself or herself physically.

Praise your child: For playing with other children in a friendly way and settling verbal disagreements themselves.

Model: Problem-solving without hitting or yelling. Spouse abuse condones physical fighting among children. Also avoid favoritism, which contributes to sibling fighting.

Spits

Rule: "Don't spit. It doesn't look nice."

Discipline technique: If your child spits on another person, use immediate time-out. If your child spits for attention-seeking purposes, restrict the places where it is permitted (such as in the toilet, sink, or outdoors). If your child spits anywhere else, place him or her in time-out.

Praise your child: For not spitting in situations where he or she previously spit.

Model: Nonspitting behavior in your own life. Take a position against chewing (smokeless) tobacco.

Yells, Threatens, Insults, or Swears (Verbal Aggression)—See THE TERRIBLE TWOS AND STUBBORN TODDLERS and TEMPER TANTRUMS, pages 331 and 333.

Misbehavior Toward Siblings or Peers

Fights Physically—See HURTING ANOTHER CHILD, page 342.

Hurts the Baby—See SIBLING RIVALRY TOWARD A NEWBORN, page 126.

Teases or Calls Names

Examples: Calling a child who is not good in school "dummy," one who is not athletic a "klutz," or one who has a bedwetting problem "smelly." These derogatory comments can be harmful to the self-esteem, especially if they are true.

Rule: "Teasing and name-calling are not allowed, because they are unfair and hurt someone's feelings."

Discipline technique: Immediate time-out.

Model: The parent should avoid teasing as well.

Tells on Another ("Tattletale")

Definition: Children report their siblings' or others' misbehavior to get them into trouble—a form of one-upmanship.

Rule: "Don't tell me about your brother's misbehavior unless it's dangerous. It hurts your friendship." This rule is based on the premise that bad news gets around, and if it's important, you'll hear about it.

Discipline technique: Give verbal disapproval: "I don't want to hear about it." You can also remind your child: "Tattletales don't have friends," and "Brothers are supposed to stand up for each other."

Praise your child: For looking after, standing up for, or telling you something good about the sibling or friend.

Model: Being supportive of others and avoiding gossip.

Takes Toys Away from Others

Rule: "Don't grab toys that other people are playing with."

Discipline technique: Use logical consequences and return the toy immediately to the child who owns it or had it. Never let the aggressive child keep a toy he or she has taken away. If the misbehavior recurs, use time-out.

Praise your child: For asking another child if he or she may use a toy, and also for returning a toy when requested.

Doesn't Share Toys

Premise: Children can't be expected to share toys until 3 or 4 years of age. Generosity has to be the child's decision. But you can plant the idea with statements such as "If you share with other children, they will usually share with you."

Discipline technique: A child should not be punished for not sharing his or her toys. Some problems can be prevented by allowing your child to take only one toy to the playground until she reaches an age where she can share. When she's not playing with her toy, pick it up so that other children won't take possession of it. For toys that belong to the family rather than an individual, temporarily put it away if two children can't take turns with it.

Praise your child: For any sharing. Encourage your child to share.

Model: Sharing in your home. Sharing your food, drink, and possessions with your child. Lending household objects to friends. Mention to your child that this is sharing.

Is a Poor Friend or Poor Sport

Examples: Some children are bossy and dominant with their friends, causing the friends to leave unhappily. Others show off so much that their friends find them boring. Others are poor sports or bad losers and try to change the rules of a game or sport.

Discipline technique: Natural consequences. Peer pressure will eventually shape your child's behavior into what is acceptable in the peer group. In the meantime your child will lose some friends until he or she has learned how to treat other children better. Occasionally ask your child: "What could you do to be a better friend?" Overall, let peers work out these disagreements themselves.

Praise your child: For being courteous, agreeable, and a good sport about losing.

Model: Stop being critical and bossy of your child if this applies. Don't argue with referees at your child's athletic events.

Misbehavior Toward Pets

Hurts Pets

Rule: "Don't hurt your pet, because animals feel pain and sadness just like people." Sometimes preschoolers are unduly rough with pets because they equate them with toys.

Discipline technique: Verbal disapproval followed by time-out.

Praise your child: For playing gently with a pet.

Model: Gentleness with animals.

Doesn't Feed the Pet

Rule: "Pets must be fed or they will starve."

Discipline technique: Give an "I" message, such as: "I really feel sorry for Charlie when you don't feed him." In addition, help your child come up with a reminder system, such as a small note on his mirror to help him remember to feed the pet. Sometimes delaying a privilege and linking it with the chore can be helpful (e.g., "No dinner for you until Charlie's been fed.").

Praise your child: For feeding the pet in a timely manner.

Model: Feeding your child in a timely manner.

Destructive Behavior Toward Property

Touches Things That Shouldn't Be Touched

Examples: Stereo, television, plants, breakables, or valuables.

Rule: "Don't touch the stereo, because it is only for grown-ups. Ask me for help if you want it turned on."

Discipline technique: Mainly restructure the environment. Put away valuable or dangerous objects, use gates, and lock doors to make certain areas off-limits. For objects that can't be removed, use clear verbal disapproval. If this fails, use temporary time-out.

Caution: Much of this exploratory behavior is normal and contributes to your child's development. In general, encourage this normal curiosity. Allow exploration of some closets or shelves. For example, give your child a drawer of his own in the kitchen where he can keep some utensils you no longer use. As he becomes older, teach your child to explore objects with his eyes rather than his hands.

Praise your child: For asking you to turn on the television or stereo.

Damages or Destroys Property Deliberately

Imitators: Some children take toys or other objects apart out of curiosity. Sometimes children break something accidentally. Since people are more important than property, these children need sympathy and help with their dilemma, not punishment.

Rule: "Don't break things, because they cost money and/or are hard to fix."

Discipline technique: Time-out. In addition, use logical consequences. If the object belongs to the child, don't replace it. If the object is yours and your child is over age 6, have him or her pay for part of it out of allowance money.

Praise your child: For taking good care of your possessions and his or her own.

Model: Show care in handling other people's belongings.

Jumps on Furniture

Rule: "Don't jump on the furniture or bed, because you might break it or get hurt."

Discipline technique: Redirect your child to some other play—if possible, one that involves jumping.

Praise your child: For playing in the bedroom without jumping on the bed.

Draws on the Walls

Rule: "Don't put any marks on the walls, because it's hard to get them clean."

Discipline technique: Logical consequences of having your child clean up the mess he or she has caused, as well as temporarily removing the privilege of using paints, crayons, or markers.

Praise your child: For drawing on paper.

Steals

Definition: Taking toys, food, or money from parents, friends, or a store.

Goal: Parents should try to teach ownership. Children are not developmentally able to learn the difference between what is "mine" and what is "yours" before age 4 or 5. Prior to that age they consider everything "mine" or that they have "borrowed it." Fortunately, they can't conceal stealing well before this age. Parents must also teach that it is wrong to borrow something without the owner's consent.

Rule: "Don't take things that don't belong to you, because they belong to somebody else, who will miss them and feel sad."

Discipline technique: Logical consequences.

- Don't accept fabrications of where your youngster found the new possession.

- Have your child take the stolen object back to the teacher, storekeeper, friend, or other rightful owner. The embarrassment of doing this with you present often prevents future stealing.

- If the object has been broken or the food has been consumed, help your child think of ways to earn money to pay the owner back.

- Be suspicious when your child suddenly "finds" a new possession. And it's good if you catch your child stealing at a young age. The sooner he learns that stealing doesn't work, the easier it will be for him to give it up.

- Give your child opportunities to earn money so he or she has less need to steal.

- Also try to teach that people can't have everything they want.

Praise your child: For honesty.

Model: Honesty.

Breaks or Throws Toys

Rule: "Don't break toys, because they cost money. Don't throw toys, because you might break something in the house."

Discipline technique: Logical consequences. If the toy is not broken, take it out of circulation for 2 days. The toy has to go back into circulation in order to teach proper behavior. If the toy is broken, delay the repair for at least 2 days. Teach that things can't be fixed until you have some free time. If the toy can't be repaired, either don't replace it or have your child use his or her own money to replace it.

Praise your child: For taking good care of possessions.

Misbehavior in Public Places

Touches Objects That Shouldn't Be Touched

Example: Grabs food off the shelves in a grocery store.

Rule: "Don't touch anything without my permission, because everything here belongs to the store and some things can break."

Discipline technique: Mainly, distract your child on arrival by getting her a snack, such as animal cookies. You can also keep her involved by giving her safe foods to carry or having her push the grocery cart. If she's sitting in the grocery cart seat, hand her foods to place in the basket. Also, talk with your child as you shop so that she feels involved. Finally, avoid taking your 2-year-old to a store with lots of breakables, such as a glass shop.

Praise your child: For helping.

Has a Temper Tantrum in a Public Place

Example: Often, children have temper tantrums when they beg for a toy or candy at the store and are not given it.

Rule: "We buy only food at the grocery store, not toys."

Discipline technique: Ignore your child and remain firm. If your child is having a temper tantrum in a safe place, walk on and he will stand up and follow you. If your child is near breakable objects or is a reckless child, take him outside for time-out. If he is annoying other people (as in a restaurant or church), also take him outside.

Model: No yelling or tantrums in the store.

Runs Away from the Parent in a Store

Rule: "Stay close to me in the store so you won't get lost."

Discipline technique: Time-out. First try putting your child in the grocery cart for 2 or 3 minutes if she doesn't stay near to you. If she won't stay in the grocery cart, take her outside and put her in time-out facing the wall of the building or sitting inside your car while you stand by. Consider buying a harness and bringing it with you to the store. Harness your child only if she wanders off. Remove it every 5 minutes, giving her a chance to prove that she can control herself in a public setting. As a last resort, leave your child at home with a sitter and be sure to tell her before you go to the grocery store that she can't come this time because she didn't stay near to you.

Praise your child: For following you through the store.

Resists Going to the Doctor's Office

Does your child dread going to the doctor's office? If so, the following tips may make it easier:

- Schedule an appointment at a time when your youngster won't be needing a nap. Also feed him beforehand so he won't be hungry.
- Bring a stuffed animal, security blanket, pacifier, or snack with you to keep him busy in the waiting room. These may also help him quiet down during parts of the exam.
- To make the physical exam go easier, practice at home holding still for looking in the ears, opening his mouth really wide, and taking deep breaths through an open mouth. By all means, don't let anyone tickle him; this will interfere with ever getting a good exam of the abdomen.

Finally, if he is over 2 years of age and fearful because of previous shots or procedures, try to help him reassociate the doctor's office with more pleasant events. Whenever you are in the neighborhood, drop in to say hello to the nurses and doctors. Just stay for a few minutes, but encourage your youngster to give people some hugs. Then give him a treat. This approach will gradually make him look forward to the visits.

Interrupting Others

Demands Constant Entertainment and Attention

Example: Some children demand that their parents play with them all the time. When a parent is reading, watching TV, fixing her hair, or thinking, the child complains of boredom, or sadness, or wants to be picked up. This situation is an example of the invasion of parents' rights, assuming the parent talks to the child and plays with the child at other times. Even parents of 1- and 2-year-olds can reasonably insist on several 15-minute blocks of personal time each day while the child is awake.

Rule: "Don't interrupt me when I'm busy."

Discipline technique: First, redirect your child by stating: "I'm going to read the newspaper now. What are you going to do?" Suggest some toys, books, or crayons. If your child keeps talking, say: "I can't listen now. We'll play when I'm done with the newspaper." If your child continues to talk or makes demands, either ignore the child or make temporary use of time-out.

Praise your child: For entertaining himself or herself when you are busy.

Interrupts the Parent on the Telephone

Rule: "Don't interrupt me when I'm on the telephone, because I can't hear what the other person is saying."

Discipline technique: Redirect your child by giving him or her some toys to play with. Have your child select these special toys in advance and keep them near the telephone. If your child continues to be disruptive, put the caller on hold (or hang up) and place your child in time-out. Then return to the telephone.

Praise your child: For being quiet and waiting while you are on the telephone. Smile at your child while you are on the telephone. Do something afterward with your child.

Prevention: Place most of your telephone calls during your child's nap or after bedtime. Keep calls to less than 5 minutes when your child is awake.

Interrupts Guests

Premise: After an initial greeting and some brief attention, your child should not be allowed to crawl on guests or interrupt adult conversations.

Rule: "Don't interrupt me when I'm talking to my friend, because it makes it hard for us to talk."

Discipline technique: For a younger child, distract him with special toys or games. For an older child, tell her she has to find something to do. If your child persists in interrupting, don't feel guilty about sending her to her room or, if it's near bedtime, to bed. Children should be able to take a backseat to guests. Other adults will approve of your insisting on this.

Praise your child: For good behavior when guests are over.

Interrupts Family Conversations with Incessant Talking and Questioning

Rule: "Don't talk when other people are talking. Don't change the topic." Although we like children to talk, they need to wait their turn if someone else is talking.

Discipline technique: Ignore the child who is interrupting and continue your conversation with the other person. If the interruption continues, tell the interrupting child that you will be glad to talk with him when you are finished talking with the other person. Suggest he listen or do something else for now. If he continues to be disruptive, send him to time-out.

Praise your child: For not interrupting and for waiting.

Model: Not interrupting other people and listening carefully when they speak.

Delaying or Ignoring Others

Doesn't Come When Called

Example: This condition is also called "parent deafness" or "tuning out the parents." This behavior occurs when children don't want to listen or follow through with a parent's suggestion. A child does not need his hearing tested if the "deafness" only occurs in selected circumstances.

Rule: "Listen to what I say, because I'll only tell you once."

Discipline technique: If you have something important to tell your child, go to her and elicit eye contact before giving your instruction. If she doesn't follow through, use logical consequences, such as cold food for getting to dinner late.

Praise your child: For coming when called.

Model: Discontinue shouting from the other room. Discontinue lectures or repeated reminders. Listen carefully to your child and respond promptly.

Doesn't Come Home on Time

Rule: "Come home on time."

Discipline technique: Logical consequences of grounding for 1 day or having your child come home earlier in the future.

Praise your child: For keeping deadlines.

Model: Being punctual.

Doesn't Get Ready on Time

Rule: "Don't be late when we have to go somewhere."

Discipline technique: Give your child some lead time. If the activity is not essential, have your child miss that activity. If the activity is important, use manual guidance to interrupt your child's dawdling.

Praise your child: For being ready on time.

Model: Don't make your child wait for you. Show your child how you get ready in a hurry.

Dressing Misbehavior

Doesn't Cooperate When the Parent Tries to Dress the Child or Change a Diaper

Rule: "Hold still when I'm trying to dress you."

Discipline technique: Give your child strong disapproval if she doesn't cooperate while you're getting her dressed. Don't smile, talk to her, or allow this behavior to become a game.

Praise your child: For helping you get her dressed.

Won't Dress Himself Though Able To

Premise: Once a child is old enough to dress himself, the parent should never need to dress him again. Avoid situations where you feel that you are pressured into becoming involved in the dressing process.

Rule: "You're old enough to dress yourself."

Discipline technique: If you're going to stay at home, don't allow your child to watch TV or go outdoors until he is completely dressed. Also, avoid buying clothing that is hard to get on.

Procrastinates Dressing When the Parent Is Trying to Leave

Examples: You need to take your child to school, day care, the store, or on some other errand. Your child won't dress herself (despite being able to) and eats breakfast slowly.

Rule: "You must be ready to leave the house by eight-thirty each morning, because we can't be late to school."

Discipline technique: Logical consequences.

- Give your child 10 minutes' warning before departure, preferably using a kitchen timer. Encourage your child to "beat the timer."
- If your child is not dressed at departure time and you are driving somewhere, put her clothes and shoes in a bag and take her to the car dressed as she is. If she likes, she can get dressed in the car after you have arrived at your destination and have removed the seat belt. If your child is going to school, try to get there a few minutes late to provide some additional pressure to speed up on the next morning. If your child misses a school bus, take her to school yourself, but be sure again that she's a few minutes late.
- Provide breakfast in the morning, but if your child is not finished with breakfast at the time of departure, that is her problem.

• Don't nag during the time your child is stalling and dawdling. By all means don't dress your child at the last minute.

Praise your child: For trying to dress herself, completely dressing herself, dressing herself promptly, or being ready to leave for school or other appointments on time.
Model: Dress before breakfast. Show your child how you sometimes dress in a hurry.

Doesn't Dress Appropriately for the Weather

Rule: "It's up to you to dress so that you won't be too hot or too cold. This is today's weather forecast."
Discipline technique: Natural consequences.
Model: Preparedness for weather variation during the day.

Washing and Bathing Misbehavior

Procrastinates About Washing, Bathing, or Toothbrushing

Rule: "We wash our hands before meals. We have a clean face and smell good before going places. We brush our teeth after meals and before bed."
Discipline technique: Logical consequences. Your child is not allowed to have his dinner until he has washed his hands. Your child is not allowed to go to school until he is clean, even if this means he will be late for school. You decide whether or not his body or teeth are clean enough, by doing a re-check after your child has had an opportunity to brush his teeth or wash again. For infants, use more distraction (such as storytelling) and enthusiasm to make your child feel positive about the cleaning process.
Praise your child: For spontaneously brushing teeth or washing. Also compliment him on how he looks and smells afterward.
Model: Have good personal hygiene habits.

Wets or Soils During the Day—See Toilet-Training Resistance, page 290.

Smears Fecal Material

Definition: A child in diapers takes fecal material and smears it on the bed, walls, bathroom, and so on. Rather than being deliberate, usually this behavior arises from a chance discovery by a bored child, perhaps one who is left in bed too long. Unlike the parents, the child is usually not repulsed by feces.

Rule: "Don't get any poop on your bed or the walls. Poop is messy. Poop goes in the toilet."

Discipline technique: For fecal smearing, give clear verbal disapproval without yelling or showing anger. Clean up your child without any entertainment or conversation. Then clean the room, with your child's help if possible. Avoid any severe punishment, because if you overrespond to the first few times your child does this, you may initiate a power struggle. If you are also toilet-training your child at this time, reduce any pressure about his or her performance.

Prevention: Supervise your child more closely. Don't leave him alone for more than 10 minutes at a time. When he awakens from his nap, lift him out of bed promptly. Leave him some toys in the bed to play with if he awakens early. Put his diapers on tightly with packaging tape so he can't easily get his hands inside.

Praise your child: For telling you when his pants are full and he needs to be changed.

Miscellaneous

Won't Talk When Able To

Definition: Some children point at things, pull on their parents' sleeves, and play dumb rather than talking.

Rule: "If you want something, tell me."

Discipline technique: Ignore your child after stating once: "I don't know what you want unless you tell me."

Praise your child: For talking. If he has speech delays, teach him some basic sign language.

Won't Confess or Apologize

Definition: Children can't be made to confess or apologize. This expectation is too high for many normally stubborn children.

Discipline technique: Rather than turning this into a power struggle, eliminate it as a problem by not asking for apologies or confessions.

Model: Demonstrate that you can sometimes apologize, such as stating: "I'm sorry that I said such-and-such when I corrected you."

Lying

Premise: Children usually lie to try to avoid punishment. Hence the saying "Ask me no questions and I'll tell you no lies." These are called self-protective lies. During the first 5 years of life, children go through a normal phase of trying to cover up by lying. They stop lying when they learn it doesn't convince anyone. Excessive lying is almost always due to harsh punishment, frequent punishment, trying to please adults with high expectations, or a parent's preoccupation with lying.

Rule: "Don't lie. Tell me the truth."

Discipline technique:

• Punish your child based on the available evidence. For example, if a dish is broken and your child has just been in the kitchen, you don't need Sherlock Holmes. Don't ask your child what happened, when you already know what he did. Children aren't good at testifying against themselves.

• For misbehavior without any evidence (e.g., you think your child watched a TV show you told her not to), overlook it. Trying to investigate it will just bring you grief.

• When you confront your child about misbehavior and she spontaneously denies she had anything to do with it, show your disapproval. Tell her, "I really feel bad when you lie to me and I hope you'll tell me the truth next time." Then give her a double time-out if she lies compared to the amount of time she has to spend there if she doesn't lie (i.e., 2 minutes instead of 1 per year of age).

• Don't try to catch your child in a lie or make her confess. These just lead to bigger and better lies.

Praise your child: For telling the truth.

Model: Being truthful yourself and lying as little as possible (including tactful lies).

INFANTS, TODDLERS, AND PRESCHOOLERS

THUMBSUCKING

Definition

Babies have a natural desire to suck. Thumbsucking is a common way babies seem to comfort themselves. Thumbsucking usually begins by 3 months of age.

A child usually sucks his thumb when he is tired, bored, sick, or upset or when he is not using his hands to play. A child may suck a finger(s) or fist instead of a thumb. Sometimes a security object, such as a blanket, may become part of the thumbsucking habit.

Causes—An infant's desire to suck on the breast or bottle is a drive that is essential for survival. More than 80 percent of babies do some extra sucking when they are not hungry. With ultrasound many babies even can be seen sucking in the uterus. Thumbsucking also appears to help a child comfort herself and often increases when breast- or bottle-feedings decrease. It does not mean that a child is insecure or has emotional problems.

Expected Course—The sucking need is strongest during the first 6 months of a child's life. In a study by Dr. T. Berry Brazelton, only 6 percent of thumbsucking babies continued the habit past 1 year of age and only 3 percent continued beyond the age of 2 years. A more recent study, however, found that 15 percent of 4-year-olds still sucked their thumbs. Those children who continued sucking their thumbs after the age of 4 often have become involved in a power struggle in their early years with a parent who tried to stop their thumbsucking. Occasionally the thumbsucking simply persists as a bad habit.

The American Dental Association advises that a child can probably suck his thumb until he is 4 or 5 years old without damaging his teeth or jawline. However, thumbsucking must be stopped before a child's permanent teeth come in (at age 6 or 7) because it can lead to an overbite (buck teeth). Another reason to encourage children to give up the habit before they enter school is to prevent the teasing they would otherwise receive.

By adolescence, most normal children abandon thumbsucking because of peer pressure.

How to Help Your Child Overcome Thumbsucking

If Your Child Is Less than 5 Years Old—Thumbsucking should be considered normal before the age of 4 years and usually ignored, especially when your child is tired, sick, or stressed. Help your child overcome any stressful situations. However, if the thumbsucking occurs when your child is bored and he is over 1 year old, try to distract him. Give him something to do with his hands without mentioning your concern about the thumbsucking. Occasionally praise your child for not thumbsucking. Until your child is old enough for you to reason with, any pressure you apply to stop thumbsucking will only lead to resistance and lack of cooperation.

After 5 Years of Age—Most 5-year-olds have reached the age of reasoning and are developmentally ready to cooperate with their parents and work on a bad habit. They must have an understanding of cause-and-effect relationships, the ability to discriminate between right and wrong, and the capacity to practice some degree of self-control and self-denial.

First get your child's commitment to giving up thumbsucking by showing her what thumbsucking is doing to her teeth and body. Show her the gap between her upper and lower teeth with a mirror. Have her look at the wrinkled rough skin (callus) on her thumb. Discuss the unhealthy aspects of placing the thumb in the mouth when there are germs or dirt on it. Appeal to her sense of pride. At this point most children will agree that they would like to stop thumbsucking.

If your child expresses the desire to stop, the next step is careful planning. Young children may become frustrated easily and will want to stop trying. To help the child succeed, parents will want to be available for the first difficult days and focus on keeping the child distracted from the sucking behavior by planning some activities to occupy his hands such as drawing, craft projects, puzzles, and games. If the hands are busy they won't be going in the mouth.

Because most children with sucking habits are unaware of the activity, it will be important to use some sort of reminder on the thumb. Character Band-Aids work well for daytime, but children generally need assistance placing the bandage comfortably on the top part of the thumb. However, it is important that it be the child's choice to wear the reminder and not be enforced by the parents. Introduce the reminder as a special helper to let the child know when the thumb is trying to sneak in the mouth. Limit television watching for the first couple of weeks and avoid other situations that stimulate the sucking habit.

Older children may also want an outlet for dealing with the urge to suck their thumb. You can suggest she do something else with her thumb, such as holding her thumb inside a closed fist for 10 seconds or twiddling her thumbs. Although self-reminders are the most effective, parental reminders may occasionally be helpful if the child approves. Ask your child if it will be all right if you remind her when she forgets. Do this gently with comments such as "Guess what?" and put an arm around your child as she remembers that she has been sucking on her thumb again.

Thumbsucking During Sleep—Most children depend heavily on the sucking activity to relax and fall asleep at naptime and bedtime. The sleeping habit is the strongest part of the behavior and takes the longest to eliminate. It will be important to address the sleeptime sucking at the same time you are working on the daytime habit to minimize frustration and enhance success.

Parents will also want to plan to be available at bedtime for the first week to help the child adjust to falling asleep without sucking. Your child can be told that the sleeptime thumbsucking is not his fault, because "that old thumb just sneaks in," and the child doesn't even know it because he is sleeping. He will need a powerful reminder, one that covers the entire hand. A long cotton tube sock is the most effective reminder. A glove or puppet sock are other options. Help your child look upon this method as a clever and fun idea rather than any kind of penalty. Again, parents should assist with putting on the bedtime reminders but not enforce cooperation. It is important to remember that parents cannot eliminate the habit for their child. The habit belongs to the child, and the child must willingly cooperate and accept responsibility if the habit is to be eliminated.

Incentives—Praise your child whenever you notice she is not sucking her thumb in situations where she previously did. This will build her self-confidence. Give her a star on her chart and a reward (such as a dime, a snack, or an extra story) at the end of any day during which she did not suck her thumb at all.

Consult with a Thumbsucking Expert—When the permanent teeth come in, thumbsucking carries the danger of causing an overbite. Eventually an overbite will require orthodontic braces, which are expensive.

An expert on thumbsucking is called a certified oral myologist (CMO). They are trained to help children stop their sucking habits quickly using motivational programs. If the other techniques mentioned here are not successful, ask your doctor about CMOs or call the International Association of Orofacial Myology at 1-303-765-4395.

What to Avoid—The following techniques are generally not helpful and may prolong the thumbsucking habit because the child looks upon them as punishment:

• Dental appliances. This is usually a reminder bar that is placed in the upper part of the mouth.
• Elastic wrap or splints. Placing these around the elbow to keep it from bending often causes some discomfort. It can also cause temporary blueness, swelling, and numbness of the arm in the morning.
• Bitter-tasting medicines applied to the thumbnail. If the parent applies the medicine without the child's permission, the child will usually just wash it off or switch to another finger. Only if your child wants to use it as a reminder might it be helpful.

Prevention of Prolonged Thumbsucking

If your baby needs to suck a lot, try to interest him in a pacifier instead of his thumb when he needs to be comforted but is not hungry. However, avoid overusing it. Unlike thumbsucking, pacifier use can be controlled as your child grows older because you can take away the pacifier. Children older than 1 year who use pacifiers do not switch to sucking their thumbs when they give up the pacifier. Children are always able to give up their pacifiers by age 4 or 5 years.

Thumbsucking lasting beyond age 5 can usually be prevented if you avoid pulling your child's thumb out of his mouth at any age. Also, don't comment in your child's presence about your dissatisfaction with the habit. Scolding, slapping the hand, or other punishments will only make your child dig in his heels about thumbsucking. If you can wait, your child will usually give up the thumbsucking naturally. If you turn the issue into a showdown, you will lose, since the thumb belongs to your child.

Call Your Child's Physician During Office Hours If

- Your child is over 4 years old and sucks her thumb constantly.
- Your child is over 5 years old and doesn't stop when peers tease her.
- Your child is over 6 years old and sucks her thumb at any time.
- Your child's teacher has expressed concern about thumbsucking in class.
- Your child also has emotional problems.
- The permanent teeth appear to be crooked.
- The thumbsucking does not improve after trying this approach.
- You have other concerns or questions.

Recommended Reading

Norman R. Van, *Helping the Thumbsucking Child* (Garden City Park, N.Y.: Avery Publishing Group, 1999).

PACIFIERS

Babies vary in how much extra sucking they do when they are not feeding. This extra sucking is a beautiful self-comforting behavior. Some babies almost constantly suck on their thumb or fingers. If you have a baby like this, you may want to try to interest him or her in a pacifier. The pacifier has to be introduced during the first month or two of life for it to be accepted as a substitute for the thumb. While the orthodontic type of pacifier is preferred because it allegedly prevents tongue-thrusting during sucking, the regular type also is fine. By trial and error, let your baby choose the shape.

Advantages of a Pacifier over Thumbsucking—The main advantage of a pacifier is that if you can get your child to use one, he won't be a thumbsucker. Thumbsucking can cause a severe overbite if it is continued after the permanent teeth come in. The pacifier exerts less pressure on the teeth and causes much less overbite than the thumb. In addition, the pacifier's use can be controlled as your child grows older. You can decide when it's reasonable to discontinue it. By contrast, thumbsucking can't be stopped when you want it to, because the thumb belongs to your child.

When to Offer the Pacifier—Start the pacifier by 1 to 2 months of age if your infant shows a tendency to become a thumbsucker. Otherwise one is probably not needed. Some babies can soothe themselves without sucking. The peak age for thumbsucking (or using a pacifier) is 2 to 4 months. During the following months, the sucking drive normally decreases. A good age to make it less available is when your child starts to crawl. A pacifier can interfere with normal babbling and speech development. This is especially important after 12 months of age, when speech should take off. It's hard to talk with a pacifier in your mouth. To prevent problems with pacifiers, make sure your child doesn't become overly attached to one (e.g., walks around with one in his mouth). Consider the following recommendations for preventing excessive use and a "pacifier habit":

• During the first 6 months of life, give the pacifier to your baby whenever she wants to suck but isn't hungry. But don't use it whenever your baby cries. See CRYING BABY (COLIC), page 253, to review other causes of crying besides hunger and sucking needs.

• After 6 months of age (or when your infant starts crawling), offer the pacifier less often. Keep it out of sight when not in use. If you allow her to use it all the time, her interest in it will increase rather than decrease. If your child seems to want a security object while awake, offer her alternatives such as a stuffed animal.

• When your older infant is unhappy, try to hold and cuddle her more rather than using the pacifier for this purpose. Some infants like massage. Try not to use the pacifier while you are comforting her.

• Reminder: If your baby likes the pacifier, don't forget to take it with you when you travel. Keeping a spare pacifier in the car is helpful. For air travel, sucking a pacifier during descent can prevent ear pain.

Pacifiers and Sleep—Never use a pacifier as a sleep transition object. (Exception: temporarily for calming colicky newborns.) It will become a bad habit that requires you to locate the pacifier following normal awakenings at night. When your infant starts to fall asleep, the pacifier will start to fall out and your child will awaken and try to grasp it with his mouth. Also, following normal awakenings at night, infants can't find, pick up, and re-insert a pacifier until 10 or 12 months old.

Help your child learn to put himself to sleep. Keep the pacifier out of the crib.

Pacifier Safety—Some cautions regarding the pacifier should be observed.

- Use a 1-piece commercial pacifier, not a homemade one. Avoid using one that comes apart (such as made from the nipple and taped to a plastic bottle cap). These can be pulled apart, become caught in your baby's throat, and cause choking.
- Don't put the pacifier on a string around your baby's neck, which could cause strangulation. Use a "catch-it-clip."
- Don't use pacifiers with a liquid center. (Some have been found to be contaminated with germs.)
- Don't coat the pacifier with any sweets, which may cause dental cavities if teeth have erupted.
- Don't coat the pacifier with honey, which may cause a serious disease called botulism in children less than 1 year of age.
- Rinse off the pacifier each time your baby finishes using it or if it drops to the floor.
- Replace the pacifier if it becomes damaged.

Stopping Use of the Pacifier—If the pacifier's use has been restricted to times you are holding your child, she will usually lose interest in it by 9 to 12 months of age. If she has been allowed to use it frequently and is very interested in it, you can usually obtain her permission to give it up completely by the age of 3 or 4. Pick a time when your child is not coping with new stresses or fears. Sometimes giving it up on a birthday, holiday, or other celebration makes it easier.

Make the transition as pleasant as possible. Sometimes incentives are needed. If your child seems strongly attached, offer to replace the last pacifier with a new stuffed animal or encourage her to trade it for something else she wants. Never force her to give up the pacifier through punishment or humiliation.

Give your child a choice such as throwing it away, leaving it out for Santa Claus or the "pacifier fairy," etc. Saving it somewhere in the house is usually not a good idea, because your child will be more likely to ask for it during periods of stress. At such times, offer to cuddle your child instead. Help your child talk about how she misses the pacifier. Praise your child for this sign of growing up.

BREATH-HOLDING SPELLS

Symptoms and Characteristics

- Preceded by an upsetting event, such as being frustrated, angry, injured, or frightened
- Child gives out 1 or 2 long cries
- Then holds his breath in expiration until the lips become bluish
- Then passes out (most children stiffen, and some have a few twitches or muscle jerks)
- Then resumes normal breathing and becomes fully alert in less than 1 minute
- Onset between 6 months and 2 years of age
- Occurs only when child is awake

If your child's symptoms are different, call your physician for help.

Cause—Five percent of normal children have an abnormal reflex that allows them to hold their breath long enough to actually pass out. Holding the breath (when angry) and becoming bluish without passing out is a common reaction and not considered abnormal.

Expected Course—The attacks occur from 1 or 2 times a day to 1 or 2 times a month, and are gone by age 4 or 5 years. They are not dangerous, and they don't lead to epilepsy or brain damage.

Call Your Child's Physician

Immediately If

- There is no breathing or air flow for more than 1 minute (call 911).
- Your child was unconscious for more than 1 minute (by the clock).
- Your child is less than 6 months old and turns blue.
- Your child turns whitish rather than bluish.

During Office Hours If

- Any muscle jerks occurred during the attack.
- More than 1 spell occurs per week (so we can prevent them from becoming more frequent).
- You have other questions.

Home Care for Breath-Holding Spells

Treatment During Attacks—These attacks are harmless and always stop by themselves. Breath-holding spells look terrible and cause some parents to panic. They are harmless, however, so try to be calm. Have your child lie flat (rather than holding him upright) to increase blood flow to the brain. (This position may prevent some of the muscle-jerking.) Apply a cold, wet washcloth to your child's forehead until he or she starts breathing again. Time the length of a few attacks, using a watch with a second hand, since it's difficult to estimate the length of an attack accurately.

Don't start resuscitation or call 911; it's unnecessary. Also, don't put anything in your child's mouth; it could cause choking or vomiting. Above all, don't shake your baby, because it could lead to bleeding in the brain (subdural hematomas).

Treatment After Attacks—Give your child a brief hug and go about your business. A relaxed attitude is best. If you are frightened, don't let your child know it. If your child had a temper tantrum that progressed to a breath-holding spell because she wanted her way over something, don't give in to her after the attack. Breath-holding attacks should not result in any payoff for your child, any more than a temper tantrum should.

Prevention of Breath-Holding Spells—Most attacks from falling down or a sudden fright can't be prevented; neither can most attacks that are triggered by anger. However, some children can be distracted from their breath-holding if you intervene before they become blue. Tell your child to come to you for a hug or to look at something interesting. Ask her if she wants a drink of juice.

If your child is having daily attacks, he probably has learned to trigger some of the attacks himself. This can happen when parents run to the child and pick him up every time he starts to cry or when they give him his way as soon as the attack is over. Avoid these responses, and your child won't have an undue number of attacks.

Prevention of Injuries—The main risk of breath-holding spells is sustaining a head injury. If your child starts to have an attack while standing near a hard surface, go to her quickly and help lower her to the floor.

Call Your Child's Physician Later If

- The attacks become more frequent.
- You have other questions about breath-holding.

SEX EDUCATION FOR PRESCHOOLERS

By age 4, most children develop a healthy sexual curiosity. They ask a variety of questions and need honest, brief answers. If they don't ask sexual questions by age 5, it is your job to bring up this subject. If you don't, they may acquire a lot of misinformation from their schoolmates.

Promoting Good Sex Education

- Teach the differences in anatomy, and the proper names for body parts. This is easy to do during baths with siblings or friends.
- Teach about pregnancy and where babies come from. The easiest way is to get a pregnant friend to volunteer and have your child feel her baby moving about.
- Explain the birth process. Tell your child that the baby comes out through a special passage called the vagina. Help him understand the process by seeing the birth of some puppies.
- Also, explain sexual intercourse. Many parents who discuss everything else keep postponing this topic. Get past this hurdle by reading your child some picture books on sex education. If you cover these topics by age 5, your child will find it easy to ask you more about them as he grows older.

Normal Sexual Play

A common part of normal sexual development between ages 3 and 5 is for children to get undressed together and look at each other's genitals. This is their attempt to learn about sexual differences. There's no reason why you can't turn this discovery into a positive one.

- After your child's friends have gone home, read him a book about sex education. Help him talk about how boys' and girls' bodies differ.
- Tell your child that genitals are private. That's why we wear clothes. Clarify some basic rules. It's okay to see other people's genitals but not to touch them or stare at them. It's not acceptable to show someone your genitals deliberately.
- In the future, supervise the play a little more closely. If the children occasionally expose their bodies to each other, just ignore it. But if it seems to be becoming more frequent, tell the children it's not polite and has to stop. If this doesn't get your message across, give them a 5-minute time-out in separate rooms, or send the visiting child or children home for the day. But don't give any major punishment or act horrified.

• It's up to parents to put the brakes on undressing games. If you don't, they usually escalate into touching and poking. But keep your response low-key.

Nudity and Your Child

Feelings about nudity vary from family to family. Exposure to nudity with siblings or the parent of the same sex is fine and continues indefinitely (e.g., in locker rooms). But nudity with the parent or sibling of the opposite sex probably should be phased out between ages 4 and 5. Some reasons for this are the following:

• Your child will soon be entering school, and nudity is clearly not accepted there.

• Most families in our society practice modesty, so a child who is too interested in looking at other people's bodies or exposing his own can get into trouble.

• It is usually more comfortable for children to learn genital anatomy from siblings and agemates than from seeing their parents nude.

If you agree with these comments, then between ages 4 and 5 begin to teach a respect for privacy.

• Stop any showering and bathing with your children (especially those of the opposite sex).

• Discontinue having siblings of the opposite sex bathe or shower together.

• Close the bathroom door when you use the toilet, unless you are toilet-training a younger child.

• Close the bedroom door when you get dressed and suggest they do the same.

Wasn't that easy?

Call Your Child's Physician During Office Hours If

• Your child won't stop touching other children's genitals.
• Your child won't stop exposing his or her genitals.
• Your child has an excessive interest in sex or nudity.
• You have other questions or concerns.

MASTURBATION IN PRESCHOOLERS

Symptoms and Characteristics

Masturbation is self-stimulation of the genitals for pleasure and self-comfort. Children may rub themselves with a hand or other object. During masturbation, a child usually appears dazed, flushed, and preoccupied. Masturbation is more than the normal touching and inspection of the genitals commonly observed in 2-year-olds during baths. The frequency varies from once a week to several times per day. Masturbation occurs more commonly when a child is sleepy, bored, watching television, or under stress.

Cause—Occasional masturbation is a normal behavior of many infants and preschoolers. Up to a third of children in this age group discover masturbation while exploring their bodies. It continues simply because it feels so good. Some children masturbate frequently because they are unhappy about something, such as having their pacifier taken away. Others are reacting to punishment or pressure to stop completely. Masturbation has no medical causes. Irritation in the genital area causes pain or itching; it doesn't cause masturbation.

Expected Course—Once masturbation begins, it will seldom stop completely. It may decrease in frequency if associated power struggles or unhappiness are remedied. By age 3 or 4, most children can learn some discretion and masturbate only privately. Masturbation becomes almost universal at puberty with normal surges in hormones and sexual drive.

Common Misconceptions—Masturbation does not cause any physical injury or harm to the body. It is not abnormal or excessive unless it is deliberately done in public places after age 5 or 6. It does not mean your child will be oversexed, promiscuous, or sexually deviant. Masturbation can cause emotional harm (such as guilt and sexual hang-ups) only if adults overreact to it and make the child feel dirty or wicked.

Coming to Terms with Masturbation in Preschoolers

Set Realistic Goals—It is impossible to eliminate masturbation. Accept the fact that your child has learned about it and enjoys it. All that a parent can control is where it occurs. A reasonable goal is to permit it only in the bedroom or bathroom. Clarify for your child: "It's okay to do that in your bedroom." Don't ignore it completely or your child will think he or she can do it freely in any setting, leading to criticism by other adults.

Ignore Masturbation at Naptime and Bedtime—Leave your child alone at these times. Stay out of your child's room. Avoid surveillance or checking up. Do not forbid lying on the abdomen and do not ask if your child's hands are between the legs.

Distract or Discipline Your Child for Masturbation Outside Her Bedroom—Intervene as soon as possible. First try to distract your child with a toy, game, or other activity. Suggest your child run an errand within the house. If that fails, explain to your child: "I know that rubbing yourself feels good, but you can't do that around other people. It's okay to do it in your room or the bathroom, but not in the rest of the house. It's something we do when we're alone." Eventually this will help your child become sensitive to other people's feelings. Often this can't be accomplished readily before age 4 or 5. The younger child may need to be sent to his or her room to masturbate.

Discuss This Approach with All of Your Child's Caregivers—If your child masturbates at day care or preschool, ask that they try to keep their responses consistent with yours. First they should try to distract the child. If that is not effective, they should catch the child's attention with comments such as "We need to have you join us now." Masturbation should be tolerated at preschool only at naptime.

Increase Physical Contact with Your Child—Some children will masturbate less if they receive extra hugging and cuddling throughout the day. Try to be sure that your child receives at least 1 hour per day of special time together and physical affection from the parents.

Common Mistakes—The most common mistake that parents make is to try to completely eliminate masturbation. This leads to an all-out power struggle that the parents inevitably lose. Parents must also discontinue any physical punishment, yelling, or lecturing about masturbation. They should not label masturbation as bad, dirty, or sinful (the "moral approach"). They should avoid tying the hands or using any kind of restraints. All of these approaches lead only to resistance and, possibly, later sexual hang-ups.

Call Your Child's Physician During Office Hours If

- Your child continues to masturbate when other people are around.
- You suspect that your child has been taught to masturbate by someone.
- Your child tries to masturbate others.

- You feel your child is unhappy.
- You cannot accept any masturbation by your child.
- This approach does not bring improvement within 1 month.
- You have other questions or concerns.

SPEECH PROBLEMS: NORMAL VERSUS STUTTERING

As children learn to speak they may naturally have some difficulty. Usually these problems are transient and part of your child's normal development. However, sometimes children will develop a more serious problem such as true stuttering.

Normal Articulation Problems

Normal dysarthria (poor pronunciation or enunciation) is the imprecise production of speech sounds that happens to many children as they learn to speak. Normal dysarthria occurs between the ages of 1 and 4 years. Children say many words that their parents and others can't understand. The cause of normal dysarthria is usually genetic. About 70 percent of children have the ability to pronounce words clearly from the time they start to speak. The other 30 percent have many words that their parents and others can't understand. Normal dysarthria is not a brief phase but instead shows very gradual improvement over several years as a child develops. The speech of at least 90 percent of the children who have dysarthria becomes completely understandable by age 4. The speech of 96 percent of these children becomes completely understandable by age 5 or 6.

Normal Fluency Problems

Speech normally is fluid, with words flowing smoothly as the child speaks. Normal dysfluency (pseudostuttering) is the occasional repetition of sounds or syllables that children make when they are learning to speak, between 18 months and 5 years of age. It occurs in many children. Normal dysfluency occurs because the mind is able to think of words faster than the tongue can produce them. It increases when the child is tired or overexcited. Normal dysfluency only lasts for 2 or 3 months if handled correctly.

True Stuttering

Some characteristics of true stuttering include:

- Frequent repetitions of sounds, syllables, or short words
- Frequent hesitations and pauses in speech
- Absence of smooth speech flow
- Tense facial expressions or facial tics
- A fear of talking

True stuttering (stammering) occurs in only 1 percent of children. Stuttering is 4 times more likely in boys than in girls. In most cases, true stuttering is an inherited problem. It can also occur when a child with normal fluency or enunciation problems is pressured to improve and in the process becomes sensitive to his inadequacies. Soon thereafter the child begins to anticipate speaking poorly and struggles to correct it. The child becomes tense when he speaks, and the more he attempts to control his speech, the worse it becomes. Without treatment, true stuttering will become worse and persist into adulthood.

Helping Your Child Cope with Normal Dysfluency and Normal Dysarthria

The following recommendations should prevent normal dysfluency or dysarthria from developing into stuttering.

Encourage Conversation—Sit down and talk with your child at least once a day. Keep the subject matter pleasant and enjoyable. Avoid asking for verbal performance or reciting. Keep the speaking time low-key and fun.

Help Your Child Relax When Stuttering Occurs—Mild stuttering that's not causing your child any discomfort should be ignored. When your child is having trouble speaking, however, say something reassuring such as "Don't worry, I can understand you." If your child asks you about his stuttering, reassure him, "Your speech will get easier and someday the stuttering will be gone."

Don't Correct Your Child's Speech—Avoid expressing disapproval, such as by saying, "Stop that stuttering" or "Think before you speak." Remember that this is your child's normal speech for his age and is not controllable. Do not try to improve your child's grammar or pronunciation. Also avoid praise for good speech because it implies that your child's previous speech wasn't up to standard.

Don't Interrupt Your Child's Speech—Give your child time to finish what he is saying. Don't complete sentences for him. Don't allow siblings to interrupt one another.

Don't Ask Your Child to Repeat Himself or Start Over—If possible, guess at the message. Listen very closely when your child is speaking. Only if you don't understand a comment that appears to be important should you ask your child to restate it.

Don't Ask Your Child to Practice a Certain Word or Sound—This just makes the child more self-conscious about his speech.

Don't Ask Your Child to Slow Down When He Speaks—Try to convey to your child that you have plenty of time and are not in a hurry. Model a slow, relaxed rate of speech. A rushed type of speech is a temporary phase that can't be changed by orders from the parent.

Don't Label Your Child—Labels tend to become self-fulfilling prophecies. Don't discuss your child's speech problems in his presence.

Ask Other Adults Not to Correct Your Child's Speech—Share these guidelines with baby-sitters, teachers, relatives, neighbors, and visitors. Don't allow siblings to tease or imitate your child's stuttering.

Help Your Child Relax and Feel Accepted in General—Try to increase the hours of fun and play your child has each day. Try to slow down the pace of family life. If there are any areas in which you have been applying strict discipline, back off.

Call a Speech Therapist or Your Child's Physician During Office Hours If

- Your child has true stuttering.
- Your child has any dysfluency after age 5.
- Your child has facial grimacing or tics associated with his speech.
- Your child has become self-conscious or fearful about his speech.
- The dysfluency doesn't improve after trying this program for 2 months.
- Speech is also delayed (no words by 18 months or no sentences by 2½ years).
- Speech is more than 50 percent unintelligible to others and your child is over age 2.
- Speech is more than 25 percent unintelligible to others and your child is over age 3.
- Speech is more than 10 percent unintelligible to others and your child is over age 4.
- You have other questions or concerns.

SCHOOL-AGE CHILDREN

SCHOOL PHOBIA OR AVOIDANCE

Symptoms and Characteristics

- Your child experiences vague physical symptoms such as stomach aches, headaches, sore throats, nausea, or dizziness.
- Your child has missed 5 or more days of school for these symptoms.
- The symptoms mainly occur in the morning.
- The symptoms worsen at the time of departure for school or on arrival at school.
- There are usually minimal symptoms on weekends and holidays.
- Your child misses you while at school and wants to go home.
- The symptoms began during kindergarten or first grade.
- The symptoms start in September or October.
- Your child otherwise seems healthy and vigorous.

If your child's symptoms are different, call your physician for help.

Causes—A school-phobic child is usually afraid of leaving home in general, rather than afraid of anything in particular at school. For example, he may experience homesickness when staying at a friend's house. Often the first test of a child's independence comes when he must attend school daily. Aside from poor attendance, these children usually are good students and well behaved at school. The parents are typically good parents who are conscientious and loving. Such parents may also be overly protective and close, and the child finds it difficult to separate from them (separation anxiety). He may lack the self-confidence that comes from handling life's normal stresses without his parents' help.

Sometimes a change of schools, a strict teacher, hard tests, a learning problem, or a bully add to the problem. When such factors are present, they are usually just part of the problem, and your child should still go to school while they are being explored and remedied.

Expected Course—Without intervention, the physical symptoms and the desire to stay home become more frequent. The longer your child stays home, the harder it will be for him or her to return. Your child's future social life and education may be at stake. If full school attendance is enforced, the problem will improve dramatically in 1 to 2 weeks.

Call Your Child's Physician During Office Hours If

- You think the cause of the symptoms may be physical rather than emotional.
- Your child is over 12 years old.
- Your child is withdrawn in general or seems depressed.
- Your child is on homebound teaching.
- You have other questions.

Overcoming School Phobia

Insist on an Immediate Return to School—The best therapy for school phobia is to be in school every day. Normal fears are overcome by facing them as soon as possible. Daily school attendance will cause most of your child's physical symptoms to improve magically. At least they will become less severe and occur less often. Your child will eventually enjoy school again. But in the beginning, your child will test your determination to send her every day. You must make school attendance a nonnegotiable, ironclad rule. It won't be effective if handled in a hesitant way. Be optimistic with your child and reassure him that he will feel better after he gets to school.

Be Extra Firm on School Mornings—In the beginning, mornings may be a difficult time. Never ask your child how she feels, because it may just encourage her to complain. If your child is well enough to be up and around the house, she is well enough to go to school. If your child spontaneously complains of physical symptoms but they are the usual ones, she should be promptly sent to school with minimal discussion. When there is doubt about your child's health, try to err on the side of sending her to school. If things change during the day, the school nurse can reevaluate your child.

If your child is late, she should go to school anyway. In case your child misses the school bus, you should have a prearranged alternative plan of transportation. If your child wanders home during lunch or recess, she should be sent back promptly. Sometimes a child may cry and scream and absolutely refuse to go to school. In that case, after talking with your child about her fears, she has to be taken there. One parent may be better at enforcing this than the other. Sometimes a relative can take charge of this for a few days.

Have Your Child See His Physician on Any Morning He Stays Home—If your child has a new physical symptom or seems quite sick, you will probably want him to stay home. However, keep in mind that anxiety can cause a wide variety of symptoms. If you are puzzled, your child's physician will usually be able to determine the exact cause. Call the physician as soon as the office opens. The physician will try to see your child that morning. If the symptom is from a disease, appropriate treatment can be started. If the symptom is from anxiety, your child should be back in school before noon. Working closely with your child's physician in this way can solve even the most difficult problems.

Some symptoms that might keep your child at home are: fevers, vomiting (more than once), frequent diarrhea, a frequent cough, a widespread rash, earaches, or toothaches. The physician should be called about all of these problems, and many need to be seen. On the other hand, children with a sore throat, moderate cough, runny nose, or other cold symptoms (but without fever) can be sent to class. Children with mild stomachaches, headaches, or leg pains can also usually go to school. Children should not be kept home for "looking sick," "poor color," or "tiredness."

Ask the School Staff for Assistance—Schools are usually very understanding about school phobia once they are informed of the diagnosis, because this problem is such a common one. Usually the school nurse will let your child lie down for 5 to 15 minutes in her office and regroup (if the child's symptoms act up at school), rather than sending him or her home. It is often helpful if you talk to your child's teacher about the situation. If your child has special fears like reciting in class, the teacher will usually make special allowance for these.

Talk with Your Child About School Fears—At a time other than a school morning, talk with your child about her problems. Encourage her to tell you exactly what upsets her. Ask her what is the worst possible thing that could happen to her at school or on the way to school. If there's a situation you can change, tell her you will work on it. If she's worried about the physical symptoms becoming worse at school, reassure her she can lie down for a few minutes in the nurse's office as needed. After listening carefully, tell her you can appreciate how she feels, but it's still necessary to attend school while she's getting better.

Help Your Child Spend More Time with Other Children—Outside of school hours, school-phobic children have a tendency to prefer to be with their parents, play indoors, be alone in their rooms, watch a lot of TV, and so on. Many of them cannot stay overnight at a friend's home without developing overwhelming homesickness. They need encouragement to have more peer contact and less parent contact. This is a difficult task for parents who enjoy their child's company, but it is the best course of action in the long run. Your child can be encouraged to join clubs and athletic teams. Noncontact sports like baseball may be preferred initially. Your child can be sent outside more, or to other children's homes. Your child's friends can be asked to join the family for outings or for overnight stays. Help your child learn to stay overnight with relatives and friends. If he or she can handle weekend camping, a summer camp experience can be a turning point.

Call Your Child's Physician Later If
- The school phobia is not resolved by 2 weeks of using this approach.
- The school phobia recurs.
- Your child continues to have other fears or separation problems.

Prevention of Separation Anxiety and School Phobia
- School phobia tendencies can be reduced or prevented by helping your child develop a sense of independence. Acquiring independence must occur in gradually increasing amounts; your child can't avoid it and then suddenly catch up.
- Start baby-sitter contact by 6 months of age at the latest. Being apart from you and then having you return builds security and confidence in your child. Baby-sitter contact is also important for helping your child develop a sense of trust in other adults.
- Begin peer contact by at least 1 year of age, even though the children don't play cooperatively. From 3 years of age onward, your child should be able to interact with peers without your being present. This is a good age for starting shared playgroups for children.

- Enroll your child in a preschool by 3 or 4 years of age. This is especially helpful for children who show tendencies to be overly dependent on their parents. Always refer to the school as a "fun place" and the teachers as "nice people."

- Help your child adjust to kindergarten. Over half of children entering kindergarten have transient discomfort and crying for 2 to 5 days. Their symptoms resolve as long as the child returns to school each day and the teacher is supportive. You can sometimes help with the transition by temporarily staying at school (but in the background) for the first hour. By all means, don't take your child out of school, even if he or she is among the 5 percent that urgently want to leave and never return. These children (sometimes labeled "immature" by the teaching staff) need preschool and kindergarten the most.

ATTENTION-DEFICIT/HYPERACTIVITY DISORDER (ADHD)

Characteristics

- Short attention span. Normal attention span is 3 to 5 minutes per year of age. A child in kindergarten needs a 15-minute attention span, and first- and second-graders need a 20-minute span to do the work. (Note: The attention span while watching TV doesn't count.)

- Symptoms of short attention span include the following: The child hasn't learned to listen when someone talks, wait his or her turn, complete a task, or return to a task if interrupted. (Caution: These characteristics can be normal until 3 or 4 years of age.)

- The short attention span has been verified by two or more adults (e.g., parent and teacher).

- Some children (80 percent of boys and 50 percent of girls) also have associated hyperactivity (increased motor activity) with symptoms of being restless, impulsive, and in a hurry.

- Some children (20 percent) also have an associated learning disability. The most common one is an auditory processing deficit (i.e., they can't understand complex instructions).

- Intelligence is usually normal.

- The problem occurs mostly in males.

Similar Conditions—Disruptive children, children who don't mind, and aggressive children are sometimes included under the broad definition of hyperactivity. Many problem 2-year-olds are referred to as being "hyperactive." These children should be looked upon as children with behavior problems and approached with appropriate discipline techniques (see THE TERRIBLE TWOS AND STUBBORN TODDLERS and TEMPER TANTRUMS, pages 331 and 333).

Causes—Attention-deficit/hyperactivity disorder (ADHD) is the most common learning disability. It occurs in 5 to 7 percent of children. What causes ADHD? Current theory suggests that ADHD (like other learning disabilities) is probably due to subtle differences in brain chemistry and function. Genetics are a strong factor. Variations in temperament may also contribute. Environmental factors (e.g., inadequate sleep or breakfast) can accentuate the symptoms of ADHD. ADHD is not caused by poor parenting.

Expected Course—The children with ADHD on a developmental basis can expect an excellent outcome if the parents and teachers provide understanding and direction, and preserve the child's self-esteem. Many of these children as adults have adequate attention spans but remain restless, have to keep busy, and, in a sense, have not entirely outgrown the problem. However, not only does society learn to tolerate such traits in adults but in some settings the person with endless energy is prized. Children with severe ADHD may need vocational counseling as adults.

Call Your Child's Physician for Referral to a Child Psychiatrist or Psychologist If

- Your child shows unprovoked aggression and destructiveness.
- Your child has repeated accidents.
- Your child has been suspended or expelled from school.
- Your child can't make or keep any friends.
- You have "given up" hope of improving your child.
- You can't stop using physical punishment on your child.
- You are at your wits' end.

Premise: All children with ADHD should already have been evaluated by their physician and, if of school age, by the school's special-education teacher or psychologist.

Guidelines for Living with a Child Having Attention-Deficit/Hyperactivity Disorder

Medications alone are not the answer. Since ADHD is a chronic condition, these children also need special interventions at home and school. To help with impulsive behaviors, work on structuring your child's home life and improving discipline. Behavior problems can be addressed at any time after 1 year of age. If your child also has a poor attention span, specific interventions to help him learn to listen and complete tasks ("stretch" his attention span) can be initiated.

Accept Your Child's Limitations—Accept the fact that your child is intrinsically active and energetic and possibly always will be. The hyperactivity is not intentional. Don't expect to eliminate the hyperactivity but merely bring it under reasonable control. Any criticism or other attempt to change an energetic child into a quiet or model child will cause more harm than good. Nothing is more helpful for the hyperactive child than having a tolerant, patient, low-key parent.

Provide an Outlet for the Release of Excess Energy—Excessive energy can't be bottled up and stored, but some of it can be "run off" each day. Daily outdoor activities such as running, sports, and long walks are good outlets. A fenced yard helps. In bad weather your child needs a recreational room where he can play as he pleases with minimal restrictions and supervision. If no large room is available, a garage will sometimes suffice. Your child's toys should not be excessive in number, for this can accentuate his distractibility. They should also be ones that are safe and relatively unbreakable. Encourage your child to play with one toy at a time.

Although the expression of hyperactivity is allowed in these ways, it should not be needlessly encouraged. Don't initiate roughhousing with your child. Siblings should be forbidden to say "Chase me, chase me," or to instigate other noisy play. Rewarding hyperactive behavior can lead to its becoming your child's main style of interacting with people.

Follow a Structured Daily Routine—Household routines help the hyperactive child to accept order. Make wake-up, mealtimes, snacks, chores, naps, and bedtime as consistent as possible. Try to keep your environment on the quiet side, to encourage thinking, listening, and reading at home. In general, leave the radio and TV off. Predictable daily events help your child become more predictable in his or her responses.

Try Not to Let Your Child Become Overexhausted—When a hyperactive child becomes exhausted, his self-control often breaks down and the hyperactivity becomes worse. Try to have your child sleep or rest when he is exhausted. If he can't seem to "turn off his motor," hold and rock him in a rocking chair. ADHD symptoms are made worse by sleep deprivation and hunger. Be sure your child has an early bedtime and a big breakfast on school days.

Avoid Taking Young Children to Formal Gatherings—Settings where hyperactivity would be extremely inappropriate (such as concerts or restaurants) can be completely avoided except for special occasions. To avoid some friction you also may wish to reduce the number of times you allow your child to accompany you to stores and supermarkets. Not only will you be able to shop more efficiently, but the store manager will also be grateful. After your child becomes older and develops adequate self-control at home, he can gradually be introduced to these situations.

Maintain Firm Discipline—These children are usually difficult to manage. They need more carefully planned discipline than the average child. Rules should be formulated mainly to prevent harm to your child and to others. Aggressive behavior should be no more accepted in the hyperactive child than in the normal child. Unlike the expression of hyperactivity, you can try to eliminate aggressive behaviors, such as biting, hitting, and pushing. Unnecessary or unattainable rules should be avoided—don't expect your child to keep his hands and feet still. Hyperactive children tolerate fewer rules than the normal child. Set down a few clear, consistent, important rules and add other rules at your child's pace. Avoid constant negative comments like "Don't do this" and "Stop that."

Enforce Rules with Nonphysical Punishment—Physical punishment should be avoided in these children, since we want to teach them to be less aggressive rather than to make aggression acceptable. You will need an isolation or time-out room to back up your attempts to enforce rules if a show of disapproval doesn't work. This room can be your child's bedroom or a time-out chair. Your child should be sent there for about 1 minute per year of age. Without a time-out room, overall success is unlikely. Because of your child's short attention span, apply punishment for misbehavior immediately. Your child also needs adult models of control and calmness. Try to correct your child in a friendly, matter-of-fact voice. If you yell, your child will be quick to imitate you (see TIME-OUT TECHNIQUE FOR DISCIPLINE, page 320).

Stretch Your Child's Attention Span—While the attention span may never be normal, it can usually be improved. Encouraging an increased attention span and persistence with tasks is helpful in preparing your child for school. Don't wait until your child is of school age and expect the teacher to suddenly change him. By age 5 he needs at least a 15-minute attention span to perform adequately in school.

Set aside several brief periods each day to teach your child listening skills through reading. Start with picture books, and gradually progress to reading stories. Coloring of pictures can be encouraged and praised. Games of increasing difficulty can be taught to your child, starting with building blocks and progressing to puzzles, dominoes, card games, and dice games. Matching pictures is an excellent way to build your child's memory and concentration span. Later, consequence games such as checkers or tic-tac-toe can be introduced. When your child becomes restless, stop, and return for another session later. This process is slow but invaluable in preparing your child for school.

Buffer Your Child Against Any Overreaction by Neighbors— Neighbors with whom your child has contact should be enlisted as helpers. If your child is labeled by some adults as a "bad" kid, it is important that this not carry over into his or her home life. At home the attitude that must prevail is that your child is a "good child with excess energy." It is extremely important that you don't give up on him. Your child must always feel loved and accepted within the family. As long as a child has this, self-esteem and self-confidence will survive. If school is not rewarding, help your child gain a sense of success through a hobby in an area of strength.

From Time to Time, Get Away from It All—Exposure to some of these children for 24 hours a day would make anyone a wreck. Periodic breaks help parents to tolerate hyperactive behavior. In a family in which only the father goes out to work, when he comes home he should try to look after the child, not only to give his wife a deserved break but also to understand better what she must contend with during the day. A baby-sitter an afternoon a week and an occasional evening out with her partner can refresh an exhausted mother. Preschool is another helpful option. Parents need a chance to rejuvenate themselves so that they can continue to meet their child's extra needs.

Utilize Special Programs at School—Try to start your child in preschool by age 3 to help him organize his thoughts and ability to focus.

On the other hand, consider enrolling your child in regular school a year later (i.e., at age 6 rather than 5) to allow the added maturity to help him fit in better with his classmates. Once your child enters school, the school is responsible for providing appropriate programs for your child's attention-deficit/hyperactivity disorder and any learning disability he might have. Some standard approaches that teachers use to help children with ADHD are smaller class size, isolated study space, spaced learning techniques, and inclusion of the child in tasks like erasing the blackboard or passing out books as outlets for excessive energy. Many of these children spend part of their day with a learning-disability teacher who helps improve their skills and confidence.

If you feel your child has ADHD and he has not been tested by the school's special-education team, you can request an evaluation. Usually you can obtain the help your child needs by working closely with the school through parent-teacher conferences and special meetings. Your main job is to continue to help your child improve his attention span, self-discipline, and friendships while at home.

Medications Are Usually Helpful—Stimulant drugs can improve the powers of concentration. If your child's teacher and you both feel your child's short attention span is interfering with school performance, discuss the pros and cons of medication with your child's physician. In general, medications are not prescribed before school age. They should also not be prescribed until after your child has received a medical and school evaluation, an individualized educational plan (IEP) is in effect at school, and the preceding guidelines are in effect at home. While medications are helpful, they need to be part of a broader treatment program including special education and behavioral management.

SCHOOLWORK RESPONSIBILITY: HOW TO INSTILL IT

Taking responsibility for schoolwork helps children grow up to be responsible adults who keep their promises, meet deadlines, and succeed at their jobs. Responsible children finish schoolwork, homework, and long-term projects on time. They remember their assignments and turn in papers. They occasionally ask for help (e.g., with a spelling list) but usually like to think through their work by themselves.

How to Encourage Schoolwork Responsibility

The following suggestions should help you cultivate the trait of responsibility in your child and avoid problems with schoolwork that may be difficult to correct later on:

Encourage Learning and Responsibility in the Preschool Years— Listen attentively to your child's conversation. Encourage him to think for himself. Take your child to the library and read to him regularly. Watch educational programs together and talk about them. Be a role model of someone who reads, writes letters or e-mails, finds learning exciting, enjoys problem-solving, and likes to try new things. Ask your preschool child to help you with chores (e.g., clearing the table or putting away clean clothes).

Show Interest in Your Child's School Performance—Ask your child about his school day. Look at and comment positively on the drawings or graded papers he brings home. Praise your child's strong points on his report card. Show interest in the books your child is reading. Help your child attend school regularly; don't keep him home for minor illnesses. Go to regular parent-teacher conferences and tell him about them. If you feel discouraged, rather than convey this to your child, schedule an extra conference with his teacher.

Support the School Staff's Recommendations—Show respect for both the school system and the teacher, at least in your child's presence. Verbal attacks on the school may pit your child against the school and give him an excuse for not working. Even when you disagree with a school policy, encourage your child to conform to school rules, just as he will need to conform to the broader rules of society.

Make It Clear Schoolwork Is Between Your Child and the Teacher—When your child begins school, she should understand that homework, schoolwork, and marks are mainly between her and her teacher. The teacher, not the parents, should set goals for better school performance. Your child must feel responsible for successes and failures in school. People take more pride in accomplishments if they feel fully responsible for them. Parents who feel responsible for their child's school performance open the door for the child to turn her responsibilities over to them. Occasionally, elementary-school teachers may ask you to practice something (e.g., math facts) with your child or see that your child completes work that was put off at school. When your child's teacher makes such requests, it's fine for you to help, but only as a temporary measure.

Stay Out of Homework—Asking if your child has homework, helping nightly, checking the finished homework, or drilling your child in areas of concern all convey to your child that you don't trust him. If you do your child's homework or project for him, your child will have less confidence that he can do it himself next time. If your child asks for help with homework, help with the particular problem only. Your help should focus on explaining the question, not on giving the answer or taking over. A good example of useful help is reading your child's spelling list to him while he writes the words, but then letting him check his own answers. A chief purpose of homework is to teach your child to work independently.

Negotiate a Homework Start Time—Eventually children learn how to pick the best time to do their homework. Initially, however, many will need help blocking out the time. Talk it over; don't dictate it. Then provide a desk, a comfortable chair, and good lighting in a quiet place with minimal distractions. That means the TV, radio, and stereo are off. A good after-school rule is "No TV or video games until homework is completed." For long-term assignments, help your child organize his work the first few times if he seems overwhelmed. Help him estimate how many hours he thinks the project will take. Then help him write a list of the days at home he will work on the project.

Accept Your Child's Word That Homework Is Completed—Don't check it for accuracy. Your child needs to learn to proof his own work. If the work is incomplete or incorrect, the teacher will point this out and your child will learn from the experience. If it becomes a chronic problem, you will hear about it and can then become more involved with monitoring completion.

Provide Home Tutoring for Special Circumstances—Occasionally a teacher will request parental assistance when a child has lots of makeup work following a prolonged absence or a transfer to a new school. If your child's teacher makes such a request, ask her to send home notes about what he or she wants you to help your child with (e.g., multiplication for 2 weeks). By using this approach you are still not taking primary responsibility for your child's schoolwork, because the assignments and request for help come from the teacher. Provide this home instruction in a positive, helping way. As soon as your child has met the teacher's goal for improvement, remove yourself from the role of tutor. In this way you have provided temporary tutoring to help your child over an obstacle that the school staff does not have the time or the resources to deal with fully.

Request Special Help for Children with Learning Problems— Some children have learning problems that interfere with learning some of the basic skills (e.g., reading). The comments so far have assumed that your child has no learning limitations. If a child with a reading disability slips too far behind in class, the child may lose confidence in his ability to do schoolwork. If you have concerns about your child's ability to learn, set up a conference with your child's teacher. At that time, request an evaluation by your school's special-education team. With extra help, children with learning disabilities can preserve their self-esteem and sense of competency.

HOMEWORK PROBLEMS (School Underachiever)

Characteristics
- Performs below his or her potential at school
- Has average or better intelligence, with no learning disabilities
- Doesn't finish schoolwork or homework
- "Forgets" to bring homework home
- "Forgets," loses, or doesn't turn in finished homework
- "Doesn't remember" what parents have taught
- Gets a poor report card
- Doesn't want any help

Causes—Some children get into bad habits with their homework because they become preoccupied with TV programs or video games. Some middle-school children become sidetracked by their hormones or by sports. Other children who find schoolwork difficult would simply rather play. If parents help these children cut back other activities to reasonable amounts and count on the teacher to grade the child's efforts on schoolwork and homework, most of these children will improve. Motivation for good grades eventually comes from a desire to please the teacher and be admired by peers, enjoyment in knowing things, ability to see studying as a pathway to a future career, knowledge that she needs a 3.0 average to get into college, and her own self-reproach when she falls short of her goals.

When parents overrespond to this behavior and exert pressure for better performance, they can start a power struggle around schoolwork. "Forgetfulness" becomes a game. The child sees the parents' pressure as a threat to his independence. More pressure brings more resistance. Poor grades become the child's best way of proving that he is independent of his parents and that he can't be pushed around. Good evidence for this is the child doing worse in the areas where he receives the most help. If parental interference with a child's schoolwork continues for several years, the child becomes a school "underachiever."

Helping Your Child Regain Responsibility for Schoolwork

Get Out of the Middle—Clarify that completing and turning in homework is between your child and the teacher. Remember that the purpose of homework is to teach your child to work on his own. Don't ask your child if he has any. Don't help with homework except at your child's request. Allow the school to apply natural consequences for poor performance. Walk away from any power struggles. Your child can learn the lesson of schoolwork accountability only through personal experience. If possible, apologize to your youngster, saying, for example, "After thinking about it, we have decided you are old enough to manage your own affairs. Schoolwork is your business, and we will try to stay out of it. We are confident you will do what's best for you."

The result of this sink-or-swim approach is that arguments will stop, but your child's schoolwork may temporarily worsen. Your child may throw caution to the winds to see if you really mean what you have said. This period of doing nothing but waiting for your child to find her own reason for doing well in school may be agonizing. However, children need to learn from their mistakes. If you can avoid "rescuing" your child, her grades will show a dramatic upsurge in 2 to 9 months. This planned withdrawal of parental pressure is best done in the early grades, when marks are of minimal importance but the development of the child's own personal reason for learning is critical.

Avoid Reminders—Repeatedly reminding your child about schoolwork promotes rebellion. So do criticizing, lecturing, and threatening your child. Pressure is different from parental interest and encouragement. If pressure works at all, it works only temporarily.

We can never force children to learn or to be productive. Learning is a process of self-fulfillment. It is an area that belongs to the child and one that we as parents should try to stay out of, despite our yearnings for our children's success.

Coordinate with Your Child's Teacher—Schedule a parent-teacher conference. Discuss your views on schoolwork and homework responsibility. Tell your child's teacher you want your child to be responsible to the teacher for homework. Clarify that you would prefer not to check or correct the work, because this has not been helpful in the past. Tell them you want to be supportive of the school and could do this best if the teacher sent home a brief weekly progress report. If the teacher thinks your youngster needs extra help, encourage her to suggest a tutoring program. In middle school, peer tutoring is often a powerful motivator.

Limit TV Until Schoolwork Improves—While you can't make your child study, you can increase the potential study time. Eliminate all TV and video game time on school nights. Explain to your child that these privileges will be reinstated after the teacher's weekly report confirms that all homework was handed in and the overall quality of work (or grades) is improving. Explain that you are doing this to help him better structure his time.

Consider Adding Incentives—Most children respond better to incentives than to disincentives. Ask your youngster what he thinks would help. Some good incentives for improved schoolwork are taking your child to a favorite restaurant, amusement park, video arcade, sports event, or the movies. Sometimes earning spending money by working hard on studies will interest your child. The payments can be made weekly, based on the teacher's progress reports. A's, B's, and C's can receive a different cash value. What your child buys with this money should be his business (music, toys, etc.). Rewarding hard work is how the adult marketplace works.

Consider Removing Other Privileges for Falloff in Schoolwork— You have already eliminated school night TV-viewing because it obviously interferes with studying. If the school reports continue to be poor, you may need to eliminate all TV and video games. Other privileges that may need to be temporarily limited should be those that matter to your child (e.g., telephone, bike, outside play, or visiting friends). If your teenager drives a car, this privilege may need to be curtailed until his grades are at least a 3.0 (B) average. For youngsters who have fallen behind in their work, grounding (i.e., no peer contact) for 1 to 2 weeks may be required until they catch up. Avoid severe punishment, however, because it will leave your youngster angry and resentful. Canceling something important (like membership in Scouts or an athletic team) or taking away something they care about (like a pet) because of poor marks is unfair and ineffective. Being part of a team is also good for motivation.

Call Your Child's Teacher for a Conference If

- Your child's schoolwork and grades do not improve within 2 months.
- Homework is still an issue between you and your child after 2 months.
- You think your child has a learning problem that makes school difficult.

Call Your Child's Physician During Office Hours If

- You think your child is preoccupied with some stresses in his life.
- You think your child is depressed.
- You have other questions or concerns.

Note: If these attempts to motivate your child fail, he may need an evaluation by a child psychologist or child psychiatrist.

TELEVISION: REDUCING THE NEGATIVE IMPACT

TV has a tremendous influence on how children view our world. Youngsters spend more hours watching TV from birth to age 18 than they spend in the classroom. The positive aspects include seeing different lifestyles and cultures and entering school more knowledgeable than children did before the era of TV. Television also presents some positive, even heroic role models. In addition, TV has great entertainment value, providing humor, excitement, and other types of diversion. While TV can be a good teacher, many children watch TV excessively and therefore experience some of its negative consequences.

Harmful Aspects of TV

- TV displaces active types of recreation. It decreases time spent with peers, when games and other creative activities are experienced. It decreases daydreaming and thinking time. It takes away the practice time required to become competent in sports, art, or music. Television is especially dangerous for children who already tend to be shy or withdrawn.

- TV interferes with conversation and discussion time, especially if kept on during meals. It reduces social interactions with family and friends.

- TV discourages reading. Reading requires much more brain activity and thinking than television. Reading improves a youngster's vocabulary. A falloff in reading scores may be related to excessive TV time.

- Heavy TV viewing (more than 4 hours a day) definitely reduces school performance. This much TV interferes with study, reading, and thinking time. If watching television prevents adequate sleep, the children will not be alert enough to learn well on the following day.

- TV discourages exercise. An inactive lifestyle leads to poor physical fitness. If accompanied by frequent snacking, watching TV contributes to weight problems. A recent study found that for each additional hour of television watched per week, the tendency toward obesity was increased by 1 percent.

- TV advertising encourages a demand for material possessions. Particular toys are highlighted in such a way that young children pressure their parents to buy them. TV portrays materialism as the "American way."

- TV advertising teaches poor eating habits. Sweets (such as sugared cereals) tend to be emphasized for young children.

- TV advertising teaches a magical trust in health products, drugs, and vitamins. TV suggests that there is a pill for every symptom.

- TV fosters a poor reality base. Young children through age 10 have some difficulty separating fact from fantasy. Television frequently presents a distorted view of the world in which most problems have easy solutions. Game shows may give children the sense that they can suddenly become rich and that hard work and delayed gratification is unnecessary.

- TV depicts unrealistic stereotypes of human beings. Minority groups, elderly people, common occupations, and middle-class lifestyles are underrepresented.

- TV is sexually seductive. Television programs and commercials depict relationships that rapidly progress to sexual activity. The risks and ethics of promiscuity are seldom addressed. Some programs (such as music videos) may portray sexual violence toward women. Many of the lead characters also smoke and drink heavily.

• TV violence creates its own set of problems. Crime and violence occur on television 10 times as often as in real life. Viewing violence may cause pessimism regarding personal safety and the future. Several studies have shown that TV violence can lead to apathy toward violence. TV violence may numb the normal sympathy toward victims of human suffering. Young children may be more aggressive in their play after seeing violent television shows. While TV violence does not increase aggressive behavior toward people in most children, it does so in disturbed or impulsive children.

The Prevention of TV Addiction

Encourage Active Recreational Outlets—Help your child become interested in sports, games, hobbies, and music. Occasionally just turn off the television and take a walk or play a game with your child.

Read to Your Children—Begin reading to your child by 6 months of age and encourage him to read on his own as he becomes older. Some parents help children earn TV or video game time by equivalent reading time. Help him improve his conversational skills by spending more of your time talking with him.

Limit TV Time to 2 Hours per Day or Less—Allowing children to view excessive amounts of television is probably an even greater problem in our country than watching violence on TV. Another alternative is to limit TV to 1 hour on school nights and 2 or 3 hours per day on weekends. You occasionally may want to allow extra viewing time for special educational programs. If you cut back your child's TV watching, don't be surprised if he initially complains. Excessive TV watching is a habit that, once established, is hard to break. Suggest other activities to fill the free time.

Don't Use TV as a Distraction or a Baby-sitter for Preschool Children—Preschoolers' viewing should be limited to special TV shows and videotapes that are produced for young children. Use your VCR to save good programs for rainy days. Because the difference between fantasy and reality is not clear for this age group, regular TV shows may cause fears.

If Your Child Is Doing Poorly in School, Limit TV Time to a Half Hour Each Day—Make a rule that homework and chores must be finished before television is watched. If his favorite show is on earlier, try to record it for later viewing.

Set a Bedtime for Your Child That Is Not Altered by TV Shows That Interest Her—Children who are allowed to stay up late to watch television are usually too tired the following day to remember what they were taught in school.

Don't Allow a TV Set in Your Child's Bedroom—This eliminates your control over bedtime and what your child is viewing. If your teen is responsible, consider changing the rule at age 15 or so.

Turn Off the TV Set During Meals—Family time is too precious to be squandered on TV shows. After your children are grown up and have left home, you will probably regret it if your mealtimes were not protected and your children were allowed to disappear into their private TV worlds while they ate. In addition, don't use television as a background sound in your house. If you don't like a quiet house, leave a radio or CD player on playing music without lyrics. Television is too engrossing a medium. It demands to be seen as well as heard. Also turn off the TV set during study time or when you have visitors.

Teach Critical Viewing—Turn the TV on only when a specific program is going to be watched. Don't turn it on at random and scan for something interesting. Teach your child to look first in the program guide. On some nights, nothing worthwhile or entertaining is on television.

Teach Your Child to Turn Off the TV Set at the End of a Show—If it is allowed to stay on, your child will probably become interested in the following show and then it will be difficult to turn it off.

Encourage Your Child to Watch Some Shows That Are Educational or Teach Human Values—Point out characters who care about others. Encourage watching documentaries, real-life dramas, or programs about great artists. Look at what public television has to offer (including the absence of advertising). Use programs about love, sex, family disputes, drinking, and drugs to open family discussions on these difficult topics.

Try to Be Present with Your Child the First Time He or She Watches a New Program—Help decide whether or not this is a program you wish to allow your child to watch on a weekly basis.

Forbid Violent TV Shows—This means you have to know what your child is watching and turn off the TV set when you don't approve of the program. Develop separate lists of programs that are okay for older and younger kids to watch. Make your older children responsible for keeping the younger ones out of the TV room at these times. If not, the show is turned off. The availability of cable or satellite television and videocassette or DVD players means that any child of any age has access to the uncut versions of R-rated films. Many children under 13 years of age develop daytime fears and nightmares after watching vicious movies. Children in elementary school should not be allowed to watch R-rated movies or music video channels.

Discuss the Consequences of Violence If You Allow Your Older Child to Watch Violent Shows—Point out how violence hurts both the victim and his family. Be sure to discuss any program that has content which upsets your child.

Discuss Commercials with Your Children—Help them identify high-pressure selling and exaggerated claims. If your child wants a toy that is a look-alike version of a TV character, ask him how he would use it at home. The response will probably convince you that the toy will be added to a collection of rarely used toys rather than become a catalyst for much active play. Point out foods that cause cavities or high cholesterol.

Discuss the Differences Between Reality and Make-Believe—This type of clarification can help your child enjoy a show and yet realize that what is happening doesn't happen in real life.

Set a Good Example—If you are a TV addict, you can be sure your child will become one. The types of programs you watch also sends a clear message to your child. Consider starting yourself on a TV diet.

TV Program Ratings

Most television programs are now rated. The TV ratings are:

- Y (made for all children)
- Y7 (made for children 7 or older)
- Y7-FV (made for children 7 or older, includes fantasy violence)
- G (general audience, appropriate for all ages)
- PG (parental guidance suggested, may be inappropriate for young children)
- TV-14 (parents strongly cautioned, may be inappropriate for children under 14)
- TV-MA (mature audience only, may be unsuitable for children under 17)

Most newer television sets include a V-chip so that you can block TV shows with certain ratings. But remember, ratings are just guidelines. They cannot replace your good judgment. An educational animal show may have the same rating as a violent cartoon.

VIDEO GAMES

Home video games are very popular and have a significant influence on our children. Over 85 percent of students say they play video games regularly. Over 30 percent of American homes have a video game system hooked up to the television. Millions more own portable game systems. Over 20 percent of homes have broadband access to video games. And while these games are still heavily played by males, the number of female players is rapidly growing as well. Video games have a positive and a negative side. With proper supervision, they can be a fun and educational form of play.

Video Games Versus Television

Compared to watching television, video games are a better form of entertainment. Video games are interactive. Your child's mind has to be turned on and working. The following are some benefits of playing video games:

• Promotes paying attention to details (e.g., to clues), memory, sequencing, and strategizing
• Promotes eye-hand (visual motor) coordination
• Improves visual perception (spatial awareness)
• Promotes use of imagination
• Provides entertainment children and adults can share

Disadvantages of Video Games

The drawbacks of video games are similar to the ones we see with TV (see page 394):

• Video games can dominate your child's free time and study time. Video games can eliminate time needed to develop competence in sports, music, or art. If reading and homework are displaced, school performance can be affected.
• Video games can be a solitary activity, reducing social interactions with family and friends. Your youngster can become a junior hermit interacting with friends only to pump them for pieces of information about hidden passages or secret trap doors. Encourage playing video games with other children.
• Violent video games can teach an acceptance of violent behavior in real life.

- Overall, realize that your child is overdosing on video games if his grades have fallen, he doesn't finish his homework, he doesn't get adequate sleep, he doesn't play outdoors, he has become a loner, or he is preoccupied with karate chops or other aggressive behavior that is part of one of his video games.

Take a Stand on Video Games

Don't expect your youngster to limit the time allocated to this mesmerizing form of entertainment. Given his own way, he might play video games every waking moment. You are responsible for protecting your child from harm. You must decide on rules that are appropriate for your child. If the rules are broken, the game (or control panel) needs to be put away for 1 or more days.

- *Allow video games only after homework and chores are completed.* Access to video game time can even be presented as an incentive for finishing these tasks properly.
- *Limit video game time.* Two hours a day or less is a reasonable goal. An alternative is to limit it to 1 hour on school nights and 2 or 3 hours a day on weekends. Some parents allow the system to be used only on weekends. If your child is doing poorly in school, temporarily eliminate video game time on school nights. Some parents have their children earn video game time by putting in equivalent reading time.
- *Don't allow your child to postpone bedtime because he wants to finish a video game.* Remember that children who are allowed to stay up late are usually too tired the next day to remember what they are taught in school. When bedtime is drawing near, give your child a 10-minute warning.
- *Don't allow a video game set in your child's bedroom.* This eliminates your control over bedtime and what kinds of games your child is playing. If your teen is responsible, consider changing the rule at age 15 or so.
- *Encourage your children to settle their own disputes over using the video game.* When possible, stay out of disagreements, as long as they remain verbal. Children can't go through life having a referee to resolve their differences. If the argument becomes too loud, remove the control panel until your children work out a schedule.
- *Help your child buy video games that are not excessively violent.* Encourage him to buy or rent sports, puzzle, maze, or adventure games. Avoid games that contain lots of murder, combat, and destruction. Since your child is an active participant in the mayhem on video games, research

suggests they have a greater impact on his aggressive behavior than violent TV shows, in which he is strictly an observer. If your child borrows or rents a new video game, have a rule that you have to approve of its contents before he uses it. Look at game ratings, but also preview the game before letting your child play. Ratings are not a perfect system for screening things you don't want your child to hear or see.

• *If you own a computer, take advantage of some of the educational games.* These tap the motivational power of the arcade games to help your child learn. They combine academics and entertainment. They also teach computer skills. If you have a choice, buy computer games rather than video games.

• *Try to channel your child's free time into a variety of activities.* Video games are not bad for children. They can teach skills. They are more educational than TV. And, if you try to forbid video games, your child will play them at an arcade or another child's home. So help your child learn to use them in moderation after the first weeks of normal infatuation have passed. Encourage more reading, music, hobbies, sports, and playing with friends.

R-RATED MOVIES: PROTECTING YOUR CHILD

The following symptoms have all been reported in children after watching violent, R-rated movies:
• Bedtime fears
• Recurrent nightmares
• Daytime flashbacks of something frightening
• Disruption of concentration and study
• A fearful view of the world

Since these movies were made to frighten teenagers and adults, this information should come as no surprise to you. Frequent exposures to violent material can also cause a child to become insensitive to human suffering. The impact of these movies on disturbed children may go a step further: Some of them try to imitate the movies.

Causes—Most bad reactions are to R-rated movies containing horror, graphic violence, or sexual violence. The content of violent movies has changed over the last 20 years. Mutilation is the message. Thanks to improved special effects, we can now see the details of torture or brutality in slow, agonizing close-up. Recent movies show a head being chopped off, a brain being blown up, the disfigurement of a face with a knife, a neck being slashed, or a hypodermic needle being plunged into an eyeball.

The 12-and-under age group is most at risk for severe reactions. Most elementary-school children don't have the adult defense mechanisms needed to cope with these movies. They are most threatened by movie villains who seem real and play on their deepest fears (e.g., surprise attack, kidnapping, torture, or death). They are especially vulnerable if they identify with the victim in the movie. Some of these mad slashers (unlike real people) are portrayed as indestructible and leave the young viewer feeling helpless. Children less than 7 or 8 also think concretely: If it can happen on the screen, it could happen to them tonight.

Access to these violent movies has also changed. The uncut versions of violent movies are now readily available through cable or satellite TV and video rentals. Parents say, "I didn't know she was watching that. I can't keep track of everything she sees." A popular party game in middle school involves renting a horror movie and seeing how much of it your friends can watch before becoming ill.

Most of the research done on the impact of violence on children has used TV violence. This research shows that TV affects children's behavior. No research review committee will ever approve a study in which children are exposed to R-rated movies. You don't have to be a psychiatrist to know that viewing graphic violence in movies (which is much more powerful than anything on TV) is harmful to children. Yet some parents allow it.

Expected Course—Without treatment, these fears and preoccupations can last 1 to 6 months. With treatment, they usually improve over a few weeks.

Protecting Your Child from Movie Violence

Understand the Movie Rating System—Don't lump all R-rated movies together. The R rating means that children under 17 are not admitted without a parent. It is given for nudity, profanity, violence, or a combination of the above. Nudity, depending on the context, may be harmless. Profanity in the movies has contributed to the common use of profanity on elementary-school playgrounds, and this trend is probably irreversible. It is violence in movies that has the most disturbing impact on children. In fact, if one reads the ratings carefully, the degree of violence is also often listed (e.g., graphic violence or rape).

Forbid All R-Rated Movies Before Age 13—Never allow a child who is less than 13 years of age to see any R-rated film, no matter how liberal you may be about nudity and profanity. Between 13 and 17, the maturity and sensitivity of your child must be carefully considered in deciding when he is ready to deal with some of these movies. Don't allow your child to see movies with personal or sexual violence (graphic violence) before age 17. These movies are not a required part of life experiences at any age.

Select Your Child's Movies—Don't let your child see a movie unless you know the rating and have read a review. Don't give in to their pressure to see something that is potentially harmful (that's an adult decision). Keep a list of movies you approve of.

Monitor What Your Child Is Watching on TV—Don't allow him to turn on the cable movie channel unless he has your permission to view a specific program. Even some of the edited versions of movies on network TV can be too frightening for young children. Don't let your younger children watch the programs that you have approved only for your older children (including the evening news). Young children who have viewed fires, tornadoes, earthquakes, warfare, or terrorism on the news have become worried about their personal safety.

Warn Your Child About Violent Movies Outside the Home—Protect your youngster from being unintentionally victimized by film violence. Be especially vigilant about slumber parties or Halloween parties. Tell your child to call you if the family he is visiting or a babysitter is showing any scary movies. Teach him to walk out of movies that make him scared or upset. Warn him to obey theater policies and not to sneak into R-rated movies.

Discuss Any Movie That Upsets Your Child—Respect your child's fears; don't make fun of them. Help him talk about what scared him. Help him gradually come to grips with the situation.

Prevention—Protect your child's mental health from unnecessary fears. R-rated movies are never harmless for children in elementary school. Use the movie ratings and your common sense to choose age-appropriate movies for your child. Never let your child see anything that frightens you.

TICS (Twitches)

Symptoms and Characteristics

- Tics (also called habit spasms) are rapid, repeated muscle twitches.
- Eye-blinking, facial-grimacing, forehead-wrinkling, head-jerking, and shoulder-shrugging are the most common types.
- Most tics last only 1 second.
- Tics increase with stress.
- Tics decrease with relaxation.
- Tics disappear during sleep.
- Tics occur in 20 percent of children.
- They occur in boys 3 times more frequently than in girls.
- The peak age is 6 to 10 years.

Causes—Most motor tics are due to inherited biochemical differences, not emotional problems. Flurries of tics, however, reflect the spilling over of emotional tension and mean your child is under pressure. All tics are involuntary, not deliberate.

Tics usually occur in normal, bright, sensitive children. Tics are more severe in children who are shy or overly conscientious. Tics can be accentuated by critical parents who nag, pressure for achievement beyond the child's ability, or draw negative comparisons to siblings.

Expected Outcome—If tics are ignored, they will usually disappear in 2 months to 1 year's time. If extra effort is made to help the child relax, they will usually improve more quickly. Without intervention, most children with tics have spontaneous improvement or clearing at adolescence. Approximately 3 percent of children with tics develop incapacitating tics if they are not handled appropriately.

How to Help Your Child with Tics

Help Your Child Relax in General—Tics are a barometer of inner tension. Make sure your child has free time and fun time every day. If he or she is overscheduled with activities, try to lighten the commitments.

If your child is unduly self-critical, praise him more and remind him to be a good friend to himself.

Identify and Remove Specific Environmental Stresses—Keep a tic diary. Whenever your child has a flurry of tics, write down the date, time, and the preceding event. From this diary, you should be able to identify some of your child's pressure points. (Note: Your child shouldn't be aware you are keeping this diary.) In any event, reduce the amount of criticism that your child receives about grades, music lessons, sports, keeping his or her room clean, table manners, and so forth. Avoid stimulant medications (such as decongestants), which can lower the threshold for tics.

Ignore Tics When They Occur—When your child is having tics, don't call his or her attention to them. Reminders imply that they are bothering you. If your child becomes worried about the tics, then every time they occur, the child will react with tension rather than acceptance. The tension in turn will trigger more tics (a vicious cycle). Don't allow siblings or others to tease your child about the tics. Be sure that relatives, friends, and teachers also abide by this approach. When tics occur, people should focus on reducing any pressure they may be causing the child.

Don't Talk About Tics When They Are Not Occurring—Stop all family conversation about tics. The less said about them, the less your child will be apprehensive about their occurring. If your child brings up the topic, say something reassuring, such as "Eventually your face muscles will learn to relax and the tics will go away."

Avoid Any Punishment for Tics—Some parents have the mistaken idea that tics are a bad habit that can be broken. This idea is absolutely false. Also, having children practice tic control in front of a mirror usually makes them realize they can't control the tics. Any facial exercises or massage should also be discontinued, because they just draw undue attention to the problem.

Call Your Child's Physician During Office Hours If

- The tics interfere with friendships or studies at school.
- The tics involve sounds, words, or profanity.
- The tics involve coughing.
- The tics involve parts of the body other than the head, face, or shoulders.

- The tics become frequent (more than 10 each day).
- The tics have lasted for more than a year.
- The tics are not better after trying this program for 1 month.
- You have other questions or concerns.

NAIL-BITING HABIT

Most school-age children nibble their nails occasionally. Some 40 percent of youngsters and 20 percent of adults are chronic nail biters. Some children just bite their cuticles. Before clippers and knives were invented, everyone may have chewed off their fingernails. In general, this is a harmless habit. Occasionally a child will cause some bleeding or minor infection of the cuticle. Trying to break a nail-biting habit by reminding, nagging, scolding, or punishment never works. Unless a child wants to stop, intervention won't be effective. The following measures may help:

- Keep the edges of the fingernails filed, since rough edges are irresistible to the nail-biter.
- For children younger than 4 or 5 years, distract them when they are biting their nails.
- For children over 4 or 5 years of age, tell them that nail-biting doesn't look good. If they wish to continue, it should be done in a private place. In general, don't try to change a nail-biting habit unless the child wants some help.
- For children over age 4 or 5 years who want to give up the nail-biting habit, other habits can be substituted. The child can be encouraged to chew gum or fidget with worry beads (smooth stones) or a toy. The child should also be provided with a good clipper for cutting the cuticles and a good file for smoothing off rough nails.
- Identify and relieve any obvious tensions that are present in the home. Some children chew their nails mainly when under pressure or stress. For most nail-biters, however, stress is not an important factor.
- In general, since this is a harmless habit, the parent should ignore it and trust that eventually peer pressure at school, or concern about appearance during the teenage years, will reduce its frequency.

FAMILY ISSUES

THE WORKING MOTHER: JUGGLING CHILDREN, HOME, AND CAREER

The Decision to Work

Reasons for Working—At this time only 10 percent of American households have a full-time homemaker-mother. More than 60 percent of mothers with infants are working outside the home. The frequency is even higher for mothers of preschoolers.

The reasons for working outside the home are many. In some families, it is financial need, as in a single-parent family. Other mothers work because two incomes are needed to sustain a middle-class lifestyle. For some mothers it is the personal preference for work over housekeeping and mothering. For others it is essential for staying up-to-date in a fast-changing career, as well as for the fulfillment work brings. It has often been said that a satisfied parent makes a better parent.

The question of returning to work versus staying at home has no easy or correct answer. The decision is one that each parent must make based on her particular circumstances. Children can do well with either approach; the family's needs are the main issue.

Pros and Cons for Your Child—If you can provide your child with a consistent nurturing caretaker, there is no evidence that your return to work will cause your child any harm. Children of working mothers develop as well emotionally as do other children. Working does not weaken the mother-child bond. In fact, there are some benefits for your child in having a working mother. These include increased independence, responsibility, and maturity. Young children of working mothers learn to trust other adults and to negotiate with peers. (The stay-at-home mother must provide extra adult and peer contact to achieve similar social skills.) Other advantages include, for girls, having higher career aspirations and, for boys, learning that fathers share in housework. Each parent must decide how important it is for her to be present during her child's early years. Research does not document any dire consequences to the children of working mothers, except that day care brings increased infections (but usually minor ones, such as colds).

Timing the Return to Work—A mother should try to remain at home for 6 to 8 weeks after the birth of her baby in order to recover physically from normal childbirth and establish breast-feeding. A preferred maternity leave might extend to 4 months after the birth, at which time the mother would have developed greater confidence regarding her mothering skills and have a baby who sleeps through the night. Unfortunately, few mothers can return to work at the time of their preference. Many mothers need to return to work because of financial realities and the limits of subsidized leave. At this time only 40 percent of jobs provide any paid maternity leave, and a smaller percentage guarantee job security through unpaid leave until the baby is 4 months of age. In fact, the United States is the only advanced nation without federal legislation guaranteeing maternity leave. (Over 100 nations do have such leave.)

The optimal length of maternity leave is unknown and should probably be based upon individual preference. Some authorities suggest that mothers should attempt to be a full-time parent during the first 2 or 3 years of their babies' lives. In the best of all worlds I would agree, but the advantages of this commitment remain unproven. Mothers should not feel guilty about returning to work when their babies are 2 to 4 months of age. But during the early years, try to find part-time or at-home employment.

Child-Care Resources

Types of Child Care—Several types of child care are available in most communities. During the first 2 years of life, children often do better with individual care or family day care because they need more cuddling and personal attention. The child-care arrangements are listed in descending order of preference for younger infants.

- *Individual care in your own home.* This is the preferred arrangement for infants. The care is usually provided by a grandmother or professional sitter. Often the parents will need to advertise in the local newspaper.

The applicant's references need to be carefully checked, especially for characteristics that are important to you. While most professional sitters provide part-time services, some are available as live-ins (a nanny).

- *Individual care in someone else's home.* This arrangement is very similar to the previous one except that your child will not have the extra stability of being cared for in his or her own home. In addition, you will need to pack diapers, bottles, and toys, as well as to transport your child to the sitter's home.

- *Family child-care homes.* In these settings a mother may care for 2 to 5 children in her home. This is the most common type of day care used for young children and it's usually less expensive than center-based care. Disadvantages are that the children do not usually receive as much individual attention, and some of these homes are not licensed or monitored by the state.

- *Center-based child care.* In these settings 30 or more children may be cared for. Because of the numbers, many children do not adapt well to these large centers until they are over age 2 or 2½ years. Optimal day-care centers are workplace-based, but they remain uncommon in our country. Day-care centers are state-licensed and must comply with certain standards. If you are looking for a day-care center, assemble a list from friends or by looking in the Yellow Pages under "Child Care" or "Day Nurseries and Child Care."

The Substitute Caregiver: Choosing the Right Person—The most important factor in your decision about choosing a child-care resource is finding a caretaker who understands and meets children's emotional needs. Choose someone who is warm, affectionate, sympathetic, plays with the children, and has a sense of humor. Avoid someone who is harsh, fussy, nagging, regimented, or overly concerned with neatness, cleanliness, and order. Try to find someone who understands children's normal emotional development. Look for someone who listens to and complies with your expectations (e.g., no spanking, and similar toilet-training methods). Form a close partnership with your child's caregiver. Choose a center that has a staff with a positive attitude toward parents, and then support that staff for what they provide for your child. Competition and rivalry are unnecessary if you've chosen well. Be sure that no more than two consistent caregivers are assigned to your child. More than three or four parent-equivalents (including the parents) can cause confusion and lack of security for a young child.

Choosing the Right Child-Care Environment—Don't make your final decision about a child-care center until you have visited it for at least half a day. Children deserve high standards of care. During your visit review the following checklist.

- The ratio of staff to children should be 1:3 for infants (especially for those who don't feed themselves) and 1:4 to 1:6 for preschool children, depending upon their age. By and large these ratios are regulated by each state.
- Each child has a regular primary caregiver assigned.
- The staff turnover is low.
- The playground is safe.
- Sinks and toilets are adequate.
- Diapers are changed promptly, not on some schedule.
- Space and time are adequate for rest and naps.
- Young infants are put down to sleep on their backs and on a firm surface.
- Staff members wash their hands after changing diapers and before handling food.
- The staff doesn't smoke on the premises.
- Toys are age appropriate. Pictures on the walls are child-oriented and at their eye level.
- Baby walkers are not used.
- A TV or VCR with tapes is absent or viewed minimally.
- The center's atmosphere is positive when one enters it.
- The children appear happy and busy.
- The children receive individualized attention.
- The children receive plenty of verbal stimulation. (Be concerned if the setting is too quiet or too loud.)
- The preschoolers receive some learning activities.
- The staff works through praise and suggestion rather than criticism and punishment.
- Staff members are warm, affectionate, and not afraid to hug the children.
- The staff welcomes you as a visitor at any time.
- The staff welcomes your suggestions and questions.
- The staff provides feedback about each child at the time of pickup, especially if anything significant has happened.

Helping Your Child Adjust to Child Care—All parents occasionally need to leave their child with another caretaker while they go to an appointment, go shopping, or go out for an evening. Day care is simply an extension of this concept. However, your child will not be ready to adjust to a day-care setting unless the child has had previous successful experiences with a baby-sitter within your home. Also, before beginning day care, your child should have had ample opportunity to visit with other children in friends' homes. Because of the separation fears that children normally experience between 6 months and 2½ years of age, being left at day care can initially be somewhat stressful during this time. Talk about the day-care center before you actually go there. Then visit it briefly, pointing out the positive aspects.

When you take your child to day care for the first day, plan on spending that day there. Let your child gradually reach out and become involved with the other children and staff. On the second day, stay 5 or 10 minutes while your child makes a transition to interacting with a member of the day-care staff. Leave a familiar toy or security object with your child. If the day-care center is near your workplace, visit your child during the day. When you leave, do so with a cheerful attitude and let your child know you are leaving—don't sneak away. Don't be surprised if your child gets teary on the first days that you depart from the day-care center. When you pick your child up, there may also be tears. For the first week your child may talk about not wanting to return. Remain firm in your decision and your child will gradually adapt to the change. Some children take as long as 1 or 2 months to look forward to attending day care. Usually, this process cannot be hurried.

Dealing with a Sick Child—The onset of illness can be a major disruption for the working mother. Many day-care centers will not accept sick children. Your options are: staying home with your child, using your sick leave; having your spouse take time off from work and stay home with your child; or having your child stay with a friend or relative who has agreed in advance to be a backup for illness care. Rarely, a parent may have the type of job in which an employer will allow an employee to work at home for a day under these conditions.

Some communities have special child-care centers for sick children. These facilities allow children with moderate illness to receive the extra care they need outside of their own home without exposing well children to illness. These facilities rarely make enough money to cover their expenses and are often subsidized by community agencies. Some large corporations provide sick-child care in an attempt to offset the costs of working-mother absenteeism. Check with local agencies or the National Association for Sick Child Daycare (www.nascd.com) to see what's available in your community. Care for sick children generally is more expensive than regular child care.

When a child becomes sick, the parents first have to decide whether or not their child needs to see a physician. Refer to the guidelines in this book that pertain to your child's symptoms to help answer this question. If your child becomes sick during the working day and your review of his illness indicates that he needs to see a physician, try to arrange for a late-afternoon appointment by calling before 3:00 P.M. In addition, many physicians are scheduling evening clinic hours to accommodate the high numbers of working parents.

A second decision that a working parent must make is when the child is well enough to return to day care. Children with a sore throat, moderate cough, runny nose, or cold symptoms (but without a fever or breathing difficulties) can usually return to day care. In the first place, day care is where they acquired the infection. In the second place, the spread of colds cannot be prevented. The return should be based mainly on how well your child feels. Children with fevers, chicken pox, vomiting, or diarrhea cannot return to a regular day-care setting until symptoms are gone. Children with strep throat or an eye infection can usually return after 24 hours on an antibiotic. Many child-care centers have their own rules about which children will be excluded, and you should become familiar with these rules (see CONTAGIOUS DISEASES AND INCUBATION PERIODS, page 231).

Latchkey Children (Self-Care)—A latchkey child is a school-age child who is left alone either before or after school while his parent is at work. The name comes from the wearing of a house key around the neck. This practice of self-care has been estimated to occur for 3 million children between 6 and 12 years of age, and 7 million children between 12 and 18 years of age. Elementary-school-age children often develop fears from being left alone. They feel unsafe, lonely, and neglected.

The following recommendations may make the practice more acceptable.

• Children shouldn't be left alone unless they are over 10 years of age.

• They should not spend more than 2 hours per day alone—which means they should not be left alone during school holidays or when they are sick.

- They should be taught how to handle household emergencies and what telephone numbers to call for assistance.
- A safe play area should be designated.
- They should not be left with too many chores, because they need time for schoolwork and entertainment.
- Sometimes the availability of pets will provide a sense of protection and companionship.
- The parents should be available by telephone and periodically call the children during this time. Children should also have a backup adult who lives close by and whom they can call or visit if they have any questions.
- The parents should be punctual about the time at which they promise they will come home.

Since the latchkey-child practice is clearly a compromise, the availability of after-school services for these children in schools, community centers, or churches is a welcome development.

Surviving Each Day as a Working Mother

Being a working mother is always harder and more stressful than being a full-time mother, because the main caregiver and housekeeper roles are never completely absorbed by other people. The following recommendations may help you balance career and family.

Look for a Supportive Employer and Workplace—If it's financially acceptable, try to find part-time work. Some employers offer flexible schedules, with a set number of hours per week fulfilled during different times of the day. This arrangement allows a parent to leave early for a soccer game or special event at school. Other jobs allow the employee to work in her home. Job sharing by two parents, each working 20 hours per week, is another alternative. Clearly the options are changing rapidly in our country. However, many women with financial needs or career obligations continue to work 40 or more hours per week.

Avoid Sleep Deprivation—If you can't get enough sleep, nothing else will seem to turn out right. You won't have the initiative to nurture your children at the end of the day. You won't have the energy necessary to maintain a marriage or friendships. Pick a reasonable bedtime and stay with it. Cut corners in other areas but protect your sleep time. And by all means, prevent sleep problems by teaching your infant to put herself to sleep (page 258).

Provide Quality Time with Your Child—Working parents spend a lot of energy trying to make up to their children for not being with them all day. Research has shown that both the quality and quantity of time you spend with your child are important. If you interact with your child, actively listen to him, talk with him, and keep it pleasant, that's quality time. Children need some quality time with their parents every day. Let's look at how you can turn scattered moments during a typical day into quality time.

- Talk with your child during the drive to and from child care without the radio or other distraction.
- Include your child in adult activities such as shopping, cooking, and home repair. As long as you make him feel important or even helpful, this is quality time.
- When you first get home from work, try to snuggle with your kids for 5 minutes (giving them the first 30 minutes, as some experts suggest, is usually impractical unless you are still breast-feeding). Then give them something to do and look after yourself. Your day was probably much more stressful than theirs, and you may need to regroup as well as prepare dinner.
- Make dinner a pleasant, unhurried time, with the TV off.
- Use the 30 minutes before bedtime to discuss the day's events at your child's pace. End with your usual bedtime ritual.
- If you're providing some of this quality contact every day, you're doing great.
- A common mistake of working parents is to think that bed-sharing is quality time. This isn't a good choice. If your child is asleep in your bed, we could call this neutral time. If your child is awake and crying, it's aggravating for everyone. If you want to provide extra quality time with your child, set aside some special half days on the weekend for family child-centered activities.

Reduce Your Housework Time—If you can afford it, hire a housekeeper. In any case, try to simplify your home life. A spotless house must become a low priority. Do less cooking. On the weekends, make triple recipes and freeze leftovers.

Ask Other Family Members for Help—It is imperative that the spouse share with the housework and child care. The father must actively participate in what was formerly considered the mother's responsibilities. He must be more than "available" or a "backup." He must look after more than outside work and the car. Child care and housework tasks must be redistributed to prevent the mother from becoming overworked. The father can help buy a son's clothing, carpool, cook, and do housecleaning chores. School-age children can also be assigned some chores.

Watch Out for Guilt—Try to understand that the "supermom" who does and has it all is a myth. You can't do everything singlehandedly or perfectly. You need help and deserve help. Don't compare yourself to other mothers or necessarily expect support from your mother, friends, or relatives for your pursuit of a career. You don't need to apologize to anyone for not doing well enough. If you have chosen a good child-care resource, you should be comfortable during the day with your child's well-being. And despite your best efforts, your child will sometimes cry when dropped off at child care, become sick, or fall apart when picked up. Try not to rethink your career decision every time this happens.

Nurture Your Marriage—One major loss for a working mother is recreational time with her husband. Try to compartmentalize your life. You deserve a break from your endless list of unfinished work. Make a date for a night out with your husband once a week or as often as finances permit. Consider it an investment. A strong marriage is an important underpinning for a working mother. Relaxation time is essential, not frivolous or wasteful. Plan it and savor it.

Nurture Yourself as an Individual—Carve out time occasionally to go out with girlfriends, to an exercise class, to a book club, or whatever makes you feel whole again. Trade weekend child-care shifts with your spouse to free up some individual time.

Single-Parent Families: Extra Help—In the United States today over 30 percent of children live in single-parent households. Mobilizing a support system consisting of your family, friends, and neighbors is essential. Try to find a friend with a child close in age to yours. Share shopping, overnight and weekend visits, baby-sitting, carpooling, and other responsibilities with your friend. Trading services will, in this way, save you money. Sometimes, living with another single mother is mutually beneficial. It's crucial that you spend time with other adults and do something for yourself once in a while. Consider joining a support group for single parents. Look for courses on survival skills for single parents at community colleges.

DIVORCE'S IMPACT ON CHILDREN

More than 1 million children are affected by divorce each year. Over a third of U.S. marriages end in divorce. Our primary goal should be to minimize the emotional harm to these children. The main way to achieve this is to help them maintain a close and secure relationship with both parents. The following recommendations may help your child cope with divorce:

Keep Your Child Informed—Tell your child about the separation or divorce before the actual departure of one parent. Preferably, both parents and all children should be present at that meeting. The following topics may serve as a good agenda.

Reassure Your Child That Both Parents Love Him—Clarify that although you are unhappy with each other and disagree about many things, the one subject you both completely agree on is "We love you." Demonstrating this love by time together is even more important. Preschoolers need lots of cuddling from both parents, but don't start bad habits like letting your child sleep with you.

Keep Constant as Many Parts of Your Child's World as You Can— The fewer changes, the better your child will cope with the stress of divorce. Try to keep your child in the same home or neighborhood. If this is impossible, at least try to keep your child in the same school with the same teachers, friends, and sports teams (even if it's on a temporary basis). Reassure your child that although your standard of living may decrease some, you will continue to have the basic necessities of living (i.e., food, clothing, and shelter).

Reassure Your Child That the Noncustodial Parent Will Visit— Young children are confused by divorce and fear that one parent may abandon them. Children need to know that they will have ongoing contact with their father (or mother, if the father has custody). The custodial parent should strongly support the visiting schedule. Your child needs both parents. Have a scheduled, predictable time for visiting. One full day every 1 or 2 weeks is usually preferable to more frequent, rushed, brief visits. Your child will eagerly look forward to visiting, so the visiting parent must keep promises, be punctual, and remember birthdays and other special events. If there is more than one child, all should spend equal time or the same time with the noncustodial parent to prevent favoritism. Try not to do too much in one day. Even more important, both parents should work to make these visits pleasant. Allow your child to tell you he had a good time during the visit with your ex-spouse. Children should also be provided with the telephone number of the non-custodial parent and encouraged to call at regular intervals. If the noncustodial parent has moved to a distant city, telephone calls and letters become essential to the ongoing relationship.

If the Noncustodial Parent Becomes Uninvolved, Find Substitutes—Turn to relatives, neighbors, teachers, and Big Brother or Big Sister volunteers to spend more time with your son or daughter. Explain to your child, "Your dad [or mom] is not capable right now of being available for you. He's sorting out his own problems. There's not much we can do to change that." Help your child verbalize his or her sense of disappointment and loss. If your child is a teenager, writing and calling may eventually reengage the absent parent.

Help Your Child Talk About Painful Feelings—At the time of separation and divorce, many children experience symptoms of anxiety, depression, and anger, as would be seen with any crisis. They are frequently on the brink of tears, sleep poorly, have stomachaches, experience a decline in school performance, and so forth. To help these symptoms pass, encourage your child to talk about these unhappy feelings and respond with understanding and support. A divorce discussion group at school can help children counter the isolation and shame they often feel. Allow feelings to be expressed honestly. But if anger turns into acting-out behavior, limits must be imposed while you help your child put the anger into words. Books about other children of divorce who deal with feelings of sadness but ultimately emerge stronger can provide reassurance.

Make Sure Your Child Understands That He Is Not Responsible for the Divorce—Children often feel guilty, believing that they somehow caused the divorce. Your children need reassurance that they did not in any way cause the divorce.

Clarify That the Divorce Is Final—Some children hold on to a wish to reunite the parents and pretend that the separation is temporary. Clarifying that the divorce is final can help children mourn their loss and move on to more adaptive functioning.

Try to Protect Your Child's Positive Feelings About Both Parents—
If possible, mention the good points about the other parent. Don't be
overly honest about your negative feelings toward your ex-spouse. (You
need to unload these feelings on another adult, not your children.)
Devaluing or discrediting the other parent in your child's presence can
reduce your child's personal self-esteem and create greater stress.

Don't ask your child to take sides. A child does not need to have loyalty to just one parent. Your child should not have to choose between parents. Your child should be able to love both of you, even though you don't
love each other.

Maintain Normal Discipline in Both Households—Children need
consistent child-rearing practices. Overindulgence or leniency by one
parent makes it more difficult for the other parent to get the child to behave. Constant competition for the child's love through gifts or special
privileges leads to a spoiled child. Reasonable ground rules regarding
discipline should be enforced by both parents.

Don't Argue About Your Child in the Child's Presence—Children
are quite upset by seeing their parents fight. Most important, avoid any
arguments regarding visiting, custody, or child support in your child's
presence. Try to resolve your remaining differences in a civilized way.

Try to Avoid Custody Disputes—Your child badly needs a sense of stability. Challenge custody only if the custodial parent is causing obvious
harm or repeated distress to your child. False accusations of physical
abuse or sexual abuse cause great emotional anguish for the child. If possible, don't split siblings unless they are adolescents and state a clear preference for living in different settings.

Call Your Child's Physician During Office Hours If

- Your child has symptoms that interfere with schoolwork, eating, or
  sleeping for more than 2 weeks.
- You feel your child is depressed.
- Your child has any physical symptoms, due to the divorce, lasting for
  more than 6 months.
- Your child continues to believe that the parents will come back to-
  gether again, even though over a year has passed since the divorce.
- You feel the other parent is harming your child.
- Your child refuses visits with the noncustodial parent.

ADOLESCENTS: DEALING WITH NORMAL REBELLION

The main task of adolescence in our culture is to become psychologically emancipated from the parents. The teenager must cast aside the dependent relationship of childhood. Before he can develop a new adult relationship with his parents, the adolescent must first distance himself from the parents of his past and gain control of his life. This process is characterized by a certain amount of intermittent normal rebellion, defiance, discontent, turmoil, restlessness, and ambivalence. Emotions usually run high. Mood swings are common. Even teenagers who have a mild transition into adolescence hurt their parents' feelings repeatedly with clear messages of "Leave me alone" and "I don't need you."

This stage usually starts at ages 12 to 14. Under the best of circumstances, this adolescent rebellion continues for approximately 2 years. Not uncommonly it continues for 4 to 6 years. Rebellion can be accentuated or prolonged for the teenager who is doing poorly in school and is unsure of his or her adult role. The teen with a difficult temperament (who had a terrible phase of negativism in the preschool period) is also likely to have a difficult adolescence. Parental high standards or expectations cause teens to overreact as well. Defiance will become very intense if the parent tries to eliminate any signs of normal rebellion and regain control over the teenager.

Practical Approaches to Living with an Adolescent

Treat Your Teenager as an Adult Friend—Whatever relationship you would like to have with your child as an adult, start working on it by age 12. Treat your child the way you would like him or her to treat you as an adult. Your goal is mutual respect, support, and having fun together. Strive for relaxed, casual conversations during bicycling, hiking, playing catch, fishing, cooking, working, driving, and especially at mealtime. Use praise and trust to help build self-esteem. Recognize and validate your child's feelings by listening carefully and making nonjudgmental comments. Remember that listening doesn't mean you have to solve your teen's problems. The friendship model is the best basis for family functioning. In this model people do things for each other out of caring and loyalty. (It doesn't mean bending your behavior or values in an attempt to be popular with your teenager.)

Avoid Criticism About No-Win Topics—Most negative parent-adolescent relationships are caused by too much criticism and pressure to change. Much of the objectionable behavior merely reflects conformity with the current preferences of the youngster's peer group. Peergroup immersion is one of the essential stages of adolescent development. Dressing, talking, and acting differently from adults help your child feel independent from you. So back off, as your teenager would say.

Try not to attack your teenager's clothing, hair style, makeup, music, dance steps, friends (unless they're in trouble with the law), recreational interests (such as movies, television, or hobbies), room decorations, how money or free time is spent, speech, posture, manners, religion, and philosophy. Allowing your teen to rebel in these minor areas often prevents testing in major areas—such as experimentation with drugs, truancy, or stealing. Intervene and try to make a change only if the behavior is harmful, illegal, or infringes on your rights (see CLARIFY THE HOUSE RULES AND CONSEQUENCES, page 421). Another error is to criticize your teen's mood, attitude, or facial expression. A negative or lazy attitude can only be changed through good example and praise. The more you dwell on these nontraditional (even strange) behaviors, the longer they will last.

Let Society's Rules and Consequences Teach Responsibility Outside the Home—Your teenager must learn from trial and error. As she experiments, she will learn to take responsibility for her decisions and actions. The parent should speak up only if the adolescent is going to do something dangerous or illegal. Otherwise, the parent must rely on self-discipline, positive peer pressure, and logical consequences (the school of hard knocks).

City curfew laws will help to control late hours. The requirement for punctual school attendance will influence when your teen goes to bed at night. If she has trouble getting up in the morning, buy her an alarm clock. School grades will usually hold your teenager accountable for homework and other aspects of school performance. (Prevent confusion by making clear your support for the rules imposed by the school and community. But it's not your job to check the homework.) If your teen has bad work habits, she will lose her job. If she selects an excessively violent movie, she may have nightmares. If your teenager makes a poor choice of friends, she may find her confidences broken or that she gets into trouble. If she doesn't practice hard for a sport, she will get pressure from the team and coach to do better. If she misspends her allowance or earnings, she will run out of money before the end of the month. If she abuses her freedom to choose clothes, her fixed clothing allowance will be spent before she buys something she needs, such as a bathing suit. (By age 16, your teenager should have a summer job. These earnings should cover most of the year's expenses, and any allowance can be discontinued.) If your teenager's mood or attitude is negative, she will lose friends.

If by chance your teenager asks you for advice about these problem areas, try to cover the pros and cons in a brief, impartial way. Ask some questions to help her think about the main risks. Then wrap up your remarks with a comment such as "Do what you think is best." Teenagers need plenty of opportunity to learn from their own mistakes before they leave home and have to solve problems without a support system.

Clarify the House Rules and Consequences—You have the right and the responsibility to make rules regarding your house and other possessions. Written ones cut down on misunderstandings. A teenager's preferences can be tolerated within his own room but they need not be imposed on the rest of the house. You can forbid loud music or incoming telephone calls after 10:00 P.M. that interfere with other people's concentration or sleep. You can forbid a TV set in his bedroom. While you should make your teen's friends feel welcome in your home, clarify the ground rules about parties or where snacks can be eaten. Your teen can be placed in charge of cleaning his own room, washing his clothes, and ironing his clothes. You can insist upon clean clothes and enough showers to prevent or overcome body odor. You must decide whether to loan out your car, bicycle, camera, radio, TV, clothes, and other possessions. To borrow the car, he must ask in advance, tell you his destination, clean the car after using it, and promise not to drive it if he drinks any alcohol.

Reasonable consequences for breaking house rules include loss of telephone, TV, stereo, and car privileges. (Time-out is rarely useful in this age group, and physical punishment can escalate to a serious breakdown in your relationship.) If your teenager breaks something, he should repair it, pay for its repair or replacement, or work for you until his debt is paid off. If he makes a mess, he should clean it up. If your teen is doing poorly in school, you can restrict TV time. You can also put a limit on telephone privileges and weeknights out. If your teen stays out too late or doesn't call you when he's delayed, you can ground him for a day or a weekend. In general, grounding for more than a few days is looked upon as unfair and is hard to enforce.

Use Family Conferences for Negotiating House Rules—Some families find it helpful to have a brief meeting after dinner once a week. At this time your teenager can ask for changes in the house rules or bring up family issues that are causing problems. You can also bring up issues (such as the demand to drive your teen to many places and your need for his or her help in arranging car pools). The family unit often functions better if the decision-making is democratic. The objective of negotiation should be that both parties win. The atmosphere can be one of: "Nobody is at fault; we have a problem. How can we solve it?"

Give Space to a Teenager Who Is in a Bad Mood—Generally when your teenager is in a bad mood, he or she won't want to talk about it with you. If teenagers want to discuss a problem with anybody, it will probably be with a close friend. In general, it is advisable at this time to give your teen lots of space and privacy. This is a poor time to talk to your teenager about anything, pleasant or otherwise.

Use "I" Messages for Rudeness—Some talking back is normal. We want our teenagers to express their anger through talking and to challenge our opinions in a logical way. We need to listen. Expect your teenager to present his case passionately, even unreasonably. Let the small stuff go; it's only words. But don't accept disrespectful remarks such as calling you a "jerk." Unlike a negative attitude, these mean remarks should be addressed. You can respond with a comment like "I really hurt inside when you put me down or don't answer my question." Make your statement in as nonangry a way as possible. If your adolescent continues to make angry, unpleasant remarks, leave. Don't get into a shouting match or game of uproar with your teenager because this behavior is not adaptable to outside relationships. Set a good example of the ability to express disapproval without insult or attack. If angry or rude remarks come up in the context of a complaint about something, try to overlook the rudeness and directly engage your teen in a discussion of the issue. If you can focus on objective problem-solving and keep a courteous tone of voice, often your teenager will be able to regain control over his or her emotions and remarks.

What you are trying to teach is that one has the right to disagree and even to express anger. However, screaming and rude conversation are not allowed in your house. When your teen is angry about something, he or she can explain what it is, but in a calm voice. Family friends and other visitors are also to be treated with respect. You can prevent some rude behavior by role-modeling politeness, constructive disagreement, and the ability to apologize.

Call Your Teenager's Physician During Office Hours If

- You think your teenager is depressed, suicidal, drinking or using illegal drugs, or going to run away.
- Your teenager is taking undue risks (e.g., reckless driving or unsafe sex).
- Your teenager has no close friends.
- Your teenager's school performance is declining markedly.
- Your teenager is skipping school frequently.
- Your teenager's outbursts of temper are destructive or violent.
- You feel your teenager's rebellion is excessive.
- Your family life is seriously disrupted by your teenager.
- You find yourself escalating the criticism and punishment.
- Your relationship with your teenager does not improve within 3 months using this approach.
- You have other questions or concerns.

VI. Common Symptoms and Illnesses

GENERAL SYMPTOMS OF ILLNESS

FEVER

Definition of Fever

- A fever means the body temperature is above normal.
- Rectal temperature over 100.4°F (38.0°C) is a fever.
- Oral temperature over 99.5°F (37.5°C) is a fever.
- Axillary (armpit) temperature over 99.0°F (37.2°C) is a fever.
- Pacifier temperature over 100°F (37.8°C) is a fever (not reliable under 3 months old).
- Ear (tympanic) temperature over 100.4°F (38.0°C) is a fever (not reliable under 6 months old).
- Temporal artery temperature over 100.4°F (38.0°C) is a fever (not reliable under 6 months old).
- Tactile (touch) fever is the impression that your child has a fever because he feels hot to the touch. Checking this way to see if your child has a fever is more accurate than we used to think. But if you're going to call the doctor, actually measure the temperature.
- While the body's average temperature is 98.6°F (37°C) orally, it normally fluctuates during the day from a low of 97.6°F in the morning to a high of 99.5°F in the late afternoon (called normal diurnal variation).
- Mild elevations of 100.4 to 101.2°F (38 to 38.5°C) can be caused by exercise, excessive clothing, a hot bath, or hot weather. Warm food or drink can elevate an oral temperature. If you suspect one of these causes, retake the temperature in a half hour, after eliminating the possible cause.

Similar Conditions—For CONVULSIONS WITH FEVER or DELIRIUM (acting very confused) with fever, go directly to those guidelines (see pages 41 and 45).

Taking the Temperature—If you have questions about how to take your child's temperature, see page 433.

Causes of Fever—Over 90 percent of fevers are due to viral infections (such as colds, coughs, diarrhea, or rashes). Fever is a symptom, not a disease. Fever is the body's normal response to infections and it plays a role in fighting them. Fever turns on the body's immune system, thereby increasing the release and activity of white blood cells and other germ–killing substances. The usual fevers (100 to 105°F) that all children get are not harmful. Most "fevers" that stay under 101°F are simply due to hot weather or overdressing. Teething does not cause fever.

Expected Course of Fever—Most fevers associated with viral illnesses range between 101 and 104°F and last for 2 to 3 days. In general, the height of the fever doesn't relate to the seriousness of the illness. How sick your child acts is what counts. Fever causes no symptoms such as being tired or cranky until it reaches 102 or 103°F. Fever causes no permanent harm (such as brain damage) until it reaches 108°F. Fortunately, the brain's thermostat keeps untreated fevers due to infections below 105° or 106°F. While all children get fevers, only percent develop a brief febrile convulsion. Since this type of seizure generally harmless, it is not worth worrying about, especially if your child has experienced high fevers without one.

Call Your Child's Physician
Immediately If

- Your child is difficult to awaken (call 911).
- Breathing is very difficult (call 911).
- Your child is drooling saliva and is unable to swallow anything (call 911).
- Your child is under 3 months old and has a fever (over 100.4°F or 38.0°C rectally).
- The fever is over 105°F.
- Your child is crying inconsolably or whimpering.
- Your child cries if you touch him or move him.

- The neck is stiff. (Note: The inability to touch the chin to the chest is an early symptom in meningitis.)
- Any purple spots or dark red dots are present on the skin.
- A convulsion has occurred and stopped.
- Your child acts or looks very sick. (Note: If your child hasn't received acetaminophen, recheck his condition 1 hour after giving him a proper amount.)
- Burning or pain occurs with urination.

Within 24 Hours If
- Your child is 3 to 6 months old (unless fever is due to a DTaP shot).
- The fever repeatedly goes above 104°F.
- The fever has been present more than 24 hours without an obvious cause or location of infection.
- The fever went away for more than 24 hours and then returned.
- The fever has been present more than 72 hours.
- Your child has a history of febrile seizures.
- You think your child needs to be seen.

Home Care for Fever

Fever Phobia and the Overtreatment of Fever—*Fever phobia* is a term I coined in 1980 to describe the unwarranted fears many parents hold about normal fevers that all children experience. My study found that 80 percent of parents thought fevers between 100 and 106°F could cause brain damage. Some 20 percent of parents thought that if they didn't treat the fever, it would keep going higher. Neither of these statements is true. Because of these misconceptions, many parents treat low-grade fevers with unnecessary medicines and sponging. They also spend many sleepless nights worrying about their child's fever. Try to keep fever in perspective (see page 431) as you treat your child's fever.

Extra Fluids and Less Clothing—Encourage your child to drink extra fluids, but do not force him to drink. Popsicles and iced drinks are helpful. Body fluids are lost during fevers because of sweating. Bundling can be dangerous. Clothing should be kept to a minimum because most heat is lost through the skin. Do not bundle up your child; it will cause a higher fever. During the time your child feels cold or is shivering (the chills), give him a light blanket. If the fever is less than 102°F this is the only treatment needed. Fever medicines are not necessary.

Medicines to Reduce Fever—Remember that fever is helping your child fight the infection. Use drugs only if the fever is over 102°F (39°C) and preferably only if your child is also uncomfortable. Two hours after they are given, these drugs will reduce the fever 2 to 3°F (1 to 2°C). Medicines do not bring the temperature down to normal unless the temperature was not very elevated before the medicine was given. Repeated dosages of the drugs will be necessary because the fever will go up and down until the illness runs its course. If your child is sleeping, don't awaken him for medicines.

• *Acetaminophen.* Children older than 3 months of age can be given acet-aminophen (Tylenol). Give the correct dosage for your child's weight every 4 to 6 hours. See the dosage table on page 238.

• *Ibuprofen.* Ibuprofen (Advil, Motrin) is similar to acetaminophen in its ability to lower fever. Its safety record is also similar. The FDA has ap-proved it for infants over 6 months of age. One advantage ibuprofen has over acetaminophen is a longer-lasting effect (6 to 8 hours instead of 4 to 6 hours). Children with special problems requiring a longer period of fever control may do better with ibuprofen. Give the correct dosage for your child's weight every 6 to 8 hours. See the dosage table on page 240. (Caution: The dropper that comes with one product should not be used with other brands.)

• *Avoid aspirin.* Doctors recommend that children (through age 21 years) not take aspirin if they have any symptoms of a cold or viral infection, such as a fever, cough, or sore throat. Aspirin taken during a viral infec-tion, such as chicken pox or flu, has been linked to a severe illness called Reye's syndrome. If you have teens, since they tend to self-medicate, be sure they know to avoid aspirin.

Sponging for Fever—Sponging is usually unnecessary. Never sponge with-out giving acetaminophen or ibuprofen first. Sponge immediately only for semi-emergencies such as heat stroke, delirium from fever, a seizure from fever, or any fever over 106°F (41.1°C). For other children, sponge only if the fever is over 104°F (40°C), it stays above that level when you retake it 30 minutes after acetaminophen has been given, and your child is uncom-fortable. Until acetaminophen or ibuprofen has taken effect (by resetting the body's thermostat to a lower level), sponging will just cause shivering, which is the body's way of trying to raise the temperature.

Sponge your child in lukewarm water (85 to 90°F or 29 to 32°C). (Use slightly cooler water for emergencies.) Sponging works much faster than immersion, so sit your child in 2 inches of water and keep wetting the skin surface. Cooling comes from evaporation of the water. If your child shivers, raise the water temperature or wait for the medication to take effect. Don't expect to get the temperature down below 101°F. Don't add rubbing alcohol to the water; it can cause a coma or seizure if breathed in. Never leave your child alone in the tub; accidents can happen quickly. If your child is seizing or thrashing about, sponge him on some towels on the floor.

Retaking the Temperature—In general, take the temperature once a day in the morning until the fever is gone. Take it more often if your child feels very hot or is acting miserable despite receiving acetaminophen or ibuprofen; he may also need sponging. In addition, take it before calling your physician.

With most infections, the level of fever bounces around for 2 or 3 days. Shivering (or feeling cold) means the fever is going up, a flushed (pink) appearance means the fever has peaked, and sweating means it is coming down. The main purpose of temperature taking is to determine if a fever is present or absent, not to chart its every move.

Call Your Child's Physician Later If

- The fever goes over 104°F (40°C).
- The fever lasts more than 72 hours.
- You feel your child is getting worse.
- Your child develops any of the "Call your Child's Physician" symptoms.

Remember: The response, or lack of response, of the fever to medicines tells us little about the severity of the infection. If your febrile child smiles, plays, and drinks adequate fluids, you need not worry about the fever.

FEVER: MYTHS AND FACTS

Misconceptions about the dangers of fever are commonplace. Unwarranted fears about harmful side effects from fever cause lost sleep and unnecessary stress for many parents. Let the following facts help you put fever into perspective:

Myth: All fevers are bad for children.
Fact: Fevers turn on the body's immune system. Fevers are one of the body's protective mechanisms.

Most fevers are good for children and help the body fight infection. Use the following definitions to help put your child's level of fever into perspective:

100 to 102°F (37.8 to 39°C)	Low-grade fever: beneficial. Try to keep the fever in this range.
102 to 104°F (39 to 40°C)	Mild fever: beneficial.
Over 104°F (40°C)	Moderate fever: causes discomfort but still harmless.
Over 105°F (40.6°C)	High fever: higher risk of bacterial infections, so child needs to be examined. Fever level still harmless.
Over 106°F (41.1°C)	Very high fever: need to bring it down.
Over 108°F (42°C)	Dangerous fever: the fever itself can harm the brain.

Myth: Fevers cause brain damage or fevers over 104° (40°C) are dangerous.
Fact: Fevers with infections don't cause brain damage. Only body temperatures over 108°F (42°C) can cause brain damage. The body temperature goes this high only with high environmental temperatures (for example, if a child is confined in a closed car in hot weather).

Myth: Anyone can have a febrile seizure (seizure triggered by fever).
Fact: Only 4 percent of children have a febrile seizure.

Myth: Febrile seizures are harmful.
Fact: Febrile seizures are scary to watch, but they usually stop within 5 minutes. They cause no permanent harm. Children who have had febrile seizures do not have a greater risk for developmental delays, learning disabilities, or seizures without fever.

Myth: All fevers need to be treated with fever medicine.

Fact: Fevers need to be treated only if they cause discomfort. Usually that means fevers over 102 or 103°F (39 or 39.4°C).

Myth: Without treatment, fevers will keep going higher.
Fact: Because of the brain's thermostat, fevers from infection top out at 105 or 106°F (40.6 or 41.1°C) or lower.

Myth: With treatment, fevers should come down to normal.
Fact: With treatment, fevers usually come down 2 to 3°F (1.1 to 1.7°C).

Myth: If the fever doesn't come down (if you can't "break the fever"), the cause is serious.
Fact: Fevers that don't respond to fever medicine can be caused by viruses or bacteria. Whether the medicine works or not doesn't relate to the seriousness of the infection.

Myth: If the fever is high, the cause is serious.
Fact: If the fever is high, the cause may or may not be serious. If your child looks very sick, the cause is more likely to be serious.

Myth: The exact number of the temperature is very important.
Fact: How your child looks is what's important, not the exact temperature.

Myth: Temperatures between 98.7 and 100°F (37.1 and 37.8°C) are low-grade fevers.
Fact: The normal temperature changes throughout the day. It peaks in the late afternoon and evening. A low-grade fever is 100 to 102°F (37.8 to 39°C).

A reading of 99.4°F (37.4°C) is the average rectal temperature. It normally can change from 98.4°F (36.9°C) in the morning to a high of 100.3°F (37.9°C) in the late afternoon. A reading of 98.6°F (37°C) is just the average oral temperature. It normally can change from a low of 97.6°F (36.4°C) in the morning to a high of 99.5°F (37.5°C) in the late afternoon.

TEMPERATURE: HOW TO MEASURE IT

Getting an accurate measurement of your child's temperature takes practice. If you have questions about these instructions, ask your health-care provider to show you how it's done. Then ask your provider to watch you do it.

Where to Take the Temperature

A rectal (in the bottom) temperature is the most accurate. Temperatures measured by mouth, by electronic pacifier, or by ear are also accurate if done properly. Temperatures measured in the armpit are the least accurate, but they are better than no measurement. The best place to use the thermometer depends on the age of your child.

• For a baby less than 3 months old (90 days old), an armpit temperature is best because it is safest and and works fine for a quick check. If the armpit temperature is over 99°F (or 37.2°C), double-check it with a rectal temperature. It is good to double-check with a rectal temperature because if your baby has a true fever, you should see a health care provider immediately.

• For a child between 3 months and 4 or 5 years old, a rectal temperature or electronic pacifier thermometer are best. Using an ear thermometer is fine after 6 months old. An armpit temperature is fine for a quick check if done correctly.

• For a child older than 4 or 5 years old, take the temperature by mouth (orally).

How to Take a Rectal Temperature

1. If you are using a glass thermometer, shake until the mercury line is below 99°F (37.2°C). If you are using a digital thermometer, turn it on.

2. Have your child lie stomach down on your lap.

3. Before you insert the thermometer, put some petroleum jelly on the end of the thermometer and on the opening of the bottom (anus).

4. Insert the thermometer gently into the bottom about 1 inch. If your child is younger than 6 months old gently insert the thermometer only one-quarter to one-half inch. If you put the thermometer in just until the silver tip disappears, that is about one-half inch. Never try to force it past any resistance. Forcing could damage the bowel.

5. Hold your child still while the thermometer is in.

6. If you are using a glass thermometer, leave it in your child's bottom for 2 minutes before you take it out. If you are using a digital thermometer take it out when you hear the correct signal (usually a series of beeps).

7. Read the temperature on the thermometer. If you are using a glass

thermometer you may have to rotate the thermometer until you can see the end of the mercury line.

8. Fever is a rectal temperature over 100.4°F (38°C).

How to Take an Armpit (Axillary) Temperature

1. If you are using a glass thermometer, shake it until the mercury line is below 98.6°F (37°C).

2. Place the tip of the thermometer in a dry armpit.

3. Close the armpit by holding the elbow against the chest for 4 or 5 minutes. The tip of the thermometer must be covered by skin. Do not remove it before 4 minutes have passed.

4. After 4 or 5 minutes take the glass thermometer out and read the temperature by finding where the mercury line ends. You may need to rotate the thermometer until you can see the mercury. If you are using a digital thermometer remove it after you hear the signal (usually a series of beeps) and read the temperature on the screen.

5. Fever is an armpit temperature over 99°F (37.2°C). If you're not sure it is correct, check it by taking a rectal temperature.

How to Take an Oral (Mouth) Temperature

1. Be sure your child has not had a cold or hot drink in the last 30 minutes.

2. If you are using a glass thermometer, shake the thermometer until the mercury line is below 98.6°F (37°C). If you are using a digital thermometer, turn it on.

3. Place the tip of the thermometer under one side of the tongue and toward the back. An accurate temperature depends on putting it in the right place. Ask your health care provider to show you where it should go.

4. Have your child hold the thermometer in place with his lips and fingers (not his teeth). He should breathe through his nose, keeping his mouth closed. If your child can't keep his mouth closed because his nose is blocked, suction out the nose.

5. Leave the glass thermometer in the mouth for 3 minutes. Leave a digital thermometer in the mouth until you hear the correct signal (usually a series of beeps).

6. Read the temperature. If you are using a glass thermometer you may need to turn the thermometer until you can see where the mercury line ends.

7. Fever is an oral temperature over 99.5°F (37.5°C).

How to Take an Electronic Pacifier Temperature

1. Have your child suck on the pacifier until the temperature stops changing and you hear a beep. This usually takes 3 to 4 minutes.

2. Read the temperature. Fever is a pacifier temperature over 100°F (37.8°C).

How to Take an Ear Temperature

1. If your child has been outdoors on a cold day, he needs to be inside for 15 minutes before taking the temperature. (Earwax, ear infections, and ear tubes, however, do not interfere with accurate readings.)

2. Pull the ear backward to straighten the ear canal.

3. Place the end of the thermometer into your child's ear canal and aim the probe toward the eye on the opposite side of the head. Then press the button.

4. In about 2 seconds you can read the temperature.

5. Fever is an ear temperature over 100.4°F (38°C).

Types of Thermometers

Glass (with Mercury) Thermometers—This type of thermometer has been around since 1870. These are the least expensive thermometers. They have some disadvantages. They measure temperatures slowly and are often hard to read. If broken, they cause a mercury spill, which can be harmful and difficult to clean up. The American Academy of Pediatrics advises parents not to use mercury thermometers.

Glass thermometers come in two forms, oral with a thin tip and rectal with a rounder tip. This difference is not too important. If necessary, a rectal thermometer can be used in the mouth as long as the thermometer is cleaned with rubbing alcohol. An oral thermometer can be used in the rectum if you are extra careful when you put it in.

Digital Electronic Thermometers—Digital electronic thermometers measure temperatures with a heat sensor and require a button battery. They measure temperatures quickly, usually in less than 30 seconds. The temperature is displayed in numbers on a small screen. The same thermometer can be used to take both rectal and oral temperatures.

A study in *Consumer Reports* magazine found that digital thermometers were more accurate than glass thermometers. Buy one for your family. They cost about $10.00.

Ear Thermometers—Many hospitals and medical offices now take your child's temperature using an infrared thermometer that reads the temperature of the eardrum. In general, the eardrum temperature provides a measurement that is as accurate as the rectal temperature.

The biggest advantage of this thermometer is that it measures temperatures in less than 2 seconds. It also does not require cooperation by the child and does not cause any discomfort. Ear thermometers for use at home have been developed and they cost $30 to $40.

Digital Electronic Pacifier Thermometers—The new electronic pacifier thermometers have a heat sensor and are powered by a button battery. These pacifiers let you measure oral temperature in younger children. They are quite accurate if 0.5°F is added to the digital reading. It takes approximately 3 minutes to get a reading. They cost about $15.

Temperature Strips—Liquid crystal strips put on the forehead have been studied and have been found to be inaccurate. They do not detect an elevated temperature in most children with fever.

Touching the forehead is somewhat reliable for detecting fevers over 102°F (38.9°C) but tends to miss mild fevers.

Conversion of Degrees Fahrenheit (F) to Degrees Celsius (C)

Temperatures can be measured in degrees Fahrenheit (F) or degrees Celsius (C). Remember that 1°C equals 1.8°F and that 1°F equals 0.55°C. Despite attempts to learn metric, most Americans conceptualize fever in degrees Fahrenheit. The table below shows the temperatures in degrees Celsius that are equivalent to temperatures measured in degrees Fahrenheit:

95°F = 35°C
96.8°F = 36°C
98.6°F = 37°C

99°F	=	37.2°C
99.5°F	=	37.5°C
100°F	=	37.8°C
100.4°F	=	38°C
101°F	=	38.3°C
102°F	=	38.9°C
103°F	=	39.5°C
104°F	=	40°C
105°F	=	40.6°C
106°F	=	41.1°C
107°F	=	41.7°C
108°F	=	42.2°C

DECREASED APPETITE WITH ILLNESS

Symptoms and Characteristics
- Reduced food intake of recent onset
- Associated acute illness

If your child's symptoms are different, call your physician for help.

Cause—A falloff in appetite is normal with most minor illnesses. This is not harmful. It is not very helpful in assessing the seriousness or cause of the illness.

Home Care
Temporarily, serve your child his favorite foods. Let him decide how much he eats. Avoid the tendency to pressure him to eat more when he is sick. Usually, his fluid intake will remain normal and that is the only important aspect of diet during an illness. Look at other guidelines for information on the treatment of associated symptoms.

Call Your Child's Physician

Immediately If
- Your child is under 1 month old.
- Your child is not drinking adequate fluids.
- Your child has not urinated in more than 8 hours.
- Your child looks or acts very sick.

During Office Hours If

- Poor appetite lasts for more than 1 week.
- You feel your child is getting worse.

INCREASED SLEEP WITH ILLNESS

Most children sleep several extra hours a day when they are sick with any infectious illness. It helps them fight the illness and speeds recovery. Increased sleep is not very useful in judging the seriousness of the illness.

Call Your Child's Physician

Immediately If

- Your child is difficult to awaken (call 911).
- Your child could have taken any sleeping pills or other drugs (call 911).
- Your child is drowsy or confused when awake (rather than alert and thinking clearly).
- Your child is on any medicines that could cause drowsiness.
- Your child looks or acts very sick.

During Office Hours If

- Your child is otherwise not sick.
- Your child could be upset or depressed.
- You have other questions.

Home Care

Treatment—No special treatment is needed. Refer to the guidelines regarding the basic illness your child is suffering from.

- Remember that extra sleep helps recovery from any illness.

Call Your Child's Physician Later If

- The increased sleeping and tiredness last for more than 1 week.
- You feel your child is getting worse.
- Your child develops any of the "Call Your Child's Physician" symptoms.

Related Topic

DELIRIUM (see page 45)

DECREASED ACTIVITY WITH ILLNESS

Most children are less active when they are sick with an infectious illness. When they are awake, most of them prefer to be out of bed, watching television, or playing with toys.

Home Care

When children are sick, it is fine for them to choose their own level of activity. If they are feeling really bad, they will want to be in bed. Children naturally decrease their activity when they are sick. We probably don't trust this survival instinct because we know too many adults who go full speed ahead when they are sick.

Bed Rest Is Not the Answer

Mandatory bed rest is no longer recommended for treating childhood illnesses. These are the reasons:

- No evidence exists that enforced bed rest is helpful for common childhood illnesses. It doesn't reduce symptoms such as fever, despite the myth that children should stay in bed until their fever is gone. It doesn't help the body heal faster. It neither shortens the length of an illness nor prevents complications.
- The only medical conditions where bed rest is helpful are heart failure and respiratory failure. Children with these serious problems elect to remain in bed because of how badly they feel.
- Enforced bed rest is impossible to achieve. If you insist that your child stay in bed and leave the room, when you return you may find him using that bed as a trampoline.

SKIN: WIDESPREAD PINK OR RED RASHES

RASHES, UNKNOWN CAUSE (Widespread)

Symptoms and Characteristics

- Red or pink rash (erythema)
- Smooth or slightly bumpy
- Spots or solid red
- Over most of body (widespread or generalized)
- Not itchy

Similar Condition—Fever over 103 or 104°F can cause a pinkness of the skin. Sometimes it's blotchy. If it clears with fever reduction, it's normal fever erythema. If the rash is itchy, turn directly to the guideline on ITCHING, UNKNOWN CAUSE (WIDESPREAD), page 442.

Causes of Widespread Rashes—The possible causes of a non-itchy pink or red rash are many. If one of the following is suspected, save time by turning directly to that guideline.

AMOXICILLIN RASH (see page 443)
CHICKEN POX (VARICELLA) (see page 446)
HEAT RASH (MILIARIA) (see page 455)
MEASLES (RUBEOLA) (see page 458)
MEASLES VACCINE RASH (see page 460)
NEWBORN RASHES AND BIRTHMARKS (less than 2 weeks old) (see page 108)
ROSEOLA (see page 461)

SCARLET FEVER (see page 463)
SUNBURN (see page 503)

Expected Course—Depends on the diagnosis.

Call Your Child's Physician

Immediately If

- The rash is purple or blood-colored.
- It is bright red *and* tender to the touch.
- It looks like a burn.
- Your youngster is a female adolescent *and* she currently is having her menstrual period.
- Your child looks or acts very sick.

Within 24 Hours If

- Your child has a fever or sore throat.
- The rash has been present longer than 48 hours.
- Your child is taking a medicine.
- You think your child needs to be seen.

Home Care for Widespread Rashes

Treatment—Widespread rashes can occur with viral illnesses. No treatment is necessary. These rashes are unimportant and usually disappear within 48 hours.

Call Your Child's Physician Later If

- It lasts more than 48 hours.
- Your child develops any of the "Call Your Child's Physician" symptoms.

ITCHING, UNKNOWN CAUSE (Widespread)

Causes of Widespread Itching

The possible causes are many. If one of the following is suspected, turn directly to that guideline.

BITES: INSECT, BEE, OR TICK (see page 19)
CHICKEN POX (VARICELLA) (see page 446)

DRY SKIN (see page 449)
ECZEMA (ATOPIC DERMATITIS) (see page 450)
HEAT RASH (MILIARIA) (see page 455)
HIVES (URTICARIA) (see page 456)
PITYRIASIS ROSEA (see Glossary)
SCABIES (see Glossary)

Call Your Child's Physician

Immediately If
- Breathing or swallowing is difficult (call 911).
- The itching started immediately after your child took medicine, ate food he is allergic to, or was stung by an insect (call 911).

Within 24 Hours If
- The itching keeps your child from sleeping.

During Office Hours If
All other children with a widespread itchy rash need medical consultation. (Exception: If you know the cause and can eliminate it, proceed to HOME CARE, below.)

Home Care for Itchy, Widespread Rashes
The following measures may help to relieve itching regardless of the cause:
- Wash the skin once with soap to remove any irritants.
- Give your child cool baths without soap for 10 minutes every 3 to 4 hours. (Exception: If the cause is dry skin, see the guideline on page 449.)
- Follow with calamine lotion (no prescription needed) or a baking soda solution (1 teaspoon in 4 ounces water). For very itchy spots, apply 1 percent hydrocortisone cream (no prescription needed). (Exception: If the cause is chicken pox, see the guideline on page 446.)
- Encourage your child not to scratch. Cut the fingernails short.
- Since sweating aggravates itching, temporarily avoid excessive heat, sunbathing, exercise, or sleeping with several blankets.
- Since they cause dry skin, also avoid soaps and swimming pools.
- Your child should not wear itchy or tight clothes.

RASHES WHILE ON DRUGS

Most children who develop a rash while on a medication have a viral rash (viral exanthem) that is unrelated to the medicine (e.g., roseola). Another common rash is the type seen in children on amoxicillin (see AMOXICILLIN RASH, page 445). This is not an allergic rash (it's called a toxic rash), and the medicine can be continued.

Call Your Child's Physician

Immediately If

- Breathing or swallowing is difficult (call 911).
- The tongue is swollen (call 911).
- The rash is hives.
- The rash is very itchy.
- The rash is purple or blood-colored.
- The rash is bright red *and* tender to the touch.
- The rash looks like a burn.
- Your youngster is a female adolescent *and* she currently is having her menstrual period.
- Your child looks or acts very sick.

Within 24 Hours

- For all other widespread red rashes in association with drugs.

Note: Localized rashes are not due to drugs. (See the guideline on localized rashes, page 465.)

Home Care

Stopping the Medication—Once your child is labeled as being allergic to a medicine, he can never receive any drugs in that category (e.g., all penicillins) in the future. Hence this is a critical decision. Unless your physician tells you otherwise, have your child examined before stopping a medication.
Exceptions: (1) If your child has a severe rash *and* is taking antiseizure or sulfa drugs, stop the drugs. (2) If you are certain your child has hives.

Antibiotic Replacement—Anytime antibiotics are discontinued without completing the full course, the child must be seen within 24 hours to assess the need for a new antibiotic. Without this precaution, many children would have flare-ups of partially treated infections.

AMOXICILLIN RASH

Symptoms and Characteristics

- Pink or red spots
- Small, flat, and nonitchy spots
- Always on the trunk
- Spreads to the face in 50 percent of cases
- Occurs while taking amoxicillin
- Usual onset: day 5 from start of medicine (with a range of 1 to 16 days)

If your child's symptoms are different, call your physician for help.

Cause—From 5 to 10 percent of children taking amoxicillin get a skin rash. This is a harmless nonallergic rash and does not indicate any allergy to amoxicillin or penicillin.

Expected Course—The rash usually lasts 3 days, with a range of 1 to 6 days.

Call Your Child's Physician

Within 24 Hours If

- The rash looks like hives.
- The rash is itchy.
- Your child has any joint pains or swelling.
- You have other questions or concerns.

Home Care

No treatment is necessary.

Amoxicillin—Keep your child on the amoxicillin until it is gone. The rash will disappear just as quickly whether or not your child continues on amoxicillin. Your child can receive amoxicillin in the future when necessary and probably won't get a rash next time.

Call Your Child's Physician Later If

- The rash becomes itchy.
- The rash lasts more than 6 days.
- You feel it is a drug allergy.

CHICKEN POX (Varicella)

Symptoms and Characteristics

- Multiple small red bumps progress to thin-walled water blisters, then cloudy blisters or open sores, and finally dry brown crusts (all within 24 hours).
- Repeated crops of new chicken pox emerge for 4 to 5 days.
- The sores or crusts are usually less than ¼ inch across.
- The rash is on all body surfaces but usually starts on the head and back. Occasionally the rash stays localized for the first day or two.
- Fever is present. (The more extensive the rash, the higher the fever. However, your child may not have any fever on the first day of chicken pox or if the rash remains mild.)
- Sores (ulcers) can also occur normally in the mouth, eyelids, and genital area.
- Your child was exposed to a child with chicken pox 10 to 21 days previously.

If your child's symptoms are different, call your physician for help. Usually the diagnosis of chicken pox is easy.

Cause—Exposure to a highly contagious virus 14 to 16 days previously.

Expected Course—New eruptions continue to crop up daily for 4 to 5 days. The fever is usually the highest on the third or fourth day. Children start to feel better and the fever clears once they stop getting new bumps. The average child gets a total of 400 to 500 chicken pox bumps. Since chicken pox often looks terrible, reassure your child that the bumps are not serious and will go away. Chicken pox rarely leaves any permanent scars unless the eruptions become badly infected with impetigo or your child repeatedly picks off the scabs. Normal chicken pox, however, can leave temporary marks on the skin that take 6 to 12 months to fade. One attack gives lifelong immunity. Very rarely, a child may develop a mild second attack.

Call Your Child's Physician

Immediately If

- Your child is difficult to awaken or confused (call 911).
- Your child develops a patch of red, tender skin.

- Your child develops a speckled red rash that looks like scarlet fever (page 463).
- Your child has trouble walking.
- The neck is stiff.
- The breathing is difficult.
- Vomiting occurs 3 or more times.
- Bleeding occurs into the chicken pox.
- Your child acts or looks very sick.

Within 24 Hours If
- The scabs become soft and drain yellow pus.
- The scabs become larger in size. (Note: Use a nonprescription antibiotic ointment on these sores until your child is seen.)
- One lymph node becomes larger and more tender than the others.
- Your child has been exposed to chicken pox and never had the vaccine or the disease.
- You think your child needs to be seen.

Home Care for Chicken Pox

Itching and Cool Baths—The best treatment for skin discomfort and itching is a cool bath for 10 minutes every 4 hours for the first few days. Baths don't spread the chicken pox. To protect the scabs, pat rather than rub your child dry. Calamine lotion can be placed on the most itchy spots after the bath. Itchy spots can also be massaged with an ice cube for 10 minutes.

If the itching is severe or interferes with sleep, give your child a nonprescription antihistamine called Benadryl. For the proper dosage of Benadryl, see the table on page 239.

Fever—Acetaminophen may be given for a few days if your child develops a fever over 102°F (39°C). (For dosage, see the table on page 238.) Do not give ibuprofen products because of a possible link with severe strep infections. Warning: Do not give aspirin to children and adolescents with chicken pox because of the possible link with Reye's syndrome.

Sore Mouth—Since chicken pox sores also occur in the mouth and throat, your child may be picky about eating for a few days. Encourage cold fluids. Offer a soft diet (e.g., ice cream, eggs, pudding, Jell-O, mashed potatoes). Avoid salty foods and citrus fruits.

For infants, give fluids by cup rather than a bottle because the nipple can cause pain. If the mouth ulcers become troublesome and your child is over age 4, have him or her gargle or swallow 1 teaspoon of a liquid antacid 4 times per day after meals.

Sores also normally occur on the eyelids; this carries no danger to vision.

Sore Genital Area—Sores normally occur in the genital area. These can be very painful. If your child (especially a girl) complains of a lot of pain or holds back her urine, buy a local anesthetic like 2.5 percent Xylocaine ointment (no prescription needed). Apply it to the genital ulcers as often as necessary to relieve the pain (every 2 to 3 hours). The cool baths should also help.

Prevention of Impetigo (Infected Sores)—To prevent the sores from becoming infected with bacteria, trim your child's fingernails short. Also, wash the hands with an antibacterial soap frequently during the day. Discourage picking and scratching, especially of the face. For young babies who are scratching badly, you may want to cover their hands with cotton socks.

Contagiousness and Isolation—Children with chicken pox are contagious until all the sores have crusted over, usually about 6 or 7 days after the rash begins. Therefore, they should be kept out of school for about 1 week. Your child does not have to stay home until all the scabs fall off, since this may take 2 weeks.

- Avoid sunlight, since extra chicken pox will occur on sun-exposed parts of the skin.
- Most adults who think they didn't have chicken pox as a child in fact had a mild case. Only 4 percent of adults are not protected. If you lived in the same household with siblings who had chicken pox, consider yourself protected.
- Siblings will come down with chicken pox in 10 to 21 days. The second case in a family usually has many more chicken pox bumps than the first case.
- To avoid exposing other children outside the family, try not to take your child to the physician's office. If you must, leave your child in the car with a sitter while you check in.
- If a child with a serious disease or taking steroids is exposed to chicken pox, he should see his physician promptly because he may need protection with a special antiviral medicine.

- Children with chicken pox must avoid pregnant women who have not had chicken pox during the first trimester because of the risk to the fetus.

Acyclovir—Acyclovir is an oral antiviral drug that can be used to treat chicken pox. It helps only if started within 24 hours of the appearance of the first sores. According to recent research, acyclovir has mild benefits: It reduces the number of sores by 20 percent and the days of illness by 1. The complication rate for chicken pox is not reduced. If used, acyclovir needs to be taken for 5 days. The cost is about $50. The drug has few reported side effects.

Which children with chicken pox should receive acyclovir is a controversial topic. Physicians do agree that all children who have immune system defects, are taking steroids, or have a chronic skin or lung disease should receive acyclovir. Some physicians prescribe acyclovir for adults, college students, and high school students. Some also prescribe it for younger children who have social obligations (such as travel). Most physicians don't treat normal, healthy children with acyclovir.

Chicken Pox Vaccine—The chicken pox vaccine can prevent or reduce the severity of disease even if given after exposure to a child with chicken pox. The vaccine can be given as late as 5 days after exposure. Therefore, if your child has been exposed to chicken pox and has not had the vaccine or the disease, call your child's doctor during office hours.

Call Your Child's Physician Later If
- The fever lasts over 4 days.
- The itching is severe and doesn't respond to treatment.
- You feel your child is getting worse.
- Your child develops any of the "Call Your Child's Physician" symptoms.

DRY SKIN

Dry, rough skin is mainly caused by removing the skin's natural oils through too much bathing and soap (soap dermatitis). Once the oils are gone, the skin can't hold moisture. Dry climates make it worse, as does winter weather (winter itch). Genetics also plays a role in dry skin. The problem is less common in teenagers, because the oil glands are more active. Dry, rough, bumpy skin on the back of the upper arms is called keratosis pilaris. Dry, pale spots on the face are called pityriasis alba. Both are complications of scrubbing dry skin with soap. The dry areas are often itchy, and this is the main symptom.

Home Care

Soap and Bathing—For children with dry skin, avoid all soaps. They take the natural oils out of the skin. Have your child bathe or shower less often than usual—perhaps twice a week. Keep bathing time to less than 10 minutes. Avoid soaps, detergents, and bubble baths. Don't let a bar of soap just float around in the tub. For teenagers, buy a special soap for dry skin. Teenagers can get by with applying soap only to the armpits, genitals, and feet. Use no soap on itchy areas. Don't lather up—the outer arms are often affected for this reason. Rinse well.

Lubricating Creams for Dry Skin—Buy a large bottle of a lubricating cream (see ECZEMA, below, for details). Apply the cream to any dry or itchy areas several times a day, especially immediately after bathing to trap the moisture in the skin. You will probably have to continue this throughout the winter. If the itch persists after 4 days, use 1 percent hydrocortisone cream (no prescription needed) temporarily.

Humidifier—If your winters are dry, you can protect your child's skin from the constant drying effect by running a room humidifier full time. The presence of static electricity means your home is much too dry. During cold weather, have your child wear gloves outside to protect against the rapid evaporation of moisture from the hands.

Bath Oils—It does not make sense to pour bath oils into the bathwater; most of the oil goes down the drain. It also makes the bathtub slippery and dangerous. If you prefer a bath oil instead of skin lotion, it should be applied immediately after the bath. Baby oil (mineral oil) is inexpensive and keeps the skin moisture from evaporating.

Call Your Child's Physician Later If

• No improvement occurs within 2 weeks.

ECZEMA (Atopic Dermatitis)

Symptoms and Characteristics

• Red, extremely itchy rash

- Often starts on the cheeks at 2 to 6 months of age
- Most common on flexor surfaces (creases) of the elbows, wrists, and knees (infants who are crawling often have more rash on the forearms and lower legs)
- Occasionally the neck, ankles, and feet are involved.
- If scratched, the rash becomes raw and weeping.
- Constant dry skin
- Previous confirmation of this diagnosis by a physician is helpful.

If your child's symptoms are different, call your physician for help.

Cause—Eczema results from an inherited type of sensitive, dry skin and lowered itch threshold. A personal history of asthma or hay fever or a family history of eczema adds weight to the diagnosis. Flare-ups occur when there is contact with irritating substances (especially soaps and chlorine). While food allergies are not the underlying cause of eczema, in 30 percent of these infants a particular food may cause the eczema to flare up. If you suspect some food (e.g., cow's milk, soy formula, eggs, or peanut butter), feed it to your child as a single challenge after avoiding it for 2 weeks. If it plays any role, the eczema should become itchy or develop hives within 2 hours of ingestion. If this occurs, avoid this food in the future and talk to your child's physician about food substitutes.

Expected Course—This is a chronic condition and will usually not go away before adolescence. The goal is control, not cure. Eczema of the face usually clears by age 2 or 3 years. Early treatment of any itching or change in the skin is the key to preventing a severe rash.

Call Your Child's Physician

Immediately If
- The rash appears to be infected and your child has a fever.
- The rash flares up after contact with someone with fever blisters (herpes).
- Your child acts or looks very sick.

Within 24 Hours If
- The rash appears to be infected, as evidenced by pus or soft yellow scabs.
- The rash is raw and bleeding in several places.

During Office Hours If
- Your child is under 2 years of age.
- The itching interferes with sleep.
- You have other questions or concerns.

Home Care

Steroid Cream or Ointment—Steroid cream or ointment is the main treatment for the itch of eczema. Use the one your physician prescribes or nonprescription 1 percent hydrocortisone cream or ointment. Creams are better during hot weather. Apply it up to 4 times a day when the eczema flares up. When the rash quiets down, use it at least once a day for an additional 2 weeks. After that, break the itch cycle by using it immediately on any spot that itches. This cream should be applied in small amounts and rubbed in until it can't be seen. When you travel with your child, always take the steroid cream with you, and always leave it available for baby-sitters. If your supply starts to run low, buy an extra tube if it's over the counter, or get the prescription renewed.

Hydrating the Skin—Hydration of the skin followed by applying lubricating cream over the wet skin is the main way to prevent flare-ups of eczema. Your child should have 1 bath a day (especially in the wintertime) for 10 minutes. Water-soaked skin is far less itchy. Don't use any soap on the areas of rash. Eczema is very sensitive to soaps, especially to bubble bath. Young children can usually be cleaned without any soap. Teenagers need a soap to wash under the arms, the genital area, and the feet. They can use a nondrying soap for these areas. Try to keep shampoo off the eczema.

Lubricating Cream—Children with eczema always have dry skin. After a 10-minute bath, the skin is hydrated and feels good. Help trap the moisture in the skin by applying an outer layer of lubricating cream to the entire skin surface while it is damp. That means applying the lubricating cream within 3 minutes of completing the bath. Apply it after steroid cream has been applied to any itchy areas. Avoid applying any ointments, petroleum jelly, or vegetable shortening, because they can block the sweat glands, increase the itching, and worsen the rash. They cause the most trouble during hot and humid weather. Also, soap is needed to wash them off. For severe eczema or during the winter, ointments may be needed to heal the skin.

Itching—At the first sign of any itching, apply the steroid cream to the area that itches. Keep your child's fingernails cut short so they are less damaging to the skin. Also, rinse your child's hands with water frequently to avoid infecting the eczema. When itching is present, it is always worse at bedtime compared to the rest of the day, because your child has little else by way of distraction. Therefore, steroid cream at bedtime is important.

Call Your Child's Physician Later If
- The rash hasn't greatly improved within 7 days on this treatment.
- You feel your child is getting worse.
- Your child develops any of the "Call Your Child's Physician" symptoms.

Prevention of Eczema
- Try to breast-feed all high-risk infants. Otherwise, use a soy formula. Also try to avoid cow's-milk products and eggs during the first year of life. Try to avoid all nuts (including peanut butter) and seafood until 2 years old.
- Wear clothes made of cotton, or cotton combinations as much as possible.
- Avoid wool fibers and clothes made of other scratchy, rough materials. They make eczema worse.
- Avoid materials that hold in heat, such as most synthetic fibers, which can worsen the rash. Avoid overdressing.
- Avoid triggers that cause eczema to flare up, such as excessive heat, sweating, excessive cold, dry air, chlorine, harsh chemicals, and soaps.
- In dry climates, place a humidifier in your child's bedroom.
- Never use bubble bath, because it can cause a major flare-up.
- Keep your child off the grass during grass pollen season (May and June).
- Keep your child away from anyone with fever blisters. The herpes virus can cause a serious skin infection in children with eczema.

FIFTH DISEASE (Erythema Infectiosum)

Symptoms and Characteristics
- Bright red rash of both cheeks for 1 to 3 days ("slapped-cheek" appearance)
- Followed by pink "lacy" (or netlike) rash on extremities

- Lacy rash mainly on thighs and upper arms
- Lacy rash that comes and goes several times over 1 to 3 weeks
- No fever or minimal one

If your child's symptoms are different, call your physician for help. Fifth disease was so named because it was the fifth pink-red infectious rash to be described. Despite some controversy about roseola being fourth disease, the other 4 are:

SCARLET FEVER (see page 463)
MEASLES (see page 458)
RUBELLA (see page 462)
ROSEOLA (see page 461)

See those guidelines for details.

Cause—Fifth disease is caused by the human parvovirus B19. The attack rate in schools is usually 50 percent of the students.

Expected Course—This is a very mild disease with either no symptoms or a slight runny nose and sore throat. Complications in children are very rare. The lacelike rash can come and go for 5 weeks. Heat seems to be the main precipitant; therefore it returns following warm baths, exercise, and sun exposure.

Call Your Child's Physician

Within 24 Hours If
- Your child was on any medicine when the rash began.
- You think your child needs to be seen.

During Office Hours If
- A fever over 104°F is present.
- The rash is itchy.
- You have other questions or concerns.

Home Care

Treatment—No treatment is necessary. This distinctive rash is harmless and causes no symptoms.

Contagiousness—Over 50 percent of exposed children will come down with the rash in 10 to 14 days. The disease is mainly contagious during the week before the rash begins. Exposed children should try to avoid contact with pregnant women, but that can be difficult. Once the child has the slapped-cheeks rash or the lacy rash, he or she is no longer considered contagious and does not need to stay home from school.

Adults with Fifth Disease—Most adults who acquire fifth disease develop a mild pinkness of the cheeks or no rash whatever. The most common symptom in adults is joint pain, especially of the knees. These pains may take 1 to 3 months to run their course. Taking a nonprescription ibuprofen product usually relieves symptoms. An arthritis workup is unnecessary for joint pains following fifth disease.

Refer Pregnant Women Exposed to Fifth Disease to Their Obstetrician—The risk of fifth disease is to the unborn babies of pregnant women. If a pregnant woman is exposed to a child with fifth disease, she should see her obstetrician. He or she will obtain an antibody test to see if the mother already had the disease and is therefore protected. If not, the pregnancy will need to be monitored closely. Some fetuses infected with fifth disease before birth develop complications. Ten percent develop severe anemia and 2 percent may die. Birth defects, however, are never a result of this virus.

Call Your Child's Physician Later If
- You feel your child is getting worse.
- Your child develops any of the "Call Your Child's Physician" symptoms.

HEAT RASH (Miliaria)

A heat rash consists of tiny pink bumps, mainly of the neck and upper back. It is caused by blocked-off sweat glands. Lots of children get it during hot, humid weather when sweat glands are overworked. Infants can also get it in the wintertime with fever, overdressing, or ointments applied to the chest for coughs. Another name for heat rash is prickly heat.

Home Care

Treatment—Heat rash will clear up completely in 2 to 3 days with techniques that cool off the skin. Give cool baths for 10 minutes every 2 to 3 hours, without soap. Let your child's skin air-dry. Leave as many clothes off as possible. Use a fan if your child is asleep or in a playpen. Have your child lie on a towel so the head isn't constantly wet.

Calamine lotion (no prescription needed) can be applied to the worst spots. Avoid all ointments or oils, because they can block off sweat glands.

Call Your Child's Physician Later If

• The rash lasts more than 72 hours on this treatment.

HIVES (Urticaria)

Symptoms and Characteristics

• Very itchy rash
• Raised pink spots with pale centers (hives look like mosquito bites)
• Sizes of spots range from ½ inch to several inches across
• Shapes are quite variable.
• Location, size, and shape change rapidly and repeatedly.

If your child's symptoms are different, call your physician for help.

Causes—Widespread hives are an allergic reaction to a viral infection, food (especially shrimp, fruits, and nuts), drug, insect bite, or a host of other substances. Usually a child has been exposed to the substance many times in the past before developing an allergy to it. Often the cause is not found.

Localized hives are usually due to skin contact with plants, pollen, food, or pet saliva. Localized hives are not caused by drugs, infections, or swallowed foods. Hives are not contagious.

Expected Course—More than 10 percent of children get hives. Most children who develop hives have it only once. The hives come and go for 3 or 4 days and then mysteriously disappear. Large swellings are common about the eyes, lips, and genitals if hives occur there. Some young children become sensitized to mosquito or flea bites. They develop big hives (called papular urticaria) at the site of old and new bites that last for months.

Call Your Child's Physician

Immediately If
- Breathing or swallowing is difficult (call 911).
- The tongue is swollen (call 911).
- The hives started immediately after your child took medicine or was stung by an insect (call 911).
- Any abdominal pain is present.
- Your child is on any medicine.
- Your child acts or looks very sick.

Within 24 Hours If
- A fever is present.
- Joint swelling or pain is present.
- Your child had hives before *and* the cause wasn't found.
- You think your child needs to be seen.

Home Care

Treatment—The best drug for hives is an antihistamine. While an antihistamine won't cure the hives, it will reduce their numbers and relieve itching. Benadryl is a good product that is available without a prescription. The main side effect is some drowsiness. If you have another antihistamine (e.g., any drug for hay fever) at home, use it until you can get some Benadryl. Give Benadryl 4 times a day. See the dosage table on page 239.

Itching—Give a cool bath to relieve itching. Rub very itchy areas with an ice cube for 10 minutes.

Avoidance—Avoid anything you think might have caused the hives. For hives triggered by pollen or animal contact, take a cool shower or bath. For localized hives, wash the allergenic substance off the skin with soap and water. If itchy, massage the area with a cold washcloth or ice for 10 minutes. Localized hives usually disappear in a few hours and don't need Benadryl.

Common Mistakes—Many parents wait to give the antihistamine until new hives have reappeared. This means your child will become itchy again. The purpose of the medicine is to keep your child comfortable until the hives go away. Therefore, give the medicine regularly until you are sure the hives are completely gone.

Call Your Child's Physician Later If

- Most of the itch is not relieved within 24 hours on the medicine.
- The hives last for more than a week.
- You feel your child is getting worse.
- Your child develops any of the "Call Your Child's Physician" symptoms.

MEASLES (Rubeola)

Symptoms and Characteristics

- 3 or 4 days of red eyes, cough, runny nose, and fever before the rash begins
- Pronounced blotchy red rash starting on the face and spreading downward over the entire body in 3 days
- White specks on the lining of the mouth, especially by the molars (Koplik's spots)
- Exposure to a child with measles 10 to 12 days earlier

Note: Because of the measles vaccine, this disease has become rare in our country. This diagnosis must be confirmed by a physician.

Cause—A highly contagious virus.

Expected Course—Measles can be a miserable illness, and there's not much we can do to shorten it. The Koplik's spots (which cause no symptoms) appear 1 day before the rash and are gone by day 2 of the rash. The rash usually lasts 7 days (this is why it's called 7-day measles). Your child will usually begin to feel a lot better by the fourth day of the rash. Ear infections, eye infections, and pneumonia are common complications.

Call Your Child's Physician

Immediately If
- Your child is difficult to awaken (call 911).
- Your child is confused or delirious.
- Breathing is difficult *and* no better after you clear the nose.
- Your child has a severe headache.
- Your child acts or looks very sick.

Within 24 Hours If
All children with suspected measles need medical consultation. This disease must be reported to the public health department to prevent spread.

Home Care

Fever—Use acetaminophen or ibuprofen (for dosage, see tables on pages 238–40).

Cough—Use ½ to 1 teaspoon corn syrup (1 to 4 years old) or cough drops (over 4 years old). If the cough interferes with sleep, give a cough suppressant such as dextromethorphan (DM). Also, use a humidifier. (See COUGH, page 584, for further information.)

Red Eyes—Wipe your child's eyes frequently with a clean wet cotton ball. The eyes are usually sensitive to bright light, so your child may prefer the curtains drawn in his room and probably won't want to go outside for several days unless he wears sunglasses. Light exposure, however, can't damage the eyes.

Rash—The rash requires no treatment.

Diet—Offer a diet of your child's own choosing. The appetite will be poor for several days.

Contagiousness—The disease is no longer contagious after the rash is gone. This usually takes 7 days. After that, your child can see friends and go to school.

Measles Exposure—Any child or adult who has been exposed to your child and who has not had natural measles or the measles vaccine should call his or her physician. If given early, a measles vaccine is often protective.

Call Your Child's Physician Later If

- An earache develops.
- The eyes develop a yellow discharge.
- Fever is still present on the fourth day of the rash.
- You feel your child is getting worse.
- Your child develops any of the "Call Your Child's Physician" symptoms.

MEASLES VACCINE RASH

The live measles vaccine has prevented many deaths and serious complications of the natural disease. The vaccine is given to children over 12 months of age. About 20 percent of children develop some mild symptoms 7 to 10 days after the vaccine. A slight, pink rash of the trunk usually lasts 2 or 3 days. A fever is usually 101 to 103°F and lasts less than 72 hours.

Home Care

Treatment is not usually needed. The measles vaccine rash is harmless and not contagious.

Call Your Child's Physician

Immediately If

- The rash changes to purple or blood-colored spots.

During Office Hours If

- The rash becomes itchy.
- The rash lasts more than 3 days.

PURPLE SPOTS OR DOTS

If your child develops purple to bloodred spots or dots on the skin or unexplained bruises, call your child's physician *immediately*. The size of the bleeding into the skin can vary from small dots (petechiae) to large spots (purpura). These spots can be caused by a serious bloodstream infection such as meningococcemia or Rocky Mountain spotted fever (especially if your child also has a fever) or by a bleeding tendency.

(Note: Bruises due to injuries or blue birthmarks don't count.)

Related Topic

SKIN TRAUMA (see page 78)

ROSEOLA (Roseola Infantum)

Symptoms and Characteristics

- Age 6 months to 3 years
- Presence of a fine pink rash, mainly on the trunk
- Moderate to high fever during the preceding 2 to 4 days, which cleared within 24 hours before the rash appeared
- Child only mildly ill during the time with fever
- Child acts fine now

If your child's symptoms are different, call your physician for help.

Cause—Roseola is caused by the human herpesvirus type 6.

Expected Course—The rash lasts 1 or 2 days, followed by complete recovery. Some children have 3 days of fever without a rash.

Home Care

Treatment—No particular treatment is necessary, since the fever is usually gone when the rash appears. Roseola is contagious, and other children under age 3 who have been with your child may come down with roseola in about 12 days. Once the rash is gone, the disease is no longer contagious.

Call Your Child's Physician Later If

- The spots become purple or blood-colored (call now).
- The rash lasts more than 3 days.
- The rash becomes itchy.
- Any new symptoms develop that concern you.

Related Topic

RASHES, UNKNOWN CAUSE (WIDESPREAD) (see page 441)

RUBELLA (German Measles)

Symptoms and Characteristics
- Widespread pink-red spots
- Starts on the face
- Moves rapidly downward, covering the body in 24 hours
- Lasts 3 to 4 days (sometimes called "3-day measles")
- Associated enlarged lymph nodes at back of neck
- Mild fever
- Child never had the rubella vaccine.
- Diagnosis must be confirmed by a physician.

The rash is not distinctive. Many other viral rashes look like it. Physicians have difficulty being certain of this diagnosis even after examining the child.

Cause—Rubella is a viral illness. The incubation period is 14 to 21 days.

Expected Course—The disease is mild with complete recovery in 3 or 4 days. Complications are very rare except for about 10 percent of teenagers (especially girls) who develop associated joint pains. However, complications to the unborn child of a pregnant woman with rubella are disastrous and include deafness, cataracts, heart defects, growth retardation, and encephalitis. Pregnant women should avoid anyone with suspected rubella.

Call Your Child's Physician Within 24 Hours If
- Your child has a widespread, pink rash with fever.
- You think your child might have rubella.

Home Care
If your physician has confirmed that your child probably has rubella, the following may be helpful:

Treatment—None is probably necessary. Give acetaminophen or ibuprofen for fever over 102°F, sore throat, or other pains. (For dosage, see the tables on pages 238–40.)

Contagiousness—The disease is no longer contagious after 5 days.

Avoid Pregnant Women—If your child might have rubella, keep him away from any pregnant women. He is contagious for 5 days after the start of the rash.

Exposure of Adult Women to Rubella—The nonpregnant woman exposed to rubella should avoid pregnancy during the following 3 months, and the pregnant woman should see her obstetrician. If she has already received the rubella vaccine, she (and her unborn child) should be protected. If she thinks she had German measles as a child, this history is too unreliable. Even if the present exposure was minor or brief, she should have a blood test to determine her immunity against rubella.

Prevention—Get your children protected with the rubella vaccine at 12 months of age so we won't have to worry about pregnant women when kids get a pink or red rash. It's quite safe to immunize the child of a pregnant woman.

SCARLET FEVER

Symptoms and Characteristics

- Reddened, sunburned-looking skin (especially of the chest and abdomen)
- On close inspection, the redness is speckled (i.e., tiny pink dots).
- Increased redness in skin folds (especially the groin, armpits, and elbow creases)
- The rash is everywhere within 24 hours.
- Rough, sandpapery feeling to the reddened skin
- Flushed face with paleness around the mouth
- Sore throat and fever (usually preceding the rash by 18 to 24 hours)
- This diagnosis must be confirmed by a physician.

Cause—Scarlet fever is a strep throat infection with a rash. The complication rate is no different from that for strep throat alone. The rash is caused by a special rash-producing toxin that is produced by some strep bacteria.

Expected Course—The red rash usually clears in 4 or 5 days. Sometimes the skin peels in 1 or 2 weeks where the rash was most prominent (e.g., the groin). The skin on the fingertips also commonly peels. The skin may peel and flake for several weeks. The sore throat and fever clear after 1 or

2 days on an antibiotic. Your child can return to school then. The antibiotic will need to be continued for 10 days to completely eliminate the strep. The rash itself is not contagious.

Call Your Child's Physician

Immediately If
- Your child is drooling or having great difficulty swallowing (call 911).
- Your child also has a wound infection.
- Your child is a female adolescent *and* she is also having her menstrual period.
- The urine is red or cola-colored.
- Your child acts or looks very sick.

Within 24 Hours If
All other children with suspected scarlet fever need medical consultation. Your child's physician will advise you about a throat culture and antibiotics.

Home Care

Rash—The rash itself needs no treatment. It generally clears in 4 or 5 days.

Relief of Sore Throat—Acetaminophen or ibuprofen are very helpful. Children over age 1 can sip warm chicken broth or warm apple juice. Children over age 4 can suck on hard candy or lollipops.

Contagiousness—Your child is no longer contagious after he or she has been on an antibiotic for 24 hours. Therefore your child can return to school after 1 day if he or she is feeling better. The rash itself is not contagious.

Related Topic

SORE THROAT (page 570)

SKIN: LOCALIZED PINK OR RED RASHES

RASHES, UNKNOWN CAUSE (Localized)

Symptoms and Characteristics
- Red or pink rash (erythema)
- Smooth or slightly bumpy
- Spots or solid red
- On one part of body (localized or clustered)
- Not itchy

Similar Condition—If the rash is itchy, turn directly to the guideline for ITCHING, UNKNOWN CAUSE (LOCALIZED), page 467.

Causes of Localized Rashes—The possible causes are many. If one of the following is suspected, turn directly to that guideline:
- Scalp location
CRADLE CAP (see page 132)
- Face location
ACNE (see page 468)
- Finger location
If fingers are peeling, see your child's physician by appointment to rule out strep (see page 463).
- Genital location
DIAPER RASH (see page 133)
- Hand and foot location
HAND, FOOT, AND MOUTH DISEASE (see page 475)
- Nostrils (nasal openings) location

IMPETIGO (see page 476)
- Shoulder location
  TINEA VERSICOLOR (see page 487)
- Variable location
  BOILS (see page 473)
  IMPETIGO (see page 476)
  NEWBORN RASHES (less than 2 weeks old) (see page 108)
  RINGWORM (see page 484)
  SHINGLES (see page 485)

Expected Course—Depends on the diagnosis.

Call Your Child's Physician

Immediately If
- The rash is purple or blood-colored.
- It is bright red *and* tender to the touch.
- It looks like a burn.
- Red streaks that look like a spreading infection are present.
- Your child is less than 1 month old *and* has some small blisters or pimples.
- Your child acts or looks very sick.

During Office Hours If
- You think your child needs to be seen.

Home Care for Localized Rashes

Treatment—Localized red rashes can be due to a chemical or plant irritant that got on your child's skin. No treatment is necessary. Wash the rash once with soap to remove any irritating substances. Thereafter cleanse it only with water. Don't apply any medicine or petroleum jelly. If the rash seems dry, apply a moisturizing cream twice a day. If it becomes itchy, apply 1 percent hydrocortisone cream (no prescription needed) 4 times per day.

Call Your Child's Physician Later If
- The rash spreads.
- It lasts more than 1 week.
- Your child develops any of the "Call Your Child's Physician" symptoms.

ITCHING, UNKNOWN CAUSE (Localized)

Causes

The possible causes are many. If one of the following is suspected, turn directly to that guideline:

- Itching of anus
  PINWORMS (see page 613)
- Itching of elbow crease or knee crease
  ECZEMA (see page 450)
- Itching of eyes
  ALLERGIES OF THE EYES (see page 522)
  ITCHY EYE (see page 524)
- Itching of foot
  ATHLETE'S FOOT (see page 471)
- Itching of genitals
  JOCK ITCH (see page 479)
- Itching of head
  LICE (PEDICULOSIS) (see page 480)
  DANDRUFF (see page 492)
- Itching of lip
  LIP, SWOLLEN (see page 569)
- Itching in variable locations
  BITES: INSECT, BEE, OR TICK (see page 19)
  POISON IVY (see page 482)
  RINGWORM (see page 484)

Call Your Child's Physician During Office Hours If

- The itching is severe.
- The rash is larger than 2 inches in size.
- You think your child needs to be seen.

Home Care

Clarification—The itchy spot is probably due to contact with an irritant like a plant, chemicals, fiberglass, detergents, a new cosmetic, or new jewelry (called contact dermatitis). Try to figure out what caused it and avoid this substance in the future.

Treatment—Wash the area once thoroughly with soap to remove any remaining irritants. Thereafter avoid soaps in this area until the rash has cleared. Apply cold-water compresses or ice for 20 minutes every 3 to 4 hours to reduce itching. Follow this with 1 percent hydrocortisone cream (no prescription needed) 4 times per day until it feels better. Encourage your child not to scratch; cut the fingernails short.

Call Your Child's Physician Later If

- The rash spreads.
- It lasts more than 1 week.

ACNE

Symptoms and Characteristics

- Blackheads, whiteheads (pimples), or red bumps
- Face, neck, and shoulders involved
- The larger red lumps are quite painful.
- Occurs during adolescent and young adult years

Cause—Acne is due to a plugging of the oil glands. More than 90 percent of teenagers have some acne. The main cause of the changes in the oil glands is increased levels of hormones during adolescence. Heredity is also a factor. It is not caused by diet, and it is unnecessary to restrict fried foods, chocolate, or any other food. Acne is not caused by sexual activity or by dirt and not washing the face often enough. The tops of blackheads turn black because of the chemical reaction of the oil plug with the air.

Expected Course—Acne usually lasts until age 20 or even 25. It is rare for acne to leave any scars, and people worry needlessly about this.

Call Your Child's Physician Within 24 Hours If

- There are any boils.
- There are any red streaks.
- There are more than five tender, red lumps.
- You think your child needs to be seen.

Home Care

There is no magic medicine at this time that will cure acne. However, good skin care can keep acne under control and at a mild level.

Basic Treatment for All Acne

- The skin should be washed twice a day and after exercise. The most important time is before bedtime. A mild soap should be used, because overly dry skin makes acne harder to treat. Lack of washing does not cause acne. Excessive washing can make it worse.
- The hair should be shampooed daily. Also, acne can be made worse by friction if the hair is too long.
- Avoid picking and squeezing. Many young people pick at their acne when they are not thinking about it. Picking keeps it from healing. Squeezing acne causes bleeding into the skin and blotches that last a month. They should try not to touch the face at all during the day.
- Avoid looking in mirrors more than 1 or 2 minutes a day. Your youngster will just find something to pick and make the acne worse.
- Get out and meet people. Acne is not contagious.

Treatment for Pimples—Pimples are infected oil glands. They should be treated with the following:

- Benzoyl peroxide 5 percent lotion or gel. This lotion helps to open pimples, unplug blackheads, and it also kills bacteria. It is available without a prescription. Ask your pharmacist to recommend a brand. The lotion should be applied in a thin film once a day at bedtime. In redheads and blondes, it should be applied every other day initially. Apply the lotion to the entire face (except for the sensitive skin next to the eyes and mouth), not just the areas that have currently flared up. An amount the size of a pea should cover most of the face. If the skin peels or becomes red, you are using too much of the medicine or applying it too often, so slow down. After a desirable effect has been achieved, the benzoyl peroxide lotion may be needed only every other night. (Caution: benzoyl peroxide can bleach clothing and bedding, so apply it sparingly and only at bedtime.)
- Pimple opening. In general, "popping" pimples is discouraged; but teenagers do it anyway. Therefore, teach your youngster to open pimples safely without popping them. Never open a pimple before it has come to a head. Wash your face and hands first. Nick the surface of the yellow pimple with the tip of a sterile needle. The pus should run out without squeezing. Wipe away the pus and wash that area with soap and water. Scarring will not result from opening small pimples, but it can result from squeezing boils or other red, tender lumps. This should never be done, because it damages the skin.

Treatment for Blackheads (Comedones)—Blackheads are the plugs found in blocked-off oil glands. Blackheads are not infected and should be treated with the following:

- Benzoyl peroxide. This agent is the best nonprescription medicine for removing the thickened skin that blocks the openings to oil glands. It should be used as previously described. (Note: A stronger agent for stopping blackhead formation is tretinoin [Retin-A], but a prescription is required.)
- Blackhead extractor. Blackheads that are a cosmetic problem can sometimes be removed with a blackhead or comedone extractor. This instrument costs about a dollar and is available at any drugstore. By placing the hole in the end of the small metal spoon directly over the blackhead, uniform pressure can be applied that does not hurt the normal skin. This method is much more efficient than anything you can accomplish with your fingers. Soak your face with a warm washcloth before trying to remove blackheads. If the blackhead does not come out the first time, leave it alone, and consult your physician about Retin-A.

Treatment for Red Bumps—Large red bumps mean the infection has spread beyond the oil gland. If you have several red bumps, you probably also need an antibiotic. Antibiotics come as solutions for the skin or pills. Talk with your teen's doctor about this.

Results of Treatment—Even the best of medicines takes 6 to 8 weeks to improve acne. Success depends on your patience. There are no shortcuts. The proper treatment program will need to remain in effect for several years.

Common Mistakes in Treating Acne

- Alcohol wipes, medicated soaps, or abrasive soaps have no benefits, and they irritate the skin and block off more oil glands.
- Avoid rubbing the skin. Hard scrubbing of the skin is harmful because it breaks the walls of the oil glands, which leads to pimples and large lumps.
- Avoid applying any oily or greasy substances to the face. They make acne worse by blocking off oil glands. If you must use cover-up cosmetics, use water-based ones and wash them off at bedtime.
- Avoid hair tonics or hair creams (especially greasy ones). With sweating, these will spread to the face and aggravate the acne.
- Avoid any friction. Friction or pressure on the face, such as from headbands, scarves, turtlenecks, or resting the cheek or chin on the palm of the hand will worsen the acne in these areas.

- Avoid close shaves. Attempts to look extra good for a date usually nick the openings of the oil glands and cause the acne to flare up.
- Avoid self-medication with high dosages of vitamin A. Overdosage can cause brain swelling and bone pain.

Call Your Child's Physician Later If

- Acne is not improved after treating it with benzoyl peroxide for 2 months.
- Benzoyl peroxide makes the face itchy or swollen.
- You feel your child is getting worse.
- Your child develops any of the "Call Your Child's Physician" symptoms.

ATHLETE'S FOOT

Symptoms and Characteristics

- A red, scaly, cracked rash between the toes
- Rash itches and burns.
- With itching, rash becomes raw and weepy.
- Often involves the insteps of the feet
- Unpleasant foot odor
- Occurs in adolescents and adults. Prior to age 10, it's usually something else.

Similar Condition

CRACKED SKIN (see page 491)

Cause—A fungus infection that grows best on warm, damp skin. The condition is worse in summer, in people who sweat a lot (e.g., athletes), and in people who rarely take off their shoes.

Expected Course—With proper treatment, athlete's foot usually clears in 1 to 2 weeks.

Call Your Child's Physician During Office Hours If

- The rash is not confined to the instep and between the toes.
- It looks infected (yellow pus, spreading redness, red streaks).

- The feet are very painful.
- Your child is less than 10 years old.
- You think your child needs to be seen.

Home Care

Antifungal Cream—Buy Tinactin, Micatin, or Lotrimin cream at your drugstore (no prescription needed). Before applying, rinse the feet in plain water or water with a little white vinegar added. Dry them carefully, especially between the toes. Apply the cream twice a day to the rash and well beyond its borders. Continue the cream for several weeks, or for at least 7 days after the rash seems to have cleared. Successful treatment often takes 1 to 2 weeks.

Dryness—Athlete's foot improves dramatically if the feet are kept dry. It helps to go barefoot or wear sandals or thongs as much as possible. Canvas tennis shoes are good. Plastic or tight shoes are bad because they don't allow the feet to breathe. Cotton socks should be worn because they absorb sweat and keep the feet dry. Change the socks twice daily. Dry the feet thoroughly after baths and showers.

Foot Odor—Foot odor will often clear as the athlete's foot improves. Rinsing the feet and changing the socks twice daily are essential. If that doesn't work, rinse the feet in a basin of warm water containing 1 ounce of vinegar. If you can still smell your child coming, take off his tennis shoes and throw them in your washing machine with some soap and bleach.

Discourage Scratching—Scratching infected feet will delay a cure.

Contagiousness—The condition is not very contagious. The fungus won't grow on dry, normal skin. Your child may take gym and continue with sports. The socks don't need to be boiled, nor do shoes need to be discarded. Taking special precautions in community showers or swimming pools is pointless. If a preadolescent child has athlete's foot, usually a parent or older sibling also has it and requires treatment.

Prevention—Prevent recurrence by continuing the measures already described that keep your feet dry. Applying cornstarch powder to the feet once a day also helps.

Call Your Child's Physician Later If

- The athlete's foot is not improved in 1 week.

- It is not completely cured after 2 weeks of this treatment.
- Your child develops any of the "Call Your Child's Physician" symptoms.

BOILS (Abscesses)

Symptoms and Characteristics

- Tender, red lump in the skin
- Causes pain even when not being touched
- Usually ½ inch to 1 inch across

If your child's symptoms are different, call your physician for help.

Cause—A bacterial infection of a hair root or skin pore caused by staph *(Staphylococcus aureus)*. Rubbing can cause additional boils. The back of the neck is especially vulnerable because of friction from collars.

Expected Course—Without treatment, the body will wall off the infection. After about a week, the center of the boil becomes soft and mushy (filled with pus). The overlying skin then develops a pimple or becomes thin and pale ("comes to a head"). The boil is now ready for draining. Without lancing, it will drain by itself in 3 or 4 days. Until it drains, a boil is extremely painful.

Call Your Child's Physician

Immediately If

- An unexplained fever is present.
- It's on the face.
- A spreading red streak runs from the boil.
- Your child acts or looks very sick.

Within 24 Hours If

All children with boils need medical consultation to decide if antibiotics and/or lancing are needed. Boils heal faster and are less likely to recur if your child receives an antibiotic that kills the staph bacteria. Boils on the face are especially dangerous and should always be treated by a physician.

Home Care

Lancing or Draining the Boil—In general, it's better not to open a boil on your own child because it's a very painful procedure. Until the abscess comes to a head or becomes soft, apply warm compresses 3 times a day for 20 minutes. When the boil is ready, see your child's doctor. Once opened, it will drain pus for 2 or 3 days and then heal up. Since this pus is contagious, the boil must be covered by a large 4-by-4-inch gauze pad and tape. This bandage should be changed and the area washed with an antibacterial soap twice a day.

Contagiousness—The pus in boils is very contagious. Be certain that other people in your family do not use your child's towel or washcloth. Any clothes, towels, or sheets that are contaminated with drainage from the boils should be washed with a disinfectant. Any bandages with pus on them should be carefully thrown away.

Common Mistakes in the Treatment of Boils—Sometimes friends or relatives may advise you to squeeze a boil until you get the core out. The pus in a boil will come out easily if the opening is large enough. Squeezing is not only very painful, but also entails the risk of forcing bacteria into the bloodstream or causing other boils in the same area. Again, boils should be treated by a physician.

Call Your Child's Physician Later If
- The boil has come to a head and needs to be opened.
- You feel your child is getting worse.
- Your child develops any of the "Call Your Child's Physician" symptoms.

Prevention of More Boils

Boils can become a recurrent problem. The staph bacteria on the skin can be decreased by showering and washing the hair daily with an antibacterial soap. Showers are preferred to a bath because during a bath bacteria are just relocated to other parts of the skin. Often the staph bacteria are carried inside the nose. Eliminate them by applying Bacitracin ointment (no prescription needed) with a cotton swab twice a day for 2 weeks. Also discourage your child from picking the nose. A study by Dr. M. C. Weijmer found that boils are more common in people who have low serum iron levels. If your child is a picky eater or doesn't like meats, see your physician about changing the diet or adding iron supplements.

Related Topics

HAND, FOOT, AND MOUTH DISEASE

Symptoms and Characteristics
- Small ulcers in the mouth
- A mildly painful mouth
- Small water blisters or red spots located on the palms and soles, and on the webs between the fingers and toes (70 percent)
- 5 or fewer blisters per limb
- Sometimes, small blisters or red spots on the buttocks (30 percent)
- Low-grade fever
- Mainly occurs in children age 6 months to 4 years

If your child's symptoms are different, call your physician for help.

Similar Conditions—If one of the following is suspected, save time by turning directly to that guideline:

CANKER SORES (see page 565)
COLD SORES (see page 567)
THRUSH (see page 141)

Cause—Hand, foot, and mouth disease is caused by the Coxsackie A16 virus. It has no relationship to hoof and mouth disease of cattle.

Expected Course—The fever and discomfort are usually gone by day 3 or 4. The mouth ulcers resolve by 7 days, but the rash on the hands and feet can last 10 days. The only complication seen with any frequency is dehydration from refusing fluids.

Call Your Child's Physician

Immediately If
- Your child is hard to awaken (call 911).
- Your child is confused or delirious.
- Your child has not urinated for more than 8 hours.
- The neck is stiff.
- Your child acts or looks very sick.

Within 24 Hours If
- Fluid intake is poor.
- The mouth pain is severe.

- The gums are red, swollen, or tender.
- You think your child needs to be seen.

Home Care

Liquid Antacid—Use a liquid antacid for pain relief. For younger children, put ½ teaspoon antacid in the front of their mouth 4 times a day after meals. Children over age 4 can use 1 teaspoon of an antacid as a mouthwash after meals.

Diet—Change to a soft diet for a few days and encourage plenty of clear fluids. Cold drinks, Popsicles, and sherbet are often well received. For a younger child, give fluids by cup rather than from a bottle. Avoid giving your child citrus, salty, or spicy foods. Also avoid foods that need much chewing.

Fever—Acetaminophen or ibuprofen may be given for a few days for severe mouth pain or fever above 102°F (39°C). (For dosage, see tables on pages 238–40.)

Contagiousness—Hand, foot, and mouth disease is quite contagious and usually some of your child's playmates will develop it at about the same time. The incubation period after contact is 3 to 6 days. Because the spread of infection is extremely difficult to prevent and the condition is harmless, these children do not need to be isolated. They can return to school or day care when the fever returns to normal range. Although most children are contagious from 2 days before to 2 days after the rash, avoidance of other children is unnecessary.

Call Your Child's Physician Later If

- The fever lasts more than 3 days.
- You feel your child is getting worse.
- Your child develops any of the "Call Your Child's Physician" symptoms.

IMPETIGO (Infected Sores)

Symptoms and Characteristics

- Sores smaller than 1 inch in diameter
- Begin as small red bumps that rapidly change to cloudy blisters, then pimples, and finally sores

- Sores that increase in size (any wound that doesn't heal)
- Sores often covered by a soft, yellow-brown (honey-colored) scab
- Scabs possibly draining pus
- Often spread and increase in number from scratching and picking

If your child's symptoms are different, call your physician for help.

Cause—Impetigo is a superficial infection of the skin, caused by streptococcus or staphylococcus bacteria. It is more common in the summertime when the skin, which normally is a barrier to infection, is often broken by cuts, scrapes, and insect bites. When caused by a strep infection of the nose, the impetigo usually first appears near the nose or mouth.

Expected Course—With proper treatment the skin will be completely healed in 1 week. Some blemishes will remain for 6 to 12 months, but scars are unusual unless your child repeatedly picks his sores.

Call Your Child's Physician

Immediately If
- A red streak runs from the impetigo.
- The face is bright red *and* tender to the touch.
- Any big blisters (larger than 1 inch across) are present.
- The urine is red or cola-colored.

Within 24 Hours
All children with impetigo need medical consultation. Impetigo is an active bacterial infection, and the physician will decide if your child needs an antibiotic. One or 2 sores following an insect bite or cut may respond to an antibiotic ointment.

Home Care

Antibiotic—If your physician prescribes an antibiotic, be certain to take it as directed until the drug is completely gone. The following measures will also help clear up the infection.

Removing the Scabs—The bacteria live underneath the soft scabs, and until the scabs are removed, the antibiotic ointment cannot get through to the bacteria to kill them. Scabs can be soaked off initially using warm water and an antibacterial soap. Take your time. The area may need to be gently rubbed, but it should not be scrubbed. A little bleeding is common if you remove all the crust.

Antibiotic Ointment—After the crust has been removed, antibiotic ointment should be applied to the raw surface 3 times a day. Apply for 7 days, or longer if necessary. The area should be washed off with an antibacterial soap each time. Any *new* thin crust that forms should not be removed, since that would delay healing. After applying an antibiotic ointment, cover the sore with a Band-Aid to prevent scratching and spread. If your child has received oral or injectable antibiotics, the antibiotic ointment is needed for only 48 hours.

Preventing the Spread of Impetigo to Other Areas on Your Child's Body—Every time your child touches the impetigo and then scratches another part of the skin with that finger, a new site of impetigo can form. To prevent this, discourage your child from touching or picking at the sores. Keep the fingernails cut short, and wash the hands often with an antibacterial soap.

Contagiousness—Impetigo is quite contagious. Be certain that other people in the family do not use your child's towel or washcloth. Any clothes, towels, or sheets that are contaminated with drainage from the impetigo should be washed with a disinfectant or bleach. Your child should be kept out of school until he or she has been on treatment for 24 hours with oral (or injectable) antibiotics. For mild impetigo treated with an antibiotic ointment, the child can continue to attend day care or school if the sore is covered with a Band-Aid.

Call Your Child's Physician Later If
- Other people in the family develop impetigo.
- The impetigo increases in size and number of sores after 48 hours on treatment.
- The impetigo is not completely healed in 1 week.
- A fever or a sore throat occurs.
- Cola-colored urine or swollen eyelids occur.
- Your child develops any of the "Call Your Child's Physician" symptoms.

JOCK ITCH

Jock itch is also called ringworm of the crotch, or Tinea cruris.

Symptoms and Characteristics
- Pink, scaly, itchy rash
- Inner thighs and groin involved (penis is not involved; scrotum is occasionally involved)
- Occurs almost exclusively in males

If your child's symptoms are different, call your physician for help.

Cause—Jock itch is caused by a fungus, often the same one that causes athlete's foot. Sometimes it's transferred by a towel because a teenager with athlete's foot dries the groin after drying the feet.

Expected Course—With appropriate treatment, the symptoms are better in 2 or 3 days and the rash is cured in 3 to 4 weeks.

Home Care

Antifungal Medicine—Buy Tinactin, Micatin, or Lotrimin powder or spray at your drugstore. You won't need a prescription. It needs to be applied twice a day to the rash and at least 1 inch beyond the borders. Make sure you get it in all the skin creases. Continue it for several weeks, or for at least 7 days after the rash seems to have cleared.

Dryness—Jock itch will improve dramatically if the groin area is kept dry. Loose-fitting cotton shorts should be worn (avoid nylon or other synthetic-fiber underwear because these fabrics don't absorb moisture). Shorts and athletic supporters should be washed frequently. After showers and baths, all creases should be carefully dried. The rash areas should be carefully cleansed once a day with plain water. Avoid using soap on the rash.

Scratching—Scratching will delay the cure, so have your child avoid scratching the area. Also keep the fingernails cut short.

Contagiousness—The condition is not very contagious. The fungus won't grow on dry, normal skin. Your child may continue to take gym and play sports.

Call Your Child's Physician Later If
- Any pimples, pus, or yellow crusts develop.
- There is no improvement in 1 week.
- The rash is not completely cured in 1 month.

LICE (Pediculosis)

Symptoms and Characteristics
- Nits (white eggs) are firmly attached to hair shafts near the skin.
- Unlike dandruff or sand, nits can't be shaken off.
- Gray bugs (lice) are 1/16 inch long, move quickly, and are difficult to see.
- The scalp is itchy with a rash.
- The back of the neck is the favorite area.
- The nits are easier to see than the lice because they are white and very numerous.

If your child's symptoms are different, call your physician for help.

Cause—Head lice live only on human beings and can spread quickly despite good health habits and regular hair-washing. They are spread by close contact or using the hat, comb, brush, or headphones of an infected person. The nits (eggs) normally hatch into lice within 1 week. Pubic lice (crabs) are slightly different but are treated the same way. They can be transmitted from bedding or clothing and do not signify sexual contact. Pets can get a different type of lice, but they will not spread to humans.

Expected Course—With treatment, all lice and nits will be killed. A recurrence usually means another contact with an infected person or the anti-lice shampoo wasn't left on for a full 10 minutes or repeated in 7 days. Also some lice are resistant to over-the-counter shampoos and need a prescription product. There are no lasting problems from having lice and they do not carry other diseases.

Home Care

Anti-Lice Shampoos—Buy Nix 1 percent anti-lice creme rinse (no prescription needed). Pour about 2 ounces of the product into damp hair.

Add a little warm water to work up a lather. Scrub the hair and scalp for 10 minutes, by the clock. Rinse the hair thoroughly and dry it with a towel. This shampoo kills both the lice and the nits. Repeat the anti-lice shampoo once after 7 days to prevent reinfection.

Removing Nits—To make sure the nits are dead, wait at least 8 hours after using the shampoo before removing them. Remove the nits by combing with a fine-tooth comb or pulling them out individually. The nits can be loosened using a mixture of half vinegar and half water. Apply the mixture to the hair and keep your child's hair under a towel wrap for 30 minutes. Even though the nits are dead, most schools will not allow children to return if nits are present. The head does not need to be shaved to cure lice.

Lice in the Eyelashes—If you see any lice or nits in the eyelashes, apply plain petrolatum to the eyelashes twice a day for 8 days. The lice won't survive.

Cleaning the House—Lice can't live for over 24 hours off the human body. Your child's room should be vacuumed. Combs and brushes should be soaked for 1 hour in a solution containing some anti-lice product. Wash your child's sheets, blankets, pillowcases, and any clothes worn in the past 72 hours in hot water (140°F kills lice and nits). Items that can't be washed (e.g., hats, coats, or scarves) should be set aside in airtight plastic bags for 2 weeks (the longest period that nits can survive). Anti-lice sprays or fumigation of the house is unnecessary.

Contagiousness of Lice—Check the heads of everyone else living in your home. If any have scalp rashes, sores, or itching, they should be treated with the anti-lice product even if lice and nits are not seen. Bedmates of children with lice should also be treated. If in doubt, have the person checked. Your child can return to school after 1 treatment with the shampoo. Re-emphasize not sharing combs and hats. Also notify the school nurse so she can check other students in your child's class.

Call Your Child's Physician Later If
- Itching interferes with sleep.
- The rash has not cleared by 1 week after treatment.
- The rash clears and then returns.
- New eggs appear in the hair.
- The sores start to spread or look infected.

POISON IVY

Symptoms and Characteristics
- Redness, swelling, and weeping blisters
- Eruption on exposed body surfaces (such as the hands)
- Shaped like streaks or patches
- Extreme itchiness
- Onset 1 or 2 days after the patient was in a forest or field

If your child's symptoms are different, call your physician for help.

Cause—Poison ivy, poison oak, and poison sumac cause the same type of rash and are found throughout the United States (except Nevada, Alaska, and Hawaii). Over 50 percent of people are sensitive to the oil of these plants. When the plants are burned, the toxic substance becomes airborne in the smoke and soot. Some children develop a similar blistering reaction after skin contact with lime juice or celery, followed by sun exposure (called phytophotodermatitis).

Expected Course—Usually lasts 2 weeks. Treatment reduces the symptoms but doesn't cure. The best approach is prevention. Swelling or rash near the eye will not harm the eye in any way.

Call Your Child's Physician

Immediately If
- The face is red or coughing begins following exposure to smoke.
- The rash involves more than one-fourth of the body.
- Your child had a severe poison ivy reaction in the past.

During Office Hours If
- The face, eyes, lips, or genitals are involved.
- The itching interferes with sleep.
- Any big blisters are present.
- The rash is open and oozing.
- Signs of infection occur, such as pus or soft yellow scabs.
- You think your child needs to be seen.

Home Care

Cool Soaks—Soak the involved area in cool water or massage it with an ice cube for 20 minutes as many times a day as necessary. Then let it air-dry. This will reduce itching and oozing.

Hydrocortisone Cream—Buy some 1 percent hydrocortisone cream (no prescription needed). If you already have a stronger steroid (the gels are the most effective), use it. Apply the cream 4 times a day or as often as the rash begins to itch. The sores should be dried up and no longer itchy in 10 to 14 days. In the meantime, cut your child's fingernails short and discourage scratching. Keep your child busy with other activities.

Benadryl—If itching persists, give Benadryl orally (no prescription needed) every 6 hours as needed.

Contagiousness—Anything that has poison ivy oil or sap on it is contagious for several weeks. This includes the shoes and clothes you last wore into the woods, as well as any pets that may have oil on their fur. Routine laundering will remove oil from clothing, and a bath with soap will clean up the pet. The rash begins 1 to 2 days after skin contact. The fluid from the blisters, however, is not contagious. Therefore, scratching the poison ivy sores will not cause it to spread.

Call Your Child's Physician Later If

- The itching becomes severe.
- Your child develops any of the "Call Your Child's Physician" symptoms.

Prevention of Poison Ivy

- Learn to recognize poison ivy plants. They tend to grow near riverbanks. At least, avoid all plants with 3 large shiny leaves. Another clue is the presence of shiny black spots on damaged leaves. On the West Coast you will need to identify poison oak.
- If your young child gets poison ivy twice, some plants are probably growing near your home. Locate and remove them.
- Wear long pants or socks when walking through woods that may contain poison ivy.
- If you think your child has had contact with poison ivy, wash the exposed areas of skin with any available soap for 5 minutes. Strong

laundry soap has no added benefits. Do this as soon as possible, because after one hour, it is of little value in preventing absorption of the oil.

• Currently, allergy shots or pills are not of value for poison ivy.

RINGWORM

Symptoms and Characteristics
- Ring-shaped pink patch
- Scaly raised border (always has scales)
- Ring slowly increases in size
- Clearing of the center as the patch grows
- Usually ½ to 1 inch in size
- Mildly itchy

If your child's symptoms are different, call your physician for help.

Cause—A fungus infection of the skin, often transferred from puppies or kittens who have it. It is not caused by a worm.

Expected Course—Ringworm responds well to appropriate treatment. Without treatment, natural immunity will develop in about 4 months.

Call Your Child's Physician During Office Hours If
- The scalp is involved. (Reason: pills are needed for treatment.)
- More than 3 spots are present.
- You think your child needs to be seen.

Home Care

Antifungal Cream—Buy Micatin, Tinactin, or Lotrimin cream at your drugstore (no prescription needed). Apply the cream twice a day to the rash and 1 inch beyond its borders. Continue this treatment for 1 week after the ringworm patch is smooth and seems to be gone. Encourage your child to avoid scratching the area, because scratching will delay a cure.

Contagiousness—Ringworm of the skin is mildly contagious. It requires direct skin-to-skin contact. The type acquired from pets is not transmitted from human to human, only from animal to human. After 48 hours of treatment, ringworm is not contagious at all. Your child doesn't have to miss any school or day care.

Treatment of Pets—Kittens and puppies with ringworm usually do not itch and may not have any rash. Pets with a skin rash or sores should be examined by a veterinarian. Also have your child avoid close contact with the animal until he is treated. Natural immunity develops in animals after 4 months even without treatment. Call your veterinarian with other questions.

Call Your Child's Physician Later If

- The ringworm continues to spread after 1 week on treatment.
- The rash is not cleared in 4 weeks.
- Your child develops any of the "Call Your Child's Physician" symptoms.

Related Topics

IMPETIGO (see page 476)
POISON IVY (see page 482)
DRY SKIN (see pag 449)

SHINGLES (Zoster)

Symptoms and Characteristics

- A linear rash that follows the path of 1 or more nerves
- Rash occurs on only 1 side of the body.
- Rash starts with clusters of red bumps, changes to water blisters, and finally becomes dry crusts (it looks like a small group of chicken pox).
- Back, chest, and abdomen are most common sites.
- Rash usually doesn't burn or itch in children (in contrast to the adult form).
- Child does not have a fever or feel sick.
- Child had chicken pox in the past.

If your child's symptoms are different, call your physician for help.

Cause—Zoster is caused by the chicken pox virus. The disease is not caught from other people with active shingles or chicken pox. The chicken pox virus lies dormant in the body of some people and is reactivated for unknown reasons as zoster. Children with zoster are usually over 3 years old.

Expected Course—New shingles continue to appear for several days. The rash usually dries up by 7 to 10 days. Complications do not occur unless the eye is involved. If zoster involves the nose, the cornea is usually also involved. Most people have shingles just once; a second attack occurs in 5 percent of children.

Call Your Child's Physician During Office Hours If

- The rash is very painful or very itchy.
- The rash is near the eye.
- You think your child needs to be seen.

Home Care

Relief of Symptoms—Most children have no symptoms. For pain, give acetaminophen or ibuprofen as necessary. (For dosage, see the tables on pages 238–40.) Avoid aspirin for zoster because of the possible link with Reye's syndrome. Discourage itching or picking the rash. The rash does not need any cream.

Contagiousness—Children with zoster can transmit chicken pox (but not zoster) to others. Transmission occurs by touching the zoster rash. Although they are far less contagious than children with chicken pox, children with zoster should stay home from school for 7 days unless they can keep the rash covered until it crusts over. Children or adults who have not had chicken pox should avoid visiting the child with zoster (unless the rash is covered).

Call Your Physician Later If

- The rash lasts more than 14 days.
- You feel your child is getting worse.
- Your child develops any of the "Call Your Child's Physician" symptoms.

SORES

Sores are coin-sized ulcerated, weeping, or scabbed areas on the skin. Many begin as blisters which quickly break open. The possible causes are many. If one of the following is suspected, save time by turning directly to that guideline:

BURNS, THERMAL (see page 38)
CHICKEN POX (see page 446)
COLD SORES (see page 567)
IMPETIGO (see page 476)
BITES: INSECT, BEE, OR TICK (see page 19)
POISON IVY (see page 482)
RINGWORM (see page 484)

If the cause of the sores is unknown, call your child's physician during office hours for an appointment.

TINEA VERSICOLOR

Symptoms and Characteristics
- Name means "multicolored ringworm"
- Occurs in adolescents and adults
- Numerous spots and patches on the neck, upper back, and shoulders
- Spots covered by a fine scale
- Spots vary in size.
- In summer, spots are light and don't tan like normal skin.
- In winter, as normal skin color fades, spots look darker (often pink or brown) compared to normal Caucasian skin.

If your child's symptoms are different, call your physician for help.

Cause—This superficial infection is caused by a yeastlike fungus called *Malassezia furfur*. It occurs more commonly in warm, humid climates.

Expected Course—The problem tends to wax and wane for many years. Since complications do not occur, tinea versicolor is solely a cosmetic problem. Itching is uncommon.

Home Care

Selsun Blue Shampoo—Selsun Blue (selenium sulfide) is a nonprescription medicated shampoo that can cure this condition. Apply this shampoo once a day for 14 days. Apply it to the affected skin areas as well as 2 or 3 inches onto the adjacent normal skin. Rub it in and let it dry. Be careful to keep it off the eyes or genitals, since it is irritating to these tissues. After 30 minutes, take a shower. By 2 weeks, the scaling should be stopped, and the rash is temporarily cured. The normal skin color will not return for 6 to 12 months.

Prevention of Recurrences—Tinea versicolor tends to recur. Prevent this by applying Selsun Blue shampoo to the formerly involved areas once a month for several years. Leave it on for 1 to 2 hours, then shower. This precaution is especially important in the summer months, because this fungus thrives in warm weather.

Contagiousness—Tinea versicolor is not contagious. This fungus is a normal inhabitant of the hair follicles in many people. Only a few develop the overgrowth of the fungus and a rash.

Call Your Child's Physician Later If

• The rash is not improved with this treatment by 2 weeks.

• You feel your child is getting worse.

Related Topic

RINGWORM (see page 484)

SKIN: CONDITIONS WITHOUT A RASH

BLISTERS, FOOT OR HAND

Symptoms and Characteristics

- Toes or heel are most commonly involved.
- Caused by friction
- On foot, due to sports, hiking, or new shoes
- On hand, due to prolonged use of a tool (such as a shovel) or playground equipment

Home Care

Treatment—Do not open the blisters, since this increases the possibility of infection. The blisters will dry up and peel off in 1 to 2 weeks. In the meantime, take the pressure off the area by placing a foam "donut" or a Band-Aid with a hole cut in the center over the blister. Also, if the blister is on the foot, temporarily wear a more comfortable shoe. If the blister accidentally breaks open, trim off the loose skin. Keep the surface clean by washing it twice a day with an antibacterial soap and changing to clean socks (for foot blisters). The open blister can be covered with an antibiotic ointment, surrounded by a "donut" of foam rubber, and then the whole area patched over with tape. Cleanse the area with warm water and reapply the ointment each day.

Call Your Child's Physician Later If

- The blister becomes infected.

Prevention of Foot Blisters

Avoid shoes that are too tight or too loose. If your child frequently gets blisters on a certain pressure area, cover that spot with petroleum jelly or tape before athletic activities to decrease the friction on the spot. Friction can also be reduced by wearing 2 pairs of socks if the shoes are not too tight. If blisters occur under a callus, file the callus down and lubricate it so it won't contribute to the friction.

Similar Conditions That Also Have Blisters

BURNS, THERMAL (see page 38)
IMPETIGO (see page 476)
POISON IVY (see page 482)

BLUISH LIPS (Cyanosis)

If your child's lips, mouth, ears, or nail beds have become bluish or dusky, call your child's physician *immediately*. Bluish skin (cyanosis) can indicate reduced oxygen in the blood, and serious disease. If your child is bluish and very cold, check first if the normal color returns with warming. Also, normal newborns can have bluish hands and feet (acrocyanosis) from sluggish circulation until 3 or 4 days of age.

Related Topic

BREATH-HOLDING SPELLS (see page 370)

CALLUSES, CORNS, AND BUNIONS

Symptoms and Characteristics

Calluses and corns are areas of thickened, hard skin. Calluses are located on the palms or soles and are painless. They occur over areas receiving prolonged friction or pressure, as with walking barefoot or using a hand tool. Corns can be located anywhere on the foot except the sole, are caused by pressure from tight shoes, and are painful. Bunions occur on the side of the foot over the protruding bone at the base of the first or fifth toe. Occasionally a bunion will occur where the back of a shoe rubs against the back of the heel. A bunion is painful and often causes a swollen area due to damage to both the skin and underlying bone. Bunions can also result from tight shoes, especially narrow or pointed ones.

Call Your Child's Physician During Office Hours If

- A callus is quite painful.
- A callus has black dots in it (probably it's a wart).
- A bunion is extremely painful or swollen.
- An unexplained fever is present.
- You think your child needs to be seen.

Home Care

Calluses—No treatment is necessary. The callus is protective. If it cracks, see CRACKED SKIN, below. If a blister develops, see BLISTERS, FOOT OR HAND, page 489.

Corns—Change to properly fitting shoes. Temporarily protect the corn with donut-shaped foam pads or a Band-Aid with a hole cut in the center. The pain should resolve in 1 week.

Bunions—The key to recovery is changing to properly fitting (i.e., wider or longer) shoes. Your youngster may need to wear soft slippers for a week. While most tight shoes must be discarded, a prized shoe (if it is long enough) may be salvaged by having the constricting area stretched out by a shoemaker with a shoe punch. (Note: The leather-stretching chemicals give disappointing results.) Soak the feet in warm water for 15 minutes twice a day. Take acetaminophen or ibuprofen for pain. (For dosage, see the tables on pages 238–40.) Protect the area with donut-shaped bunion pads. The pain and swelling will take 2 to 3 months to resolve. Call your child's physician if it gets worse instead of better.

CRACKED SKIN

Symptoms and Characteristics

Cracked skin most commonly occurs on the soles of the feet, especially the heels and big toes (called juvenile plantar dermatosis). Deep cracks are painful and periodically bleed. The main cause is wearing wet shoes and socks, or swimming a lot. Cracks can also develop on the hands in children who frequently wash dishes or suck their thumbs. The lips can become cracked (chapped) in children with a habit of licking their lips or from excessive exposure to sun or wind.

Home Care

Even deep cracks of many years' duration can be healed in about 2 weeks if they are constantly covered with an ointment (like petroleum jelly). If the crack seems mildly infected, use an antibiotic ointment (no prescription needed). Covering the ointment with a Band-Aid, socks, or gloves speeds recovery even more. For chapped lips, a lip balm can be applied frequently. Call your child's physician during office hours if any of the cracks develop pimples or yellow drainage.

DANDRUFF

Symptoms and Characteristics

Dandruff is normal shedding of the scalp. Skin is constantly regenerating. On most of the body surface, the flakes of dead skin fall to the ground without fanfare, but they can accumulate in the hair. Some children shed skin faster than others, making the dandruff more noticeable. Keep in mind that the shedding of skin cells is a normal process that occurs throughout life on the entire body surface. It is not contagious.

Home Care

Daily Shampooing—The key to fighting dandruff is removing the flakes as fast as they form by washing the hair daily. A regular shampoo usually works very well. Brush the hair before each washing. Eventually, you may be able to wash the hair every other day without seeing dandruff, but you probably won't ever be able to wash it less often than that.

Anti-Dandruff Shampoos—If the scalp is red and irritated or the scales are quite greasy, use a medicated shampoo (one that contains selenium sulfide) for 3 days in a row and then once a week. Your pharmacist can help you select one that does not require a prescription (e.g., Selsun Blue). These shampoos not only remove the dandruff but also cut down on the rate of shedding. They are used in a special way: Lather the hair, wait 3 minutes, then rinse thoroughly. Continue to use a regular shampoo on other days.

Avoid Hair Tonics—Hair tonics and creams just cover up the problem, and the dandruff eventually comes off in bigger flakes.

Call Your Child's Physician Later If
- The dandruff is not improved after 2 weeks of treatment.

FINGERNAIL INFECTION (PARONYCHIA)

Symptoms and Characteristics
- A large pimple at the junction of the cuticle and the fingernail
- Redness and tenderness of this area
- Occasionally, pus draining from this area

If your child's symptoms are different, call your physician for help.

Causes—Those with a large pimple or draining pus are usually infected with the staphylococcus bacteria. The original cause is usually a break in the skin resulting from pulling on or chewing on the cuticle. Those limited to redness and swelling of the cuticle (without pus) usually are due to candida (yeast). The candida infections usually occur in thumb suckers or finger suckers, swimmers, or other children who have waterlogged cuticles.

Expected Course—With proper treatment, this infection should clear up in 7 days. If not, your physician will probably prescribe an oral antibiotic.

Call Your Child's Physician

Immediately If
- Fever or chills are present.
- A red streak spreads beyond the cuticle.
- The finger pad is swollen or tender.

Within 24 Hours If
- You want your physician to open the pus pockets.
- You can see pus under the base of the nail.
- The infection encircles the nail.
- This is a recurrent problem.
- You think your child needs to be seen.

Home Care

Antiseptic Soaks—For bacterial infections, soak the infected finger 3 times daily for 10 minutes in warm water and a liquid antibacterial soap. Do this for 4 days or longer if the infection has not healed.

Antibiotic Ointments—For bacterial infections, apply an antibiotic ointment 6 times a day.

Open Any Large Pimple—Open and drain any visible pus pocket using a needle sterilized with rubbing alcohol or a flame. Make a large opening where the pus pocket joins with the nail. If the pus doesn't run out, gently squeeze the pus pocket.

Yeast (Candida) Infections—For yeast infections apply Lotrimin cream 3 times daily (no prescription needed). Also, try to keep the area dry. Do not cover it with a Band-Aid.

Call Your Child's Physician Later If

- The infection is not improved by 48 hours on home treatment.
- The infection is not totally resolved within 7 days.
- Your child develops any of the "Call Your Child's Physician" symptoms.

Prevention

Discourage any picking or chewing of hangnails (loose pieces of cuticle). Instead, cut these off with nail clippers.

Related Topic

TOENAIL, INGROWN (see page 508)

SLIVERS OR SPLINTERS (Foreign Body in Skin)

Symptoms and Characteristics

A sliver is a foreign object embedded in the skin. Most of these are wood slivers (splinters) that go in very superficially. Others are thorns or glass or metal fragments. Most slivers are painful if pressed unless they are very superficial. Remember that pencil lead is actually graphite (harmless), not lead. Even colored leads are nontoxic. If appropriate, turn to the guideline on SKIN TRAUMA (SCRAPES), page 78.

Call Your Child's Physician

Immediately If

- The sliver is deeply embedded (for instance, a needle or toothpick in the foot).
- It is a fishhook or anything with a barb.
- You think you won't be able to get it out.

During Office Hours If

- It was removed but went deeply (a puncture wound) *and* more than 5 years have passed since the last tetanus booster.
- You think your child needs to be seen.

Home Care

Needle and Tweezers—Remove larger slivers or thorns with a needle and tweezers.

- Most superficial, tiny slivers do not need to be removed. They will be removed with normal shedding of the skin.
- Check the tweezers beforehand to be certain the ends (pickups) meet exactly. (If they do not, bend them.) Sterilize the tools with rubbing alcohol or a flame.
- Wash the skin surrounding the sliver briefly with soap and water before trying to remove it. Be careful not to push the sliver in deeper. Don't soak the area if the foreign body is wood (reason: can cause swelling of the splinter).
- Use the needle to completely expose the large end of the sliver. Use good lighting. A magnifying glass may help.
- Then grasp the end firmly with the tweezers and pull it out at the same angle at which it went in. Getting a good grip the first time is especially important with slivers that go in perpendicular to the skin or those trapped under the fingernail.
- For slivers under a fingernail, sometimes a wedge of the nail must be cut away with fine scissors to expose the end of the sliver.
- Superficial horizontal slivers (where you can see all of it) usually can be removed by pulling on the end. If the end breaks off, open the skin with a sterile needle along the length of the sliver and flick it out.

Cactus Spines—The following method can also be used for small Fiberglas spicules or plant stickers (e.g., stinging nettle). Usually these break when pressure is applied with a tweezers. Apply a layer of hair remover wax. Let it air-dry for 5 minutes, or accelerate the process with a hair dryer. Then peel it off with the spicules. White glue can also be tried, but it is less effective.

Call Your Child's Physician Later If

- You can't get it all out *and* the sliver is glass or metal.
- You can't get it all out *and* it's painful (i.e., not superficial).
- The site of penetration becomes infected. (See WOUND INFECTIONS, page 87.)

FRECKLES

Freckles are pigmented spots brought out by sunlight. Thus, they usually are confined to the face, neck, chest, and shoulders. They occur mainly in fair-skinned people and are due to an inherited tendency to have tanning pigment (melanin) scattered irregularly, rather than evenly, throughout the skin. They start around age 5, and although they fade somewhat each winter, they become prominent each summer.

Home Care

Sunscreens cannot prevent them, and lemon juice cannot bleach them. Therefore, the child who has freckles must learn to live with them. Family and friends can help by referring to the freckles as special and attractive. They never turn into skin cancer. People with freckles sunburn easily. They need to be extra careful about using a strong sunscreen and avoiding sun overexposure (see SUNBURN, page 503).

HAIR LOSS

Hair loss (alopecia) can occur in patches or throughout the scalp. The causes are many, including ringworm, which requires medical diagnosis and treatment.

Call Your Child's Physician During Office Hours If

All children who have hair loss should be seen by a physician, with the following exceptions:

- The hair of many newborns falls out during the first few months of life. This baby hair is replaced by permanent hair.

- Babies from 3 to 6 months of age commonly rub off a patch of hair on the back of the head due to friction from turning the head against the mattresses of cribs, playpens, and infant seats. This grows back nicely once they start sitting up.
- Hair can be lost because of vigorous brushing, hot combs, tight ponytails or braids, or exercising while wearing headphones.
- Hair follicles are very sensitive to stress, and hair may begin to fall out at about 3 months (100 days) after a severe stress (such as high fever, severe illness, psychological crisis, crash diets, surgery, or even childbirth). This is called telogen effluvium. The hair falls out in a generalized distribution over the next 3 or 4 months. After the hair stops shedding, it takes another 6 to 8 months to return to normal. Complete hair regrowth is the rule. The whole cycle takes about 12 months.

JAUNDICE

Symptoms and Characteristics

A jaundiced child has yellowish skin and sclera (the white part of the eyes). The yellow color is due to the accumulation of bilirubin pigment in the blood and skin. The most common cause of jaundice is hepatitis (a liver infection). Usually these infections are not serious, but they need to be evaluated by a physician.

While jaundice occurs in over 30 percent of newborns and is usually harmless, the follow-up of jaundiced newborns should be carried out under the direction of your baby's physician. Be certain to notify your physician if the jaundice worsens after discharge from the hospital. (See JAUNDICE OF THE NEWBORN, page 135.)

Call Your Child's Physician

Immediately If

- Your child is difficult to awaken (call 911).
- Your child is confused.
- Your child has vomited any blood.
- Your child acts or looks very sick.

Within 24 Hours If

- All children with jaundice need medical consultation. Close contacts of

children with hepatitis can usually be protected with an immune globulin injection.

Carotenemia: The Jaundice Imitator

Your child has carotenemia if the following are present:

• Yellow-orange coloration of the skin
• No yellow-orange coloration of the sclera (white part of the eye)
• High intake of yellow, orange, and green vegetables and fruits
• Your child is 6 to 18 months.

Carotenemia is harmless and temporary. The yellow color is due to a pigment (carotene) found in yellow and orange vegetables (such as squash,
carrots, and sweet potatoes) as well as fruits such as oranges, apricots,
and peaches. Carotene is also found in green vegetables (such as green
beans and peas). The intake of these vegetables and fruits needs to be reduced only if you want to change your child's skin tone. After a return to
a more normal diet, the carotenemia color will disappear in 3 or 4 weeks.
Even without dietary change, the skin color will gradually return to normal by 2 or 3 years of age.

LYMPH NODES (OR GLANDS), SWOLLEN

Symptoms and Characteristics

• Normal noninfected nodes are smaller than ½ inch across (often the size
of a pea or baked bean). The body contains more than 500 lymph nodes.
They can always be felt in the neck and groin. Normal nodes are largest
at age 10 to 12. At this age they can be twice the normal adult size.
• Active nodes with viral infections are usually ½ to 1 inch across. Slight
enlargement and mild tenderness means the lymph node is fighting infection and succeeding.
• Active nodes with bacterial infections are usually larger than 1 inch
across and exquisitely tender. If they are over 2 inches across or the
overlying skin is pink, the nodes are not controlling the infection, and
may contain pus.

Causes—Lymph glands stop the spread of infection and protect the bloodstream from invasion (blood poisoning). They enlarge with cuts, scrapes, scratches, splinters, burns, insect bites, rashes, impetigo, or any break in the skin. Cancer is an extremely rare cause in children. Try to locate and identify the cause of the swollen gland by remembering that the groin nodes drain lymph from the legs and lower abdomen, the armpit nodes drain the arms and upper chest, the back of the neck nodes drain the scalp, and the front of the neck nodes drain the lower face, nose, and throat. Most enlarged nodes in the neck are due to colds and throat infections. A disease like chicken pox can cause all the nodes to swell.

Expected Course—With the usual viral infections or skin infections, nodes can quickly double in size over 2 or 3 days and then slowly return to normal over 2 to 4 weeks. However, you can still see and feel nodes in most normal children, especially in the neck and groin. Don't look for lymph nodes, because you can always find some.

Call Your Child's Physician

Immediately If
- The node is 2 or more inches in size.
- The node is quite tender to the touch.
- The overlying skin is red.
- The node is in the neck *and* there is any difficulty with breathing, swallowing, or opening the mouth.
- The node interferes with moving the neck.
- Your child acts or looks very sick.

Within 24 Hours If
- The node is 1 to 2 inches in size.
- The cause of the swollen node is unknown.
- Your baby is under 1 month old.
- The swollen node is in the neck, and your child also has a sore throat.
- An unexplained fever is present.
- An explained fever lasts more than 3 days.
- You think your child needs to be seen.

Home Care

Treat the Cause of Swelling—In general, no treatment is necessary for swollen nodes associated with viral infections (for example, colds). For bacterial infections, the underlying disease that's causing the node to react needs to be treated. For example, remove the splinter, treat the ingrown toenail, or have a dentist treat the tooth abscess. Many children with swollen lymph nodes due to a skin infection also need an oral antibiotic.

Pain or Fever Relief—For pain or fever above 102°F, give the appropriate dose of acetaminophen or ibuprofen.

Don't Squeeze the Nodes—Poking and squeezing lymph nodes may keep them from shrinking back to normal size. Remember that it may take a month for the nodes to return to normal. They won't completely disappear. There's no need to check them more than once a month. If your child fidgets with them, discourage it if he's old enough to cooperate.

Call Your Child's Physician Later If

- The node remains larger than ½ inch for more than 1 month.
- You feel your child is getting worse.
- Your child develops any of the "Call Your Child's Physician" symptoms.

MOLES (Nevi)

Symptoms and Characteristics

Moles, or nevi, are tan, brown, or black spots on the skin. Most adults have 20 to 30 moles. They first appear around 1 year of age, and we are constantly getting new ones. They do not fade and they last throughout our lives. In general, they are harmless. Moles are no longer routinely removed just because they are in areas of friction or pressure. Even the moles removed for the changes listed below are usually not cancerous.

Call Your Child's Physician During Office Hours If

- You want a mole removed for cosmetic purposes.
- The mole is pitch-black *and* your child was born with it.
- The mole is growing rapidly in size.
- The mole has bled or become an open sore.
- The mole has changed colors (especially to red or blue).

- The surface has become lumpy (a smooth surface is normal).
- The edge (border) of the mole becomes irregular or notched.

PALE SKIN

Symptoms and Characteristics

The skin color is white or very pale.

Causes—Most of these children simply have a fair complexion. They have always been fair, have light hair, and usually have a parent with similar skin coloring. Another factor is lack of sun exposure; hence pallor (pale color) is noted more during winter months. Temporary paleness also occurs when someone is very cold; the normal color returns after warming up.

Pale skin (pallor) rarely is due to anemia (low red blood cell count). In anemia, the lips, gums, inside of the eyelids, and nailbeds are also pale. In a child with fair complexion who is not anemic, these areas should be nice and pink.

Call Your Child's Physician

Immediately If

- Your child has fainted.
- Your child becomes dizzy when standing up.
- Nosebleeds have been heavy.
- Menstrual periods have been heavy.
- Blood has been passed in stools or vomited material.
- The urine is red, pink, or tea-colored.
- The whites of the eyes are yellow.
- Your child acts or looks very sick.

During Office Hours If

- The paleness is of recent onset.
- The paleness is long-standing, but the cause is unclear.
- You think your child needs to be seen.

PIMPLES

Symptoms and Characteristics

Pimples (pustules or whiteheads) are small blisters filled with pus. They are caused by the staph bacteria (unlike acne). While they can occur on any part of the body, they commonly occur in areas of friction (as where a diaper rubs). Tight braids combined with pomades (perfumed ointments) are a common cause of pimples on the scalp. The tight braid injures the hair follicles and the pomade seals them off, thus predisposing them to infection. Pimples are a superficial skin infection and never leave scars.

Similar Conditions—If appropriate, turn directly to the following guidelines:

ACNE (see page 468)
BOILS (ABSCESSES) (see page 473)
FINGERNAIL INFECTION (PARONYCHIA) (see page 493)
IMPETIGO (see page 476)

Call Your Child's Physician

Immediately If

- Your baby is under 4 weeks old (Exception: erythema toxicum. See NEWBORN RASHES AND BIRTHMARKS, page 108.)
- An unexplained fever is present.
- Your child acts or looks very sick.

During Office Hours If

- Your child is under 1 year old.
- There are 10 or more pimples.
- The pimples are larger than ⅛ inch across.
- You think your child needs to be seen.

Home Care

Treatment—Wash the area with an antibacterial soap and water. Open any pimples that have come to a head, using a needle sterilized with rubbing alcohol or flame, and then throw the needle away. The pus should run out easily without any squeezing. Clean the open pimples with an antibacterial soap and water. Then apply an antibiotic ointment.

Common Mistakes—A common mistake is to cover pimples with a Band-Aid. This can cause them to spread. The application of petroleum jelly or any ointment not containing an antibiotic can also make them much worse.

Call Your Child's Physician Later If

- The pimples are not completely gone in 3 days.
- New pimples develop after 24 hours on treatment.
- Your child develops any of the "Call Your Child's Physician" symptoms.

Prevention of Pimples

To prevent spread, ask your child not to touch the pimples or rub the skin. Cut the fingernails short and wash the hands frequently. Give your child a shower once a day with an antibacterial soap. Be sure to use a separate washcloth and towel for this child. Wash your child's clothes and sheets with disinfectant or bleach to remove the staph bacteria from them. For pimples of the scalp, pomades should be discontinued and braiding done loosely.

SUNBURN

Symptoms and Characteristics

Sunburn is due to overexposure of the skin to the ultraviolet rays of the sun or a sun lamp. Most people have been sunburned many times. Vacations can quickly turn into painful experiences when the power of the sun is overlooked. Unfortunately, the symptoms of sunburn do not begin until 2 to 4 hours after the sun's damage has been done. The peak reaction of redness, pain, and swelling is not seen for 24 hours.

Minor sunburn is a first-degree burn that turns the skin pink or red. Prolonged sun exposure can cause blistering and a second-degree burn. Sunburn never causes a third-degree burn or scarring because it is limited to the superficial layer of skin (epidermis).

Repeated sun exposure and suntans causes premature aging of the skin (wrinkling, sagging, and brown sunspots). Repeated sunburns increase the risk of skin cancer in the damaged areas. Each blistering sunburn doubles the risk of developing malignant melanoma, which is the most serious type of skin cancer.

Call Your Child's Physician

Immediately If

- The sunburn is extremely painful *and* widespread.
- Your child is unable to look at lights because of eye pain.
- Your child has an unexplained fever over 102°F.
- Your child passes out or feels dizzy with standing.
- Your child acts or looks very sick.

Within 24 Hours If

- More than 2 blisters are present.
- Any of the blisters are broken.
- The sunburn looks infected.
- You think your child needs to be seen.

Home Care

Pain Relief—The sensation of pain and heat will probably last for 48 hours.

- Ibuprofen products begun within 6 hours of sun exposure and continued for 2 days can reduce the discomfort. (For dosage, see the table on page 240.)
- Nonprescription 1 percent hydrocortisone cream may cut down on swelling and pain, but only if used early. Apply 3 times a day. If you don't have any, apply a moisturizing cream.
- The symptoms can also be helped by cool baths or compresses several times a day. Add 2 or 3 tablespoons of baking soda to the tub.
- Showers are usually painful because of the force of the spray.
- Don't use any soap on the burned skin.
- Offer extra water on the first day to replace the fluids lost in the sunburn and to prevent dehydration and dizziness.
- Peeling will usually occur on the fifth to seventh day. Peeling and itching can be reduced by applying the 1 percent hydrocortisone cream or a moisturizing cream (see ECZEMA, page 450) to the involved skin once or twice a day. (Avoid petrolatum or other ointments because they keep heat and sweat from escaping.)

Common Mistakes in Sunburn Treatment

- Avoid applying ointments or butter to sunburn; they just make the symptoms worse and are painful to remove.

- Don't buy any of the common first-aid creams or sprays for burns. They often contain benzocaine, which can cause an allergic rash, and they don't relieve the pain of first-degree burns.
- Don't confuse sunscreens, which block the sun's burning rays, with suntan lotions or oils, which mainly lubricate the skin. Despite advertisements to the contrary, suntan oils cannot help your child tan faster or more deeply. Also, they offer no protection against sunburn.

Call Your Child's Physician Later If

- You feel your child is getting worse.
- Your child develops any of the "Call Your Child's Physician" symptoms.

Prevention of Sunburns

The best way to prevent skin cancer is to prevent sunburn. Although skin cancer occurs in adults, it is caused by the sun exposure and sunburns that occurred during childhood. Every time you apply sunscreen to your child, you are preventing skin cancer down the line.

Sunscreens—Apply sunscreen any time your child is going to be outdoors for more than 30 minutes a day. Set a good example. Apply sunscreen to your own skin as well as your child's skin.

High-Risk Children—About 15 percent of white children have skin that never tans but only burns. These fair-skinned children need to be extremely careful about sun exposure throughout their lives. If a child has red or blond hair, blue or green eyes, freckles, or excessive moles, he or she is at increased risk for sunburn and skin cancer. These children need to use a sunscreen throughout the summer even for a brief exposure. They should avoid the sun whenever possible.

Infants in the Sun—The skin of infants is thinner than the skin of older children and more sensitive to the sun. Therefore, babies under 6 months of age should be kept out of direct sunlight. Keep them in the shade whenever possible. If they have to be in the sun, sunscreens, longer clothing, and a hat with a brim are essential. When a sunscreen is needed, infants can use adult sunscreens.

Tanning—For teenagers who are determined to have a suntan, guide them as to the limits of sun exposure without a sunscreen. Try to keep sun exposure to small amounts early in the season until a tan builds up. (Caution: While people with a suntan can tolerate a little more sun, they can still get a serious sunburn.) Start with 15 or 20 minutes of sun per day and increase by 5 minutes a day. Decrease daily exposure time if the skin becomes reddened. Because of the 2- to 4-hour delay before the symptoms of sunburn appear, don't expect symptoms (such as redness) to tell you when it's time to get out of the sun. After 1 hour of sun exposure, always apply a sunscreen.

Time of Day—Avoid exposure to the sun during the hours of 10:00 A.M. to 3:00 P.M., when the sun's rays are most intense. Don't let overcast days give you a false sense of security. Over 70 percent of the sun's rays still get through the clouds. Over 30 percent of the sun's rays can also penetrate loosely woven fabrics (for example, a T-shirt).

High Altitude—Be especially careful about exposure to the sun at high altitudes. Sun exposure increases 4 percent for each 1,000 feet of elevation above sea level. A sunburn can occur quickly when a child is hiking above the timberline. Remember also that water, sand, or snow increases sun exposure. The shade from a hat or umbrella won't protect your child from reflected rays.

Eyes, Nose, and Lips—Protect your child's eyes from the sun's rays. Years of exposure to ultraviolet light increases the risk of cataracts. Buy sunglasses with UV protection. To prevent sunburned lips, apply a lip coating that contains a sunscreen. If the nose or some other area has been repeatedly burned during the summer, protect it completely from the sun's rays with zinc oxide ointment.

Sunscreens

There are good sunscreens on the market that prevent sunburn but still permit gradual tanning to occur. Choose a broad-spectrum sunscreen that screens out both UVA and UVB rays.

The sun protection factor (SPF) or filtering power of a sunscreen product determines what percentage of the ultraviolet rays get through to the skin. An SPF of 15 allows only $\frac{1}{15}$ (7 percent) of the sun's rays to get through and thereby extends safe sun exposure from 20 minutes to 5 hours without sunburning. An SPF higher than 15 protects against sunburn for more than 5 hours. However, an SPF higher than 15 is rarely needed in most parts of the United States because protection against sunburn during the 5 hours between 10 A.M. and 3 P.M. is usually sufficient.

Fair-skinned children (with red or blond hair) need a sunscreen with an SPF of 30. The simplest approach is to use an SPF of 15 or greater on all other children.

Apply sunscreen 30 minutes before exposure to the sun to give it time to penetrate the skin. Give special attention to the areas most likely to become sunburned, such as the nose, ears, cheeks, and shoulders.

Most products need to be reapplied every 3 to 4 hours, as well as immediately after swimming or profuse sweating. A "waterproof" sunscreen stays on for about 30 minutes in water. Most people apply too little sunscreen (the average adult requires 1 ounce of sunscreen per application).

SWEATING, EXCESSIVE

Symptoms and Characteristics

The parent may be concerned because a child has a wet pillow after naps. Sometimes the entire bed is wet, since sweat glands are found throughout the body's surface. Neither of these examples is necessarily abnormal.

Your adolescent may be unduly worried about underarm perspiration or sweaty palms. Teenagers may be reassured that sweating normally increases with exercise and tension, and this is never abnormal.

Similar Conditions—Sweating occurs with fever (so take your child's temperature). If fever is present, save time by turning directly to that guideline. (See FEVER, page 427.)

Causes—The purpose of sweating is to cool off the body by evaporation. The most common cause of sweating is overheating due to hot weather, a hot room, overdressing, or too many blankets. When a child is covered up in bed, the *only* way to release heat is through the head. Night sweats in a child who is otherwise well mean nothing. Some parents worry unduly about diseases from another era (such as tuberculosis or malaria).

Call Your Child's Physician During Office Hours If

- Your baby is under 1 month old.
- Your child has unexplained fevers.
- Your child has unexplained weight loss.
- You think your child needs to be seen.

Home Care

Turn down the heat in your home. Dress your child in lighter clothing for naps. Offer your child extra fluids in hot weather to prevent dehydration. Adolescents, of course, need to be introduced to underarm antiperspirants/deodorants to prevent body odor. Some also need to bathe with an antibacterial soap. For foot odors from excessive perspiration, change the socks and shoes during the day or consider special shoe liners that absorb odors.

TOENAIL, INGROWN

Symptoms and Characteristics

- Tenderness, redness, and swelling of the skin surrounding the corner of the toenail on one of the big toes.
- Occasionally drainage of pus from this area

Causes—Ingrown toenails are usually due to tight shoes (such as cowboy boots) and/or improper cutting of the toenails. Children with wide feet are predisposed, since many shoes come in only one width. Ingrown toenails take several weeks to clear up.

Call Your Child's Physician

Immediately If

- Fever or chills are present.
- A red streak spreads beyond the toe.

During Office Hours If

- Any pus or yellow drainage is present.
- The corner of the nail is impossible to locate.
- The problem is a recurrent one.
- You think your child needs to be seen.

Home Care

Soaking—Soak the foot twice a day in warm water and an antibacterial soap for 20 minutes. While soaking, massage outward the part of the cuticle (skin next to the nail) that is swollen. A "cuticle pusher" (available in most drugstores) may be helpful.

Cut Off the Corner of the Toenail—The pain is always caused by the corner of the toenail rubbing against the raw cuticle. Only this once, cut the corner off so the irritated tissue can quiet down and heal. If the corner is buried in the swollen cuticle, have your physician remove it. The main purpose of treatment is to help the nail grow *over* the nail cuticle rather than get stuck in it. Therefore, during soaks, try to bend the nail corners upward. You can try to wedge some cotton under the edge of the nail, but for practical purposes, this is impossible during the infected phase. Filing or cutting a wedge out of the center of the upper edge of the nail may help the corners bend upward.

Antibiotic Ointment—If your child's cuticle is just red and irritated, an antibiotic ointment is probably not needed. But if the cuticle is swollen or oozing, apply an antibiotic ointment (no prescription needed) 5 or 6 times a day.

Shoes—Have your child wear sandals or go barefoot as much as possible to prevent pressure on the toenail. When your child must wear closed shoes, protect the ingrown toenail as follows: If the inner edge is involved, tape cotton or a foam pad between the first and second toes to keep them from touching. If the outer edge is involved, tape cotton or a foam pad to the outside of the ball of the toe to keep the toenail from touching the side of the shoe.

Call Your Child's Physician Later If
- The problem is not much better in 1 week.
- The problem is not totally resolved in 2 weeks.
- Your child develops any of the "Call Your Child's Physician" symptoms.

Prevention of Ingrown Toenails
Prevent recurrences by making sure that your child's shoes are not too narrow. Give away those pointed or tight shoes. After the cuticle is healed, cut the toenails straight across, leaving the corners. Don't cut them too short. After baths, while the nails are pliable, lift up the corners of the nails.

WARTS

Symptoms and Characteristics

- Raised, round, rough-surfaced growth on the skin
- Skin-colored or pink
- Most commonly occur on the hands
- Not painful unless located on the bottom of the foot (plantar wart)
- Has brown dots within it and clearly has a boundary with the normal skin (unlike calluses)

If your child's symptoms are different, call your physician for help.

Cause—Warts are caused by viruses (not by playing with toads).

Expected Course—Warts are harmless. Most warts disappear without treatment in 2 or 3 years. With treatment, they resolve in 2 to 3 months. There are no shortcuts in treating warts. Itching and redness mean the wart is responding to treatment. If the treatment of warts becomes painful or expensive, it may be better to step back and wait for them to go away naturally.

Call Your Child's Physician During Office Hours If

- Some warts are on the bottom of the feet.
- Some are on the face.
- Some are on the genital area.
- A wart is open and infected-looking.
- You think your child needs to be seen.

Home Care

Cover the Wart with Duct Tape—Cover the wart with a small piece of duct tape (not regular adhesive tape). Warts deprived of air and sun exposure sometimes die without the need for treatment with acids. Remove the tape once a week. Wash the skin and rub off any dead wart tissue. After it has dried thoroughly overnight, reapply duct tape. The tape treatment may be needed for 8 weeks.

Wart-Removing Acids with Duct Tape—To get faster results, also use a nonprescription acid. Ask your pharmacist to recommend one. Apply it once a day to the top of the wart after soaking the wart in water for

5 minutes. Since you are using an acid, avoid getting any near the eyes or mouth. Keep the lid closed tightly so it won't evaporate. The acid will work faster if it is covered with duct tape.

The acid will turn the top of the wart into dead skin (it will turn white). Once or twice a week, remove the dead wart material by paring it down with a razor blade. The dead wart will be softer and easier to slice if you soak the area first in warm water for 10 minutes. If the cutting causes any pain or minor bleeding, you have cut into living wart tissue. If your child won't let you cut off the dead wart material or you are afraid you might hurt the child, file it down with an emery board or have your child's physician pare down the wart.

Contagiousness—Encourage your child not to pick at the warts, because this may cause them to spread. If your child chews or sucks the wart, cover the area with duct tape. Encourage your child to give up the habit of chewing on the wart, because doing so can lead to warts on the lips or face. Warts are not very contagious to other people. The incubation period is 1 to 4 months.

Call Your Child's Physician Later If
- New warts develop after 2 weeks of treatment.
- The warts are still present after 8 weeks of treatment.
- Your child develops any of the "Call Your Child's Physician" symptoms.

BRAIN

ALTITUDE SICKNESS

Symptoms and Characteristics
- Headache, fatigue, dizziness, nausea
- Shortness of breath and rapid heartbeat on exertion
- Insomnia or restless sleep
- Onset at 8,000 feet elevation or higher
- Onset within 6 to 8 hours of arrival at higher altitude

If your child's symptoms are different, call your physician for help.

Cause—Altitude sickness is caused by the lower level of oxygen in the air at higher altitudes. Many people travel to mountainous areas to hike or ski. Symptoms occur in 50 percent of nonacclimated people who go abruptly from sea level to 10,000 feet. The likelihood of symptoms increases with the altitude.

Expected Course—Most people with acute mountain sickness (the most common type of altitude sickness) feel normal in 2 or 3 days. With over-exertion and ascent above 10,000 feet, 4 percent of people can develop life-threatening complications such as pulmonary edema (lung failure) or cerebral edema (swelling of the brain).

Call 911 If
- Your child is confused.
- Your child can't talk normally.
- Your child can't walk normally.

- The lips are bluish.
- Breathing is labored or fast.

Call Your Child's Physician Immediately If
- The headache is severe.
- Vomiting has occurred 3 or more times.
- Your child acts or looks very sick.

Home Care

First Aid for Symptoms of Severe Altitude Sickness—Rapidly transport your child to a lower altitude. Descend at least 2,000 feet, and always go below 10,000 feet elevation. If your child cannot walk, carry him or her in a sitting position. Administer oxygen as soon as it becomes available.

Rest for Mild Symptoms—The symptoms usually respond to 2 or 3 days of rest, fluids, and a light diet. Acetaminophen can be given for the headache (aspirin may make it worse). The dizziness and headache can usually be improved by deliberately breathing faster and deeper to bring in more oxygen. Skiing, hiking, or any other type of strenuous exercise should be postponed. Once your child feels healthy again, activity should be increased gradually. Breathing from an oxygen tank can improve symptoms temporarily, but generally this is unnecessary.

Call Your Physician Later If
- The symptoms last more than 3 days.
- You feel your child is getting worse.
- Your child develops any of the "Call Your Child's Physician" symptoms.

Prevention of Altitude Sickness
- Try to stage your mountain visit. Spend a few days at 5,000 to 7,000 feet before journeying to the high country.
- Take it easy on the day of arrival. Some exercise (like short walks) is important, but take rest breaks. Gradually increase the amount of exertion during days 2 and 3.
- Avoid dehydration by drinking ample fluids.
- While mountain climbing, gain only 1,000 feet per day.
- If your child has experienced severe altitude sickness before, talk to your physician about taking Diamox tablets (a prescription medicine) preventively in the future.

Newborns and Mountain Travel

- It is destinations and overnight stays above 8,000 feet that are of concern. Brief travel over 10,000- to 11,000-foot mountain passes is safe.
- Vacationers from sea level with newborns should avoid mountain vacations above 8,000 feet for the first 1 or 2 months of life, unless the family lives there and the pregnancy took place there.
- Travel to the mountains shouldn't cause any problems if the destination is less than 8,000 feet.

Newborns and Flying

- If flying is essential, it's safe to fly after 7 days of age. Most congenital defects of importance reveal themselves in the first 3 days and almost all of them present within 1 week. This recommendation would include flights within the United States. Postpone essential transoceanic flights for 3 to 4 weeks.
- Since FAA restrictions require planes to be pressurized to at least 8,000 feet, it would be highly unusual to trigger any heart problems during the few hours aboard an aircraft.
- Because of the exposure to infection aboard aircraft, however, it's definitely preferable not to fly before 2 or 3 months of age.

DIZZINESS

Symptoms and Characteristics

Dizziness is a sensation of light-headedness, faintness, or unsteadiness. All people occasionally get temporary dizziness if they skip a meal, become a little dehydrated, get too much sun, get exhausted, stand up suddenly, stand for too long in one place, or have a viral illness. If the dizziness relates to riding in a car, going to an amusement park, or playing twirling games (turning somersaults, for instance), see the guideline on MOTION SICKNESS, page 519.

Call Your Child's Physician

Immediately If

- Your child passes out.

- Your child is unable to stand and walk.
- Your child acts or looks very sick.

Within 24 Hours If

- Ear pain or congestion is also present.
- Your child is taking any medicines that could be causing the dizziness.
- You think your child needs to be seen.

During Office Hours If

- Dizziness is a recurrent problem for your child.
- You have other questions or concerns.

Home Care

Treatment—Have your child lie down with the feet elevated for the next hour and offer something to drink. Always prevent dizziness from progressing to fainting (passing out) by reminding your child early on to lie down or sit with the head between the knees.

Call Your Child's Physician Later If

- The dizziness is still present after 2 hours of rest.
- You feel your child is getting worse.
- Your child develops any of the "Call Your Child's Physician" symptoms.

Related Topic

FAINTING (see below)

FAINTING

Symptoms and Characteristics

Fainting (syncope) is defined as falling down and being unconscious briefly (usually less than 1 minute). The four most common causes are sudden stress (such as seeing a bad accident), severe pain, prolonged standing in one position with the knees locked, or standing up suddenly (especially after bed rest). Fainting due to these conditions quickly responds to lying horizontally for a few minutes with the feet elevated.

Similar Conditions—If appropriate, turn directly to the following guidelines:

BREATH-HOLDING SPELLS (see page 370)
COMA (remaining unconscious is an *emergency*) (see page 40)
HEAT REACTIONS (see page 53)

Call Your Child's Physician

Immediately If

- The fainting followed a head injury (call 911).
- Any shaking or jerking occurred while your child was unconscious.
- The unconsciousness lasted more than 2 minutes.
- The fainting occurred during exertion or exercise.
- The cause of the fainting isn't obvious.
- Your child also looks or acts sick.

During Office Hours If

- Fainting is a recurrent problem for your child.
- You think your child needs to be seen.

Home Care

First Aid—Have your child lie down for 10 to 20 minutes with the feet elevated. Do not place a pillow under the head. Also, offer a glass of fruit juice when he is fully conscious. In hot weather, your child may also need several glasses of water and a cool compress to the forehead. If fainting was due to stress or fear, help your child talk about it. Caution: Smelling salts are unpleasant and unnecessary.

Call Your Child's Physician Later If

- Your child isn't back to normal by 1 hour.
- Your child passes out again on the same day.
- You feel your child is getting worse.

Prevention of Fainting

- To prevent recurrent fainting, drink lots of water and consume adequate salt each day.
- For fainting that occurs following prolonged standing, remind your child that keeping the knees locked interferes with recirculation of the

blood. Under these circumstances, your child should pump the blood by repeatedly relaxing and retightening the leg muscles.

• For fainting that occurs with standing up suddenly, have your child sit up first and take some deep breaths.

• Also, feeling faint at any time or place is a warning to sit or lie down quickly.

Related Topic

DIZZINESS (see page 514)

HEADACHE

Symptoms and Characteristics

Your child complains that his or her head hurts.

Similar Condition—If a blow to the head is suspected, save time by turning directly to the guideline for HEAD TRAUMA, page 72.

Causes—A mild headache commonly occurs as part of a cold or other viral illness. A high fever almost always causes a headache. Many children get a headache in the late afternoon when they are hungry.

In children and adults, the most common cause of recurrent headaches is physical, emotional, or intellectual exhaustion. These muscle tension headaches give a sensation of tightness that completely encircles the head. The neck muscles also become sore and tight. Muscle tension headaches can be caused by prolonged use of video games, computers, or typewriters. Many children get muscle tension headaches as a reaction to stresses (such as pressure for better grades or unresolved disagreements with parents). Recurrent headaches can have numerous causes and deserve a medical evaluation.

Expected Course—Many headaches clear when a fever comes down. Others come and go during an illness. Muscle tension headaches usually last 2 to 8 hours and tend to recur.

Call Your Child's Physician

Immediately If

• Your child is difficult to awaken from sleep (call 911).

• Your child is confused (call 911).

- Speech is slurred (call 911).
- The headache is severe and constant (e.g., causes constant crying).
- Vision is blurred or double.
- Walking is unsteady.
- Vomiting has occurred 3 or more times.
- The neck is stiff.
- The pupils are unequal in size.
- Your child acts or looks very sick.

Within 24 Hours If
- The headache has lasted more than 24 hours despite using a pain-relieving medicine.
- Blocked sinuses may be causing the headache.
- Headaches are a recurrent problem for your child.
- You think your child needs to be seen.

Home Care

General Treatment—Have your child lie down and rest until he or she is feeling better. If your child is hungry, offer some food. Give a pain-relieving medicine such as ibuprofen or acetaminophen and repeat it as needed. Apply a cool washcloth to the forehead.

Muscle Tension Headaches: Treatment—If your child has been evaluated by a physician and has muscle tension headaches, try the following to help ease the pain:
- When a headache occurs, your youngster should lie down and relax.
- Give acetaminophen or ibuprofen as soon as the headache begins. It's more effective if started early.
- Stretch and massage the neck muscles.
- If something is bothering your child, help him talk about it and get it off his mind.
- Teach your child not to skip meals if doing so brings on headaches.
- To prevent muscle tension headaches, teach your child to take breaks from activities that require sustained concentration. During the breaks, encourage relaxation exercises.
- If overachievement causes headaches, help your child get out of the fast track.

Call Your Child's Physician Later If
- The headache lasts for more than 24 hours despite the medicine.
- It worsens after 2 hours on pain-relieving medicine.
- You feel your child is getting worse.

Related Topic

SINUS CONGESTION (see page 561). Consider this diagnosis if the pain is on one side and near the eye, the nose is runny or blocked, and your child has previously experienced sinus problems.

MOTION SICKNESS

Symptoms and Characteristics
Motion sickness is a common condition, especially in young children. The same children who get dizzy and nauseated in the car are also prone to becoming seasick, trainsick, airsick, and sick on amusement park rides. The problem is due to an inherited sensitivity of the equilibrium center found in the semicircular canals (inner ear). It is not related to emotional problems, nor can your child control it. The sensitivity to motion is usually a lifelong problem.

Home Care

Treatment for the Nausea—Have your child lie down, and keep a vomiting pan handy. Give only sips of clear fluids until the stomach settles down. If your child goes to sleep, all the better. Usually, children don't vomit more than once, and all symptoms disappear in about 4 hours.

Prevention of Motion Sickness

Anti-Nausea Medicine—Buy some nonprescription Dramamine tablets at your drugstore. They come in 50 mg tablets or 15 mg-per-teaspoon liquid. The dosage is 1 teaspoon for children 2 to 6 years old, 1 tablet for children 6 to 12 years old, and 2 tablets for children over 12. Give the Dramamine 1 hour before traveling or going to an amusement park. The tablets give 6 hours of protection and are very helpful.

Car Trips—Have your child sit at window level. After age 12 years, have your child sit in the front seat and look out the front window. Ask your child not to look at books or play games during car travel. Keep a window cracked to provide fresh air.

Amusement Parks—Have your child avoid rides that spin (like the Tilt-A-Whirl). Some children can't even look at whirling rides without becoming sick. Your child will probably do fine on the Ferris wheel.

Sea Travel—Avoid it when practical. Otherwise, stay on deck and look at the horizon. Boating on small lakes is usually tolerated.

Air Travel—Airsickness can be helped by selecting a seat near the wings or center of the aircraft, since turbulence is felt least there.

Meals—Have your child eat light meals on these days.

SOFT SPOT, BULGING

The soft spot (called the anterior fontanel) is open during the first 12 to 18 months of life. Normally it is flat or slightly sunken. Normally it moves up and down (pulsates) with each beat of the heart, if the child is sitting up and quiet. It can be slightly elevated for a few seconds while your child is crying. If the soft spot is elevated or bulging, the brain is under pressure. Many of the causes are serious.

Call Your Child's Physician Immediately If

• Your child has a bulging soft spot.

SOFT-SPOT CLOSURE

Definition

The soft spot is a diamond-shaped area on the top of the head in newborns. This area is also called the anterior fontanel. The soft spot is located where 2 growth lines (suture lines) for the skull cross. Babies have a soft spot to allow the bone of the skull to expand as the brain grows rapidly. The soft spot normally becomes larger over the first 2 or 3 months of life and then gradually closes. It normally looks flat or slightly depressed. The soft spot should not look full or bulging. If it is bulging, it means that the brain is under some pressure and your child needs to be seen by your health care provider.

Normal Closure

A soft spot is closed when the opening can no longer be felt. The soft spot commonly closes at 18 months of age, but it could close anytime between the ages of 5 and 26 months.

If your child reaches 27 months of age and the soft spot is not closed, your child needs to be checked by your health care provider. A soft spot that closes before a child reaches 5 months of age is very rare. This is called premature closure of the fontanel and may also need to be checked by your health care provider.

Large Soft Spot

Soon after birth, the soft spot is about 1 by 1 inch. It can get as large as 2 by 2 inches. If the area is larger than this, you should have your child checked by your health care provider.

Touching the Soft Spot

It is quite safe to touch the soft spot. The open space between the bones is covered by a tough fibrous membrane that protects the brain. You can wash your baby's hair and continue with normal activities without worrying about harming the soft spot.

EYES

ALLERGIES OF THE EYES

Symptoms and Characteristics
- Itchy eyes (without pain)
- Increased tearing (without pus)
- Red or pink eyes
- Mild swelling of the eyelids
- Similar symptoms during the same month of the previous year
- Previous confirmation of this diagnosis by a physician (helpful)

If your child's symptoms are different, call your physician for help.

Similar Condition—If the nose is also involved, save time by turning directly to the guideline on HAY FEVER, page 556.

Causes—For cases that occur during the same season each year, the cause is pollens. For cases that are not seasonal, the allergic factor can be pets (cats, for instance), feathers, perfumes, mascara, eyeliner, and so forth.

Expected Course—Most eye allergies due to a pollen last for 4 to 6 weeks, which is the length of most pollen seasons. If the allergic substance can be identified *and* avoided (a cat, perhaps), the symptoms will not recur.

Call Your Child's Physician During Office Hours If
- The eye allergy keeps your child from playing or sleeping.
- The eyelids are swollen tight.
- Sacs of clear yellow fluid are present between the eyelids.
- The eyelids become matted together with pus.
  (Note: It's normal to awaken in the morning with some strands of

sticky mucus in the eye. This mucus can often be prevented by washing the pollen off the eyelids and face the night before.)

• You think your child needs to be seen.

Home Care

Removing Pollen—First wash the pollen off the face. Then use a clean washcloth and cool water to clean off the eyelids. Tears will wash the pollen out of the eyes. This rinse of the eyelids may need to be repeated every time your child comes in on a windy day. Pollen also collects in the hair and on exposed body surfaces. This pollen can easily be reintroduced into the eyes. Therefore, give your child a shower and shampoo every night before bedtime. Encourage your child not to touch the eyes unless the hands have been washed recently.

Vasoconstrictor Eyedrops—Usually, the eyes will feel much better after the pollen is washed out and cold compresses are applied. If they are still itchy or bloodshot (i.e., the blood vessels are swollen), instill some vaso-constrictive or antihistamine eyedrops (no prescription needed). Ask your pharmacist for help in choosing a reliable product. Use 1 drop every 6 to 8 hours as necessary (1 drop fills the eye even in adults). Caution: Using vasoconstrictor eyedrops daily for longer than 1 week can cause redness.

Antihistamines—If these measures aren't effective, your child probably also has hay fever (i.e., allergic symptoms of the nose). Give your child an oral antihistamine. (For dosage, see the tables on pages 238–40.)

Call Your Child's Physician Later If

• This treatment and an antihistamine do not relieve most of the symptoms in 2 or 3 days.

• Your child develops any of the "Call Your Child's Physician" symptoms.

Keep in mind that the pollen season lasts for 1 to 2 months. You need to continue the treatment for that length of time and start it again next year.

DARK CIRCLES UNDER THE EYES

Symptoms and Characteristics

The most common cause for dark, bluish circles under the eyes is congestion of the nose. The veins from the eyes drain into the veins of the nose. If the nose is blocked up, the veins around the eyes become larger and darker. To figure out what's going on, we need to look at the nose.

Usually the cause of the nasal congestion is nasal allergy or hay fever. That's why these dark circles are also called allergic shiners. Dark circles are also caused by chronic sinus infections, recurrent colds, or mouth breathing due to large adenoids. They're also more noticeable in children with a fair complexion. Overall, dark circles under the eyes are not a sign of poor health or troubled sleep.

Call Your Child's Physician During Office Hours If

- You don't know what is causing your child's dark circles.

Treatment—Treatment depends on the cause of the congestion. Turn directly to the guideline that pertains to your child:

- COLDS (see page 550)
- HAY FEVER (see page 556)
- SINUS CONGESTION (see page 561)
- TONSIL AND ADENOID SURGERY (if your child has snoring and mouth breathing) (see page 576)

ITCHY EYE

For itchy, watery, red eyes, the possible causes are many. If the itching begins suddenly and is intense, usually your child has been around something he's allergic to (e.g., a cat). If the cause is unclear, assume the itching is caused by a minor irritant. Irrigate the eyes with warm water as described on page 526. Turn directly to the guideline that pertains to your child.

ALLERGIES OF THE EYES (see page 522)
CHEMICAL IN EYE (see page 49)
RED OR PINKEYE (includes minor irritants) (see below)

RED OR PINKEYE WITHOUT PUS

Symptoms and Characteristics

- Redness of the sclera (white part of the eye)
- Redness of the inner eyelids

- A watery discharge ("watery eyes")
- No yellow discharge or matting of eyelids
- Not from crying
- Also called pinkeye, bloodshot eyes, or conjunctivitis

If your child's symptoms are different, call your physician for help.

Similar Conditions—If one of the following is suspected, save time by turning directly to that guideline:

ALLERGIES OF THE EYES (see page 522)
CHEMICAL IN EYE (see page 49)
FOREIGN BODY IN EYE (e.g., blowing dust or eyelash) (see page 50)
EYE TRAUMA (see page 66)
HAY FEVER (see page 556)
RED OR PINKEYE WITH PUS (see page 527)

Causes—Red eyes are usually caused by a viral infection, and commonly accompany colds. If a bacterial infection also occurs on top of the viral infection, the discharge becomes yellow and the eyelids are commonly matted together after sleeping. These children need antibiotic eyedrops even if the eyes are not red. The second most common cause is getting an irritant into the eyes. The irritant can be shampoo, smog, smoke, or chlorine from a swimming pool. More commonly in young kids, it comes from touching the eyes with hands carrying dirt, soap, animal saliva, or food (such as cinnamon, chili powder, or other spice). Contact with the mother's perfume or father's aftershave can also be irritating, as can rubbing faces with the family pet. The main symptom in children with irritants in the eye is constant rubbing and tearing of the eyes.

Expected Course—Viral conjunctivitis usually lasts as long as a cold does (4 to 7 days). Pinkeye is a mild infection and does not harm the vision. Red eyes from irritants usually are cured within 4 hours of washing out the irritating substance, unless reexposure occurs.

Call Your Child's Physician

Immediately If

- The outer eyelids are red or swollen.
- The eyes are constantly tearing or blinking.
- Your child is complaining of pain in the eyes.

- Vision is blurred.
- Your child acts or looks very sick.

Within 24 Hours If
- Your child is under 1 month old.
- A yellow discharge develops.
- The eyelids become matted together with pus.
- You think your child needs to be seen.

Home Care

Washing with Soap—Wash the face, then the eyelids, with a mild soap and water. This will remove any irritants.

Irrigating with Water—For viral eye infections, rinse the eyes out with warm water as often as possible, at least every 1 to 2 hours while your child is awake. Use warm (not hot) water, and use a fresh cotton ball each time. Wipe toward the inside of the eye. This usually will keep a bacterial infection from occurring. For mild chemical irritants, irrigate the eye with warm water for 5 minutes.

Vasoconstrictor Eyedrops—Viral conjunctivitis usually is not helped by eyedrops. Red eyes from irritants usually feel much better after the irritant has been washed out. If they remain uncomfortable and bloodshot, instill some long-acting vasoconstrictor eyedrops (no prescription needed). Ask your pharmacist for help in choosing a reliable product. Use 1 drop every 6 to 8 hours as necessary. Products called "artificial tears" are not helpful, since they do not contain any vasoconstrictors.

Contagiousness—If your child has pinkeye from a viral infection, the secretions can cause eye infections in other people if they get some of it on their eyes. Therefore, it is important for the sick child to have his or her own washcloth and towel. However, the infection is so mild that staying home from school or day care is unnecessary. If the pinkeye is due to irritants or chemicals, obviously your child's condition is not contagious.

Call Your Child's Physician Later If
- The redness lasts more than a week.
- Your child develops any of the "Call Your Child's Physician" symptoms.

RED OR PINKEYE WITH PUS

Symptoms and Characteristics
- Yellow discharge in the eye
- Eyelids stuck together with a little pus (especially after sleep)
- Dried eye discharge on the upper cheek
- Eyes are also usually red or pink, but may remain white
- Also called runny eyes (note: everyone can normally have a small amount of cream-colored mucus, called "sleep," in the inner corner of the eyes after sleeping)

Causes—Caused by various bacteria. After ear infections, bacterial eye infections are the next leading complication of a cold. Red eyes without a yellow discharge, however, are more common and are due to a virus (see RED OR PINKEYE WITHOUT PUS, page 524).

Expected Course—With proper treatment, the yellow discharge should clear up in 72 hours. The red eyes (which are part of the underlying cold) may persist for several more days. These infections do not harm the vision.

Call Your Child's Physician

Immediately If
- The outer eyelids are red or swollen.
- Any ulcer or sore is seen on the eyeball.
- Vision is blurred.
- Your child acts or looks very sick.

Within 24 Hours If
- You don't have any antibiotic eyedrops or ointment.
- Your infant is less than 1 month old. These children may need special cultures and an antibiotic.
- There is any suggestion of an earache.

During Office Hours If
- Your child has frequent eye infections.
- You think your child needs to be seen.

Home Care

Cleaning the Eye—Before putting in any antibiotic eyedrops, remove all the dried and liquid pus from the eye with warm wet cotton balls. This should be done as often as you see pus in the eye, sometimes every hour. Unless this is done, the medicine will not have a chance to work. Remove the dried crusts carefully so they don't scratch the eyeball.

Antibiotic Eyedrops or Ointments—A bacterial conjunctivitis must be treated with an antibiotic eye medicine. If you have an antibiotic eye medicine in your home and it has not expired, use it. If not, you must call your physician during office hours for a prescription. Some physicians will want to examine your child before prescribing.

Holding Your Child—Putting eyedrops or ointment in the eyes of younger children can be a real battle. Ideally, it's done with two people. One person can hold the child still while the other person puts in the medicine. One person *can* do it alone, sitting on the floor, holding the child's head (face up) between the knees to free both hands to put in the medicine.

Using Antibiotic Eyedrops—Put 1 drop in each eye every 4 hours while your child is awake. Do this by gently pulling down on the lower lid and placing the drops inside the lower lid. As soon as the eyedrops have been put in, have your child close the eyes for 2 minutes so the eyedrops will stay inside. If it is difficult to separate your child's eyelids, while he is lying down put the eyedrop over the inner corner of the eye. As your child opens the eye and blinks, the eyedrop will flow in. Continue the eyedrops until your child has awakened 2 mornings in a row without any pus in the eyes. If the eyedrops are stopped sooner, the infection will probably come back.

Using Antibiotic Eye Ointment (Instead of Eyedrops)—Eye ointment needs to be used only 3 times a day because it can remain in the eyes longer than eyedrops. Separate the eyelids and put in a ribbon of ointment from one corner to the other. If it is very difficult to separate your child's eyelids, put the ointment on the lid margins. As it melts from body heat, it will flow onto the eyeball and give equal results. Again, continue until 2 mornings have passed without any pus in the eye.

Contact Lenses—Children with contact lenses need to switch to glasses temporarily to prevent damage to the cornea.

Contagiousness—The pus from the eyes can cause eye infections in other people if they get some of it on their eyes. Therefore, it is very important for the sick child to have his or her own washcloth and towel. Your child should be discouraged from touching or rubbing the eyes, because it can make the infection last longer, and it puts a lot of germs on the fingers. Therefore, your child's hands should also be washed often to prevent spreading the infection. Your child can return to school after using the eyedrops for 24 hours if the pus is minimal.

Call Your Child's Physician Later If
- The infection isn't cleared up in 72 hours.
- The eyes become itchy or redder after eyedrops are begun.
- Your child develops any of the "Call Your Child's Physician" symptoms.

SWELLING OF EYELID

Symptoms and Characteristics

An insect bite near the eye can cause swelling of the eyelid. This is especially common with mosquito bites of the upper face. The eyelid is not red, but it can be pink.

Similar Conditions—If one of the following is suspected, save time by turning directly to that guideline:

EYE TRAUMA (see page 66)
ALLERGIES OF THE EYES (see page 522)
RED OR PINKEYE (see pages 524 and 527)

Call Your Child's Physician

Immediately If
- Both eyelids are swollen (exception: eye allergies).
- The swollen eyelid is tender to the touch.
- The eyelid is red.
- A fever is present.
- Your child also has sinus congestion.
- There is pain on movement of the eye.
- Your child acts or looks very sick.

During Office Hours If

- You are unsure of the cause of the swelling (i.e., you find no evidence for insect bites near the eye and it's the wrong season for mosquitoes in your community).
- You think your child needs to be seen.

Home Care for Eyelid Swelling from an Insect Bite

Treatment—Cool compresses or ice in a washcloth help. Give your child an antihistamine to decrease the swelling and help any itching. (See the dosage tables starting on page 238 for dosages.) Many common cold medicines contain antihistamines. In 2 or 3 days, the swelling from insect bites is usually gone.

Call Your Child's Physician Later If

- The swelling hasn't cleared in 3 days.
- Your child develops any of the "Call Your Child's Physician" symptoms.

Related Topic

BITES: INSECT, BEE, OR TICK (see page 19)

STYE

Symptoms and Characteristics

- A tender, red bump at the base of an eyelash
- A small pimple at the base of an eyelash

If your child's symptoms are different, call your physician for help.

Cause—A stye is an infection of the hair follicle of an eyelash, usually caused by staphylococcus bacteria.

Expected Course—It usually comes to a head and forms a pimple in 3 to 5 days. In a few more days, it usually drains and heals. Recurrences are common, especially in children who rub their eyes.

Call Your Child's Physician

Immediately If
- The infection is spreading.
- The eyelid is red or swollen.

During Office Hours If
- Styes are a recurrent problem for your child.
- There are 2 or more styes.
- You think your child needs to be seen.

Home Care

Warm Compresses—Wash the outer eyelids once daily with a baby shampoo. Apply a warm washcloth to the eye for 10 minutes 4 times a day to help the stye come to a head. Continue to cleanse the eye several times a day even after the stye drains.

Opening the Pimple—When the stye does display a center of pus, you can open it by pulling out the eyelash that goes into the pimple with tweezers. This will initiate drainage and healing. Another option is to carefully open the pimple from the side with a sterile needle. This must be done carefully. Your final option is just to continue warm compresses. Most styes will drain spontaneously in a few days after they have come to a head.

Antibiotic Eye Ointment—The ointments do not cure styes, but they may keep them from spreading and recurring. If your child has recurrent styes or more than 2 styes, call your child's physician, since this ointment requires a prescription. Most single styes respond to the treatment outlined.

Prevention of Recurrences—Ask your child not to touch the eyes, because rubbing can cause spread to other eyelashes.

Call Your Child's Physician Later If
- The stye is not draining or improved by 5 days.
- The stye is not completely healed by 10 days.
- Your child develops any of the "Call Your Child's Physician" symptoms.

EARS

EARACHE

Symptoms and Characteristics

Your child complains of ear pain. Children too young to talk may cry several times during the night and be cranky during the day. Most of these children also have symptoms of a cold and 50 percent have a fever. The peak age range for earaches is 6 months to 2 years, but they continue to be a common complaint until age 8 or 10.

Similar Conditions—If your child is doing lots of swimming and it hurts when you move the outer ear up and down, save time by going directly to the guideline on SWIMMER'S EAR (page 545).

Cause—Most earaches are due to a middle-ear infection (acute otitis media). A middle-ear infection is a bacterial infection of the space behind the eardrum. The earache is due to the bulging of the eardrum. Most children (70 percent) have one or more ear infections, and 25 percent of these will have repeated ear infections. Ear infections are the most common complication of a cold. While colds are contagious, ear infections are not.

A temporary earache can occur for 10 to 15 minutes after being outside in cold weather. When your child comes inside, the cold air inside the middle ear warms up, expands, and causes some pain. Chewing gum or drinking fluids should relieve it. However, cold wind or weather cannot cause an ear infection.

Another cause of temporary pain in front of the ear is muscle pain from excessive chewing.

Expected Course of Ear Infection—In 5 to 10 percent of children with otitis media, the pressure in the middle ear causes the eardrum to rupture and drain. The ear drainage does not mean that the ear infection is any more serious. This small tear usually heals in a few days. Most ear infections respond nicely to a course of antibiotics. At the 2-week visit for ear recheck, about 10 percent will still be infected and need a second course of antibiotics. Another 40 percent or more will have fluid in the middle ear (serous otitis) and reduced hearing. Over the following 1 to 3 months, hearing will return to normal without treatment in most of these children. A few children will need ventilation tubes placed in their eardrums (see page 547).

Call Your Child's Physician

Immediately If

- The pain is severe (e.g., a screaming child).
- The neck is stiff.
- Your child can't walk normally.
- The earache followed injury to the ear.
- Your child acts or looks very sick.

Within 24 Hours If

- All other children with earaches that last more than 30 minutes need to be examined.

Home Care

Relieving Pain

- An earache is not an emergency. Until you see the physician, give acetaminophen or ibuprofen for pain. (For dosage, see the tables on pages 238–40.) You may also put an ice bag or ice wrapped in a wet washcloth over the painful ear for 20 minutes. (Caution: Longer contact could cause frostbite.) Many physicians recommend a hot water bottle, but cold seems to provide greater relief.

Other Measures

- Do not use any ear drops unless your physician recommends them.
- If the ear is draining, wipe the material away as it appears.
- Don't plug the canal with cotton.

Air Travel with Ear Infections—Children with ear infections can travel safely by aircraft if they are taking antibiotics. Also give them an appropriate dose of ibuprofen 1 hour before takeoff for any discomfort they might experience. Most will not have an increase in their ear pain while flying.

Call Your Child's Physician Later If

- Your child develops any of the "Call Your Child's Physician Immediately" symptoms.

Prevention of Ear Infections

If your child has recurrent ear infections, it's time to look at how you can prevent some of them. The following list includes ways to help prevent getting another ear infection.

Avoid Tobacco Smoke—Protect your child from secondhand tobacco smoke. Passive smoking increases the frequency and severity of infections. Be sure no one smokes in your home or at day care.

Avoid Excessive Colds—Reduce your child's exposure to children with colds during the first year of life. Most ear infections start with a cold. Try to delay the use of large day-care centers during the first year by using a sitter in your home or a small home-based day care.

Breast-Feed—Breast-feed your baby during the first 6 to 12 months of life. Antibodies in breast milk reduce the rate of ear infections. If you're breast-feeding, continue. If you're not, consider it with your next child.

Avoid Bottle Propping—If you bottle-feed, hold your baby at a 45-degree angle. Feeding in the horizontal position can cause formula and other fluids to flow back into the eustachian tube. Allowing an infant to hold his own bottle also can cause milk to drain into the middle ear. Weaning your baby from a bottle between 9 and 12 months of age will help stop this problem.

Control Allergies—If your infant has a continuously runny nose, consider allergy as a contributing factor to the ear infections. If your child has other allergies such as eczema, talk with your child's physician about checking for a milk protein or soy protein allergy.

Adenoids—If your toddler constantly snores or breathes through his mouth, he may have large adenoids. Large adenoids can contribute to ear infections. Talk to your physician about this.

Related Topics

EAR CONGESTION

Symptoms and Characteristics
- Sudden onset of muffled hearing
- Crackling or popping noises in the ear
- A stuffy, full sensation in the ear
- No ear pain except in cases related to airplane travel

Similar Conditions—If one of the following is suspected, save time by turning directly to that guideline:

EARACHE (see page 532)
EAR DISCHARGE (see page 536)
EARWAX, PACKED (see page 537)
HAY FEVER (see page 556)

Cause—The most common cause of ear congestion is fluid in the middle ear due to intermittent blockage of the eustachian tube (the channel connecting the middle ear to the back of the nose) by a cold, hay fever, or over-vigorous nose-blowing. Sudden increases in barometric pressure, such as occur in descent from mountain driving or airplane travel, also cause ear congestion (but usually with pain, as the eardrum is pulled inward).

Call Your Child's Physician During Office Hours If
- Your child could have put something in the ear canal.
- You think your child needs to be seen.

Home Care

Treatment—Have your child chew gum, yawn frequently, and swallow (or puff out the cheeks) while the nose is pinched closed. If this isn't effective, use a long-acting decongestant nasal spray 1 hour before air travel. Ask your pharmacist to recommend a good product (no prescription needed). If your child could have water in the ear canal from a recent shower or swim, help drain it by gravity by turning the head to the side and gently pulling the ear in different directions. If your child has hay fever, an antihistamine medication should also be taken. If your child is in pain, give acetaminophen or ibuprofen (see the tables on pages 238–40 for dosage). Swimming is permitted.

Call Your Child's Physician Later If
- The ear congestion lasts more than 48 hours.
- Ear pain or fever develops.

Prevention of Ear Congestion Due to Altitude Change

Have your child repeatedly "pop" the ears by yawning or swallowing during the typical 30 minutes of descent. If this fails, attempt to blow the nose (and puff out the cheeks) against closed nostrils and a closed mouth. A baby can be given water to drink or a pacifier to suck on during descent, and the nose can be pinched closed periodically during swallowing. Ideally, the child would not sleep during descent.

People with recurrent problems should take an oral decongestant (see dosage table for pseudoephedrine on page 240) and long-acting decongestant nasal spray 1 hour before travel. If severe pain occurs despite these precautions, ask the flight attendant for a hot towel to place over the ear canal. (The heat will expand the air in the middle ear and relieve the negative pressure on the retracted eardrum.)

EAR DISCHARGE

Yellow or Cloudy Discharge

Call your child's physician during office hours. Your child probably has an ear infection with drainage through a small tear in the eardrum.

Bloody Discharge

See the guideline on EAR TRAUMA, page 66.

Earwax Discharge

For a brown or orange discharge, see the guideline on EARWAX, PACKED, page 537.

Clear Discharge

- If it followed head or ear trauma, call your child's physician immediately.

- If it followed an earache, call your child's physician within 24 hours.
- If it could be tears, bath water, or eardrops someone put in, your worries are over.

Home Care

Pending the office visit for a suspected ear infection, give acetaminophen for pain (for dosage, see the table on page 237). Wipe away the drainage as it appears. Don't pack the ear canal with cotton, because this will block the natural drainage. Don't put any cotton swabs in the ear canal.

EARWAX, PACKED

Symptoms and Characteristics

Earwax is present in everyone. The color can vary from light yellow to dark brown. It has chemicals in it that can kill germs, it keeps dust off the eardrum, and it protects the lining of the ear canal. Earwax is not abnormal or dirty.

The ear canal is designed to clean itself, unless someone pushes the earwax that's trying to get out back in. Earwax moves outward naturally during chewing and the normal growth of the ear canal's lining. Every day or two, you may notice a little earwax at the opening of the ear canal. The amount varies from person to person, and as long as it comes out, your child can't have too much of it.

Proceed with this guideline if earwax is completely blocking one of the ear canals (i.e., impacted wax). If the hearing seems normal on that side, the blockage is only partial and you can leave it alone.

Call Your Child's Physician During Office Hours If

- Any discharge comes from the ear canal other than earwax.
- The eardrum has been ruptured in the past.
- Blockage from earwax is a recurrent problem for your child.
- You think your child needs to be seen.

Home Care

Flushing Out Packed Earwax—Keep in mind that complete blockage is rare. Regular removal of earwax is not necessary to prevent wax buildup.

- If the wax is hard, soften it first. Use a 15 percent baking soda solution. Make it by adding ¼ teaspoon (1.25 ml) of baking soda to 2 teaspoons (10 ml) of water. Fill the ear canal and leave it in for 1 hour. Most of the earwax should be dissolved at this time.
- When the wax is soft, wash it out with water. A little hydrogen peroxide can be added to the water. Use a rubber ear syringe or Water Pik at the lowest setting. The water must be at body temperature to prevent dizziness. Irrigate several times, until the return is clear and the ear canal seems open when you look in with a light. Never put water in your child's ear if there is any chance the eardrum has a hole in it or your child has ventilation tubes.

Call Your Child's Physician Later If

- Your irrigation doesn't clear out the ear canal and return the hearing to normal.
- Your child develops any of the "Call Your Child's Physician" symptoms.

Prevention of Packed Earwax

Earwax can usually be removed from the opening of the ear canal with the corner of a wet cloth. Don't use your fingernail, because fingernails are usually rather dirty, and too big for the job. Nothing should be put into the ear canal to try to hurry this process along, because it usually ends up packing the wax deeper. It also runs the risk of damaging your child's eardrum if he turns his head suddenly. The most common cause of earwax buildup is putting cotton swabs into the ear canal. As your child becomes older, also remind her not to try to clean the ears.

FOREIGN BODY IN EAR

Young children often put foreign objects in their ear canals. Some common ones are erasers, beads, food, and cotton.

First Aid

If a live insect is within your child's ear canal, take your child into a dark room and shine a light by the ear. The insect will often come out on its own. If this fails, kill the intruder by pouring in some alcohol. You can use any 80 proof liquor if you have no rubbing alcohol. Then remove the insect by irrigating the canal with water and an ear syringe (or a nasal suction bulb). For other objects, make one simple attempt at removing it. Turn the involved side down. Wiggle the ear at the same time you gently shake the head, and try to get the object to fall out with the help of gravity.

Call Your Child's Physician Immediately If These Measures Fail

It is critical that you do not try to remove the object by putting tweezers, fingers, or any other device into the ear canal. Also, don't try to irrigate it out again at home. These additional attempts almost always push the object in farther and make the physician's job very difficult, even with special instruments. Watch closely that your child doesn't push it in.

ITCHY EAR

Symptoms and Characteristics

Your child repeatedly scratches his ear or complains that it itches.

Causes—Most older children who complain of itchy ear canals have a mild otitis externa from:
- Water accumulation during swimming or showers
- Soap or shampoo retention
- Irritation from hair sprays
- Canal irritation from cotton swabs (these swabs remove the earwax that normally protects the lining of the ear canal, and this leads to itching and irritation)

Similar Conditions—If one of the following is suspected, save time by turning directly to that guideline:

SWIMMER'S EAR (see page 545)
EARACHE (see page 532)
EAR DISCHARGE (see page 536)

Home Care

Treatment—White vinegar has acetic acid in it and can usually restore the ear canal to its normal chemistry. Fill one ear canal at a time with white vinegar mixed half and half with water. Do this by running the vinegar solution down the side of the opening of the ear canal so that air doesn't get trapped under it. Leave it in for 5 minutes, then remove it by putting that side of the head down and pulling the ear in different directions to help the vinegar run out. Do this twice a day for 3 or 4 days.

Call Your Child's Physician Later If

- The canal itches for more than a week.
- The ear becomes painful.
- A discharge from the ear occurs.
- A fever occurs.

Prevention of Itchy Ear

- Keep soap and shampoo out of the ear canal.
- Don't use cotton swabs in the ear canal.
- Do plug the openings with cotton prior to using hair spray.
- After swimming, get all water out of the ear canal by turning the head to the side and pulling the ear in different directions to help the water run out. Dry the opening to the ear canal carefully.

MUMPS

Symptoms and Characteristics

- Swollen parotid gland, in front of the ear and crossing the corner of the jaw (both parotid glands are swollen in 70 percent of children with mumps)
- Tenderness of the swollen gland
- Pain increased by jaw movement (chewing or even talking)
- Fever (over 100°F)
- No prior mumps vaccine
- Exposure to another child with mumps 16 to 18 days earlier

This diagnosis must be confirmed by a physician.

Cause—Mumps is an acute viral infection of the parotid, a gland that produces saliva and is located in front of and below each ear.

Expected Course—The fever is usually gone in 3 to 4 days. The swelling and pain are cleared by 7 days.

Call Your Child's Physician

Immediately If

- Your child has a stiff neck or severe headache.
- Your child is vomiting repeatedly.
- Your child has definite abdominal pain.
- Your child acts or looks very sick.

Within 24 Hours If

- All other children with suspected mumps need medical consultation.

Home Care

Pain and Fever Relief—Give acetaminophen or ibuprofen (for dosage, see the tables on pages 238–40.) Cold compresses (e.g., ice in a wet cloth for 20 minutes) applied to the swollen area may also relieve pain.

Diet

- Avoid sour foods or citrus fruits that increase saliva production and parotid swelling.
- Avoid foods that require lots of chewing.
- Consider a liquid diet if chewing is very painful.

Contagiousness—The disease is contagious until the swelling is gone (usually 6 or 7 days). Your child should be kept out of school and away from other children who have not had mumps or mumps vaccine.

Mumps Exposure—Mumps exposure can be a problem if a person has never received the mumps vaccine or had past swelling of the parotid gland (mumps). Only 10 percent of adults are susceptible, however. Adults who as children lived in the same household with siblings who had mumps can be considered protected. Adults, teens, and children who are not protected should call their physician during office hours, if they are exposed to mumps, to see if the mumps vaccine would be helpful.

Adult and teen males who get mumps have a 25 percent chance of having a swollen testicle (called orchitis) along with the other symptoms of mumps. Usually only one testicle is affected. Damage to one testicle doesn't reduce fertility. Even when both testicles are involved (10 percent), sterility is very rare.

Call Your Child's Physician Later If

- The swelling lasts for more than 7 days.
- The fever lasts for more than 4 days.
- The skin over the swelling becomes red.
- You feel your child is getting worse.
- Your child develops any of the "Call Your Child's Physician" symptoms.

Related Topic

LYMPH NODES, SWOLLEN (see page 498)

PIERCED EAR INFECTIONS

Symptoms and Characteristics

Earrings for pierced ears have become very popular in our country. Ear piercing no longer awaits the teenage years; even infants are seen with pierced ears. For safety reasons, pierced earrings should not be worn until a child is old enough (usually past age 4) to know not to fidget with them (which can lead to infections) or take them out and put them in her mouth (which can lead to swallowing or choking on them). Ideally, the ears should not be pierced until the girl can play an active part in the decision (usually past age 8).

The most common complication of pierced ears is a bacterial infection of the channel. Signs of an infection are tenderness, a yellow discharge, redness, and some swelling.

Causes—The most common causes of infection are piercing the ears with unsterile equipment, inserting unsterile posts, or frequently touching the earlobes with dirty hands. Another frequent cause is wearing tight earrings because the post is too short (earlobes come in various thicknesses) or the clasp is applied too tightly. Tight earrings don't allow air to enter the channel through the earlobe. Also, the pressure from tight earrings reduces blood flow to the earlobe and sets it up for infection. Some inexpensive earrings have rough areas on the posts that scratch the channel and allow infection to enter. Inserting the post at the wrong angle also can scratch the channel, so a mirror should be used until insertion becomes second nature. Posts containing nickel can also cause an itchy, allergic reaction.

Expected Course—If the proper precautions are taken, most mild ear-lobe infections will clear up in 1 to 2 weeks. Recurrences are common if the youngster does not become conscientious in earring care.

Call Your Child's Physician

Immediately If
• The earring clasp becomes embedded in the earlobe and can't be removed.

Within 24 Hours If
• An unexplained fever occurs.
• The lymph node in front of or behind the earlobe becomes swollen.
• Swelling or redness spreads beyond the pierced area of the earlobe.
• You think your child needs to be seen.

Home Care

Treating Mild Pierced Ear Infections—Remove the earring and post 3 times a day. Cleanse them with rubbing alcohol. Clean both sides of the earlobe with rubbing alcohol. Apply an antibiotic ointment (a nonprescription item) to the post and reinsert it. Continue the antibiotic ointment for 2 days beyond the time the infection seems cleared. Carefully review all the recommendations on preventing infections and be certain they are in effect.

Call Your Physician Later If
• The infection worsens.
• The infection is not improving after 48 hours of treatment.
• Your child develops any of the "Call Your Child's Physician" symptoms.

Prevention of Initial Infections
Avoid pierced ears entirely if your child has a tendency to bleed easily, form thick scars (keloids), or get staph skin infections. If none of these applies, have your child's earlobes pierced by someone who understands sterile technique and does them frequently. Using someone inexperienced can result in infections or a cosmetically poor result.
• The initial post should be 14 karat gold or stainless steel.
• Do not remove the post for 6 weeks.
• Apply the clasp loosely to allow for swelling.

- After washing the hands and cleaning both sides of the earlobe with rubbing alcohol, turn the posts approximately 3 rotations. Do this twice a day.
- By the end of 6 weeks, the lining of the channel should be healed and earrings may be changed as often as desired.

Prevention of Later Infections

- Remind your youngster not to touch the earrings except when inserting or removing them. The fingers are often dirty and can contaminate the area.
- Clean the earring, post, and earlobe with rubbing alcohol before each insertion.
- Apply the clasp loosely to prevent any pressure on the earlobe and to provide air space on both sides.
- Polish or discard any posts with rough spots.
- At bedtime, remove the earrings to permit air exposure and drying of the channel during the night.
- Also remind your child that dangling earrings can lead to a torn earlobe requiring plastic surgery. Avoid them during sports. Also, take precautions while dancing, hair washing, or handling young children who might yank them.

PULLING AT EAR

Symptoms and Characteristics

Young children who are pulling at or rubbing their ears, without other symptoms, do not have an ear infection. Many of them have an itchy ear canal from getting soap or shampoo in it. Some of them are responding to a piece of earwax. Some have just discovered their ears and are playing with them (4 months to 1 year old). If it occurs only when your child is sleepy, it may be a reassuring habit like clutching a security blanket.

Call Your Child's Physician Within 24 Hours If

- You think your child is in any pain.
- Your child has been crying without an obvious cause.

- Your child had trouble sleeping last night.
- A discharge from the ear occurs.
- Your child has a fever or signs of a cold.
- You think your child needs to be seen.

Home Care

Treatment—If you think your child has itchy ear canals, mix a solution of one-half rubbing alcohol and one-half white vinegar. Place 1 to 2 drops in each ear daily for 3 days.

Call Your Child's Physician Later If
- Pulling at the ear continues beyond 3 days.
- Your child develops any of the "Call Your Child's Physician" symptoms.

Prevention of Itchy Ear Canals
- Keep soap and shampoo out of the ear canal.
- Don't use cotton swabs in the ear canal, since they remove the earwax that protects the lining of the canal, and this can cause irritation or itching.
- After swimming, get all water out of the ear canals by turning the head to the side and pulling the ear in different directions to help the water run out. Dry the opening to the ear canal carefully.

SWIMMER'S EAR (Otitis Externa)

Symptoms and Characteristics
- Itchy and painful ear canals
- Child has been swimming
- Pain when the outer ear is moved up and down
- Pain when the tab of the outer ear overlying the ear canal is pushed in
- Ear feels plugged
- Slight clear discharge

If your child's symptoms are different, call your physician for help. Suspect a middle-ear infection if your child also has a cold, a fever, and no increased pain with pushing on the ear tab.

Cause—Swimmer's ear is an infection of the skin lining the ear canal. The ear canal runs from the ear opening to the eardrum, about 1 inch away. The cause is prolonged contact with water. When water gets trapped in the ear canal the lining becomes damp, swollen, and prone to infection. Ear canals were meant to be dry. Children are more likely to get swimmer's ear from swimming in lake water, compared with swimming pools or the sea. During the hottest weeks of summer, some lakes have high levels of bacteria. Narrow ear canals also increase the risk of swimmer's ear.

Expected Course—With treatment, symptoms should be better in 3 days.

Call Your Child's Physician Within 24 Hours If

- A fever is present.
- A yellow discharge issues from the ear canal.
- The canal appears full of gunk.
- The ear is very painful.
- The outer ear becomes red or swollen.
- A swollen lymph node is present behind the earlobe.
- You think your child needs to be seen.

Home Care

White Vinegar Ear Drops—For mild swimmer's ear, use half-strength white vinegar ear drops. Fill the ear canal with white vinegar diluted with equal parts of water. White vinegar has acetic acid in it and can usually restore the ear canal to its normal chemistry. Fill one ear canal at a time by running the vinegar down the side of the opening and moving the ear so that air isn't trapped under it. Leave it in for 5 minutes; then remove it by putting that side of the head down and pulling the ear in different directions to help the vinegar run out. Do this twice a day and following showers or baths. Generally, your child should not swim until the symptoms are gone. If your child is on a swim team, he or she may continue but should use a white vinegar rinse after each session. Continued swimming may cause a slower recovery but won't cause any serious complications.

Pain Relief—Use acetaminophen or ibuprofen as needed for pain relief.

Common Mistakes—Don't use earplugs of any kind for prevention or treatment. They tend to jam earwax back into the ear canal. Also, they don't keep all water out of the ear canals. Cotton swabs also should not be inserted in ear canals. Wax buildup traps water behind it and increases the risk of swimmer's ear. Rubbing alcohol is helpful for preventing swimmer's ear but not for treating it, because it would sting too much.

Call Your Child's Physician for Prescription Eardrops Later If
- The symptoms are not cleared up in 3 days.
- The pain becomes worse after 24 hours on treatment.
- Your child develops any of the "Call Your Child's Physician" symptoms.

Prevention of Swimmer's Ear
First, limit how many hours a day your child spends in the water. Another key to prevention is keeping the ear canals dry when your child is not swimming. After swimming, get all water out of the ear canals by turning the head to the side and pulling the ear in different directions to help the water run out. Dry the opening to the ear canal carefully. If recurrences are a big problem, rinse your child's ear canals with rubbing alcohol for 1 minute each time he or she finishes swimming or bathing to help it dry the ear canals and to kill germs.

VENTILATION TUBES SURGERY

Ventilation tubes are tiny plastic tubes that are inserted through the eardrum by an ear, nose, and throat surgeon. They are also called tympanostomy tubes, because they are placed in the tympanic membrane (eardrum). At least 1 million children in our country (most of them 1 to 3 years) have ventilation tubes placed each year. The ventilation tubes are used to drain fluid out of the middle-ear space and ventilate the area with air.

The eardrum normally vibrates with sound because the space behind it (the middle ear) is filled with air. If it is filled with fluid, the hearing is muffled. This happens with ear infections. Sometimes after the infection clears, the fluid remains (middle-ear effusion). This occurs if the eustachian tube (which runs from the back of the nose to the middle ear) has become blocked and no longer allows air in and fluid out. Following an ear infection, approximately 30 percent of children still have fluid in the middle ear at 1 month, 20 percent at 2 months, 10 percent at 3 months, and 5 percent at

4 months. The main concern about prolonged fluid in the middle ear is that the associated hearing deficit may have an impact on speech development. Fluid is especially likely to persist if the first bout of ear infection occurs before 6 months of age. By age 5, the eustachian tube is wider and fluid usually doesn't persist long after ear infections are treated.

Benefits of Ventilation Tubes—Ventilation tubes allow secretions to drain out of the middle-ear space and air to reenter. The risk of recurrent ear infections is greatly reduced. The hearing returns to normal with the tube in place, and speech development can get back on track. Tubes also prevent the fluid from becoming thicker (a "glue ear") and damaging the middle ear. The ventilation tubes also buy time while the child matures and the eustachian tubes begin to function better.

Risks of Ventilation Tubes—First, approximately 10 percent of children with ventilation tubes continue to have ear infections with drainage and pain. These bouts of infection, which require antibiotics, probably would have occurred anyway. Second, complications may occur around the tubes falling out too early or too late. Normally the tubes come out and fall into the ear canal after about a year. Sometimes they come out too quickly and need to be replaced by another set. Rarely, they fall into the middle-ear space and need to be removed by the surgeon. If they remain in the eardrum for over two years, the ear, nose, and throat specialist may need to remove them. Third, after they come out, some leave scarring of the eardrum or a small hole (perforation) that doesn't heal. These both can cause a small hearing loss. Because of these possible complications and the requirement for an anesthetic, physicians recommend ventilation tubes only for children who definitely need them.

Medical Indications for Ventilation Tubes—The surgical placement of ventilation tubes is usually indicated for middle-ear fluid if the following conditions are met:

• The fluid has been present continuously for over 4 months.

• Both ears have fluid.

• The fluid has caused a documented hearing loss. (While a loss greater than 20 dB can significantly affect speech, many children with fluid in their ears have nearly normal hearing.)

• The fluid has caused a speech delay (e.g., not using 3 words by 18 months or 20 words by 2 years).

Ventilation tube placement is also indicated for severe ear infections such as:

- Recurrent ear infections (defined as 3 or more within a 6-month period).
- Ear infections unresponsive to multiple antibiotics.
- Complications of ear infections such as a mastoid infection or paralysis of the facial nerve (giving a crooked smile).

Dealing with Temporary Hearing Loss—As described earlier, most children with a hearing loss due to fluid in their middle ear have it on a temporary basis. During this time when you talk with your child, get close to him, make eye contact, get his full attention, and occasionally check that he understands what you have said. If not, speak in a louder voice than you normally use. A common mistake is to assume your child is ignoring you when actually he doesn't hear you. Reduce any background noise from radio or television while talking with your child. If your child goes to school, be sure he sits in front, near the teacher. (Middle-ear fluid interferes with the ability to hear in a crowd or classroom.) Keep in mind that most children's speech will catch up following a brief period of partial hearing.

Call Your Child's Physician During Office Hours If

- You have other questions or concerns regarding ventilation tubes.

Prevention of Chronic Ear Fluid

Chronic ear fluid and recurrent ear infections are usually due to a blocked eustachian tube. In some children, however, there are contributing factors:

- Exposure to adults who smoke can cause ear problems.
- Drinking a bottle while lying down (or bottle-propping) can cause milk to enter the middle-ear space.
- Children with nasal allergies have more frequent ear fluid buildup. Consider this factor if your child has associated hay fever, eczema, asthma, or food allergies.
- Children with nightly snoring due to large adenoids (see TONSIL AND ADENOID SURGERY, page 576).

If any of these triggers are present with your child, treat or eliminate them before considering ventilation tubes.

NOSE

COLDS

Symptoms and Characteristics
- Also called an upper respiratory infection
- Runny or stuffy nose
- Usually associated with fever and sore throat
- Sometimes associated with a cough, hoarseness, red eyes, and swollen lymph nodes in the neck

If your child's symptoms are different, call your physician for help.

Cause—A cold or upper respiratory infection (URI) is a viral infection of the nose and throat. The cold viruses are spread from one person to another by the mouth (kissing) or hands. Cold germs can get on your child's hands from a cold sufferer's hands or contaminated objects. Cold viruses can live on toys, phones, doorknobs, toilet handles, tables, and other objects for up to 3 hours. The virus is then transmitted to the nose or eyes, by normal face-touching habits. Airborne droplets of germs from sneezing or coughing are a rare means of cold transmission.

Once the cold germs get a foothold in the nasal passages, they start to multiply and spread downward into the throat and windpipe, causing a sore throat and cough. Since there are up to 200 cold viruses, most healthy children get at least 6 colds a year. By adolescence, the number per year starts to taper off. Cold weather, cold winds, drafts, air conditioners, and wet feet do not increase the chances of coming down with a cold.

Expected Course—Usually the fever lasts less than 3 days, and all nose and throat symptoms are gone within 1 to 2 weeks. A cough may last 2 to

3 weeks. Colds are not serious. The main things to watch for are secondary bacterial complications such as ear infections, yellow drainage from the eyes, sinus pressure or pain (often indicating a sinus infection), or rapid breathing (often a sign of pneumonia). These complications may occur in 5 to 10 percent of colds because the viral infection temporarily lowers your child's resistance. In young infants, a blocked nose can interfere with the ability to suck. Colds usually cause more symptoms and last longer in infants.

Similar Conditions

Vasomotor Rhinitis—Many children and adults have a profusely runny nose in the wintertime when they are outdoors breathing cold air. This usually clears within 15 minutes of coming indoors. It requires no treatment beyond a handkerchief and has nothing to do with infection. If you or your child must spend all day in a cold environment (for instance, on a skiing trip), you can prevent the endless nasal drip by using pseudoephedrine or a long-acting vasoconstrictor spray beforehand (see under HOME CARE on page 552).

Chemical Rhinitis—Chemical rhinitis is a dry stuffy nose from excessive and prolonged use of vasoconstrictor nose drops (more than 5 days). It will be better within a day or two of stopping the nose drops.

Hay Fever—For a runny nose that sounds like an allergy, save time by turning directly to the guideline on HAY FEVER, page 556.

Sinus Infection—Suspect this complication of a cold if your child complains of pressure, pain, or swelling overlying a sinus, and it doesn't improve with nasal washes (page 552). Yellow or green nasal secretions are a normal part of the body's reaction to a cold. As an isolated symptom, they do not mean your child has a sinus infection. (See SINUS CONGESTION, page 561.)

Call Your Child's Physician

Immediately If
- Breathing is difficult *and* no better after you clear the nose.
- Your child acts or looks very sick.

Within 24 Hours If
- Ear pain occurs.

- Sinus pain occurs.
- The skin under the openings of the nose is raw or scabbed over (looks like impetigo).
- The eyes have a yellow discharge (not just red and watery).
- The throat is quite sore for more than 5 days (get a throat culture).
- A fever has been present for more than 3 days.
- You think your child needs to be seen.

Home Care

Remember: A good cold will be gone in a week. A bad cold will last 2 weeks. However, we can relieve many of the symptoms.

The Importance of Clearing the Nose in Young Infants—A child can't breathe through the mouth and suck on something at the same time. If your child is breast- or bottle-feeding, you must clear his nose out so he can breathe while he's sucking. Clearing the nasal passages is also important before putting your child down to sleep. Some babies can't breathe through the mouth during the first 6 months of life (obligate nasal breathers), so the nose must be kept open. Keep in mind that the treatment for a runny nose is quite different from that for a stuffy nose blocked with dried secretions.

Treatment for a Runny Nose with Profuse Clear Discharge— The only treatment needed is to clear the nose periodically. Sniffing and swallowing the secretions is better, because blowing the nose may force the infection into the ears or sinuses. Since most children developmentally are unable to blow the nose or sniff until age 3 or 4, use a soft rubber suction bulb to remove the secretions if they are bothering your child. Nasal discharge is the nose's way of eliminating viruses. Antihistamines are not recommended unless your child has a nasal allergy. However, if nasal secretions are profuse and socially inconvenient (and your child is over 1 year old), try an oral decongestant such as pseudoephedrine (see table on page 240 for dosage).

Treatment for a Blocked Nose with Dried or Thick Yellow-Green Mucus: Nasal Washes (Warm Water or Saline Nose Drops and Suctioning)
- Most stuffy noses are blocked by dry mucus. Suction alone or blowing the nose cannot remove most dry secretions. Warm tap water or saline

nose drops are better than any medicine you can buy when it comes to loosening up mucus. If you prefer normal saline nose drops, mix ½ level teaspoon of table salt in 8 ounces of water. Make up a fresh solution every few days and keep it in a clean bottle. Use a clean eyedropper or wet cotton ball to drip in drops of water.

• For the younger child who cannot blow the nose: Place 3 drops of warm water or saline in each nostril. (Caution: During the first year of life, use 1 drop at a time and do 1 nostril at a time.) After 1 minute, use a soft rubber suction bulb to suck out the loosened mucus, or a cotton swab to wipe out the mucus that's very sticky. Empty the bulb tip by squirting the secretions into a tissue. To remove secretions from the back of the nose, you will need to seal off both nasal openings completely with the tip of the suction bulb on one side and your finger closing the other side. You can get a suction bulb at your drugstore for about two dollars. Buy the short, stubby one with a clear-plastic mucus trap. If you cause a nosebleed, you are putting the tip of the suction bulb in too far.

• For the older child who can blow the nose: Use 3 drops as necessary in each nostril while your child is lying on her back on a bed with her head hanging over the side. Wait 1 minute for the water or saline to soften and loosen the dried mucus. Then have your child blow her nose. This can be repeated several times in a row for complete clearing of the nasal passages.

• Errors in using nose drops: The main errors are not putting in enough water or saline (exception: use 1 drop in infants), not waiting long enough for secretions to loosen up, and not repeating the procedure until the breathing is easy. The front of the nose can look open while the back of the nose is all gummed up with dried mucus. Obviously, putting in warm water nose drops without suctioning afterward is of little value.

• Use nasal washes at least 4 times per day or whenever your child can't breathe through the nose.

Treatment for Associated Symptoms of Colds

Fever—Use acetaminophen or ibuprofen for muscle aches, headaches, or moderate fever (over 102°F). (For dosage, see the tables on pages 238–40.) Avoid aspirin because of the possible link with Reye's syndrome. Drinking any fluid can soothe the throat.

Sore Throat—Use hard candies and saltwater gargles for children over 4 years old, and warm chicken broth for children over 1 year old.

Cough—Use cough drops for children over 4 years old, and corn syrup for younger children over 1 year old. Run a humidifier.

Red Eyes—Rinse frequently with wet cotton balls.

Poor Appetite—Encourage fluids of the child's choice. A recent study showed that eating chicken noodle soup loosened nasal mucus. The old saying "Feed a fever and starve a cold" has little merit. "Feeding a fever" isn't too far off the mark, since fevers do burn extra calories. If you try to "starve a cold," however, a child could become dehydrated.

Common Mistakes—Most cold remedies or tablets are worthless. Also, oral medicines have no ability to remove dried nasal secretions. If the nose is really congested, consider using an oral decongestant (pseudoephedrine) for a day or so. By contrast, antihistamines do not help cold symptoms. Avoid oral decongestants if they make your child jittery or keep her from sleeping at night. Prescription cold medicines offer no advantages over nonprescription products. Avoid drugs that have several ingredients; they increase the risk of side effects.

Use acetaminophen or ibuprofen for a cold only if your child also has fever, sore throat, or muscle aches.

Leftover antibiotics should not be given because they have no effect on viruses and may be harmful.

The role of steam inhalation devices in treating cold symptoms gets mixed reviews in recent research.

Call Your Child's Physician Later If
- The nasal discharge lasts more than 14 days.
- You can't unblock the nose enough for your infant to take adequate fluids.
- You feel your child is getting worse.
- Your child develops any of the "Call Your Child's Physician" symptoms.

Prevention of Colds
Over the years, we all become exposed to many cold viruses and develop some immunity to them.
- Since complications are more common in children during the first year of life, try to avoid undue exposure of young babies to other children or

adults with colds, day-care nurseries, church nurseries, and crowded shopping centers. A parent can't control the majority of contact, however.

- Since the cold viruses are commonly transmitted by hand contamination, frequent hand-rinsing and keeping the hands away from the nose and mouth are the most helpful steps in prevention.

- While coughing usually isn't contagious, sneezing is. Teach your child to cover the nose during sneezing and the mouth during coughing.

- A humidifier prevents dry mucus membranes, which may be more susceptible to infections.

- Vitamin C, unfortunately, has not been shown to prevent or shorten colds. Large doses (like 2 grams) can cause diarrhea. Many adults, however, take extra vitamin C during the first 3 days of a cold and give it to their children as well. For this purpose, an adult dose of 250 mg 3 times a day and a child dose of 125 mg 3 times a day is harmless.

Related Topics

FEVER (see page 427)
SORE THROAT (see page 570)
COUGH (see page 584)
RED OR PINKEYE WITHOUT PUS (see page 524)
RED OR PINKEYE WITH PUS (see page 527)
EARACHE (see page 532)
SINUS CONGESTION (see page 561)

FOREIGN BODY IN THE NOSE

Young children often put foreign objects in their nostrils and then forget about them. Favorites are food, seeds, nuts, paper, cotton, Styrofoam, stones, and beads. The nose is programmed to try to reject these intruders by producing a foul-smelling yellow nasal discharge. Sometimes food particles (such as rice) end up in the nose following vomiting.

First Aid

Have your child blow his nose vigorously several times while closing the other nostril. Sometimes this action will expel the object. Vomited food can be removed by repeatedly blowing the nose after splashing some water into it. If you successfully remove the object, call your child's physician later only if a yellow nasal discharge occurs.

Call Your Child's Physician Immediately If These Measures Fail

It is critical that you do not try to remove the object by putting anything into the nose, including tweezers and fingers. This almost always pushes the object in farther and makes the physician's job very difficult, even with special instruments. Watch closely to see that your child doesn't push it in.

HAY FEVER (Allergic Rhinitis)

Symptoms and Characteristics

- Clear nasal discharge with sneezing, sniffling, and nasal itching
- Symptoms occur during pollen season.
- Similar symptoms during the same month of the previous year
- Previous confirmation of this diagnosis by a physician is helpful.
- Eye allergies (itchy, watery eyes) are commonly associated.
- A tickling sensation in the back of the throat can be associated.
- Sinus or ear congestion are sometimes associated.
- No fever

If your child's symptoms are different, call your physician for help.

Cause—Hay fever is an allergic reaction of the nose (and sinuses) to an inhaled substance. The allergic sensitivity is often inherited, so other family members may also have hay fever. During April and May the most common offending pollen is from trees. From late May to mid-July, the offending pollen is usually grass. From August to the first frost, the leading cause of hay fever is ragweed pollen. Although the inhaled substance is usually a pollen, it can also be animal dander, feathers, or other agents your child is allergic to. Cats are the most allergenic of our pets. Over 30 percent of allergic people react to cats. Cat dander remains in a house for 6 to 12 months after the cat is no longer there. Cat dander will also find its way into your home on a cat owner's clothing. Hay fever is the most common allergy; over 15 percent of people have it. Skin tests or blood tests are usually unnecessary for diagnosis. These children are not allergic to hay (nor do they have a fever).

Expected Course—This is a chronic condition that will probably recur every year, perhaps for a lifetime. Therefore, learning how to control it is worth your while.

Call Your Child's Physician During Office Hours If

- Your child is also coughing a lot or wheezing.
- Sinus congestion is present more than 1 week.
- The symptoms are constant rather than seasonal.
- You think your child needs to be seen.

Home Care for Hay Fever

Antihistamines—The best drug for hay fever is an antihistamine. A good one that is found in most nonprescription products is chlorpheniramine (see the dosage table on page 239). It will relieve both nose and eye symptoms. Newer prescription antihistamines cause much less drowsiness. If your child is school-age and having side effects of drowsiness, talk with your child's doctor about them. Symptoms clear up faster if antihistamines are given at the first sign of sneezing or sniffling. For children with occasional symptoms, the antihistamines can be taken on days when symptoms are present or expected. For children with daily symptoms, the best control is attained if antihistamines are taken continuously throughout the pollen season. The bedtime dosage is especially important for helping the nose repair itself during the night.

The main side effect of antihistamines is drowsiness. If your child gets drowsy, continue the drug, but temporarily decrease the dosage. In 1 to 2 weeks the regular dosage usually will be tolerated without much drowsiness. If the drowsiness remains a problem, switch to a combination product that contains an antihistamine with a decongestant (such as pseudoephedrine).

Prescription Steroid Nasal Sprays—If not helped by antihistamines, severe hay fever can usually be controlled by steroid nasal sprays, available by prescription. Allergy shots are usually not necessary. Nasal sprays must be used when the nose is not dripping. Give your child an antihistamine to stop the dripping before you use the spray. Nasal sprays do not help eye symptoms. Therefore they are usually used along with oral antihistamines or eye drops.

Pollen Removal—Pollen tends to collect on the exposed body surface and especially in the hair. Shower your child and wash the hair any time lots of symptoms (especially itchy or burning skin) are present following heavy exposure to pollen. At a minimum, shower your child every night before going to bed. Avoid handling pets that have been outside and are probably covered with pollen.

Eye Allergies Associated with Hay Fever—If your child also has itchy, watery eyes, some additional treatment measures are in order. Wash the face and eyelids to remove the pollen. Then apply a cold compress to the eyelids for 10 minutes. An oral antihistamine will usually bring the eye symptoms under control. If not, instill 1 drop of long-acting vasoconstrictor eyedrops every 8 to 12 hours as necessary for a few days (no prescription needed). Ask your pharmacist for help in choosing a reliable product. If your child is receiving oral antihistamines, however, they also treat the eyes and eyedrops are usually unnecessary.

Common Mistakes—Nose drops or nasal sprays usually do not help hay fever, because they are washed out of the nose by nasal secretions as soon as they have been instilled. Also, if vasoconstrictive (decongestant) nose drops are used for more than 5 days, they can irritate the nose and make it more congested.

Call Your Child's Physician Later If

- The treatment does not relieve most of the symptoms.
- Your child is missing any school, work, social activities, or sleep because of hay fever.
- Your child develops any of the "Call Your Child's Physician" symptoms.

Prevention of Hay Fever Symptoms

- Reduce pollen exposure by closing car windows (if possible) during drives in the country and closing the vents, staying indoors when it is windy, closing the windows that face the prevailing winds, turning off attic fans, and not having your child near when someone is cutting the grass during pollen season (especially when the pollen count is high). Routinely keeping your child indoors during the pollen season, however, is overtreatment.
- Avoid feather pillows, pets, farms, stables, barns, stock shows, and tobacco smoke if any of them seems to bring on or accentuate symptoms of nasal allergy. If your child is allergic to one dog, usually he is allergic

to all dogs. Short hair or long hair makes no difference, since the allergy is to the dog saliva and skin cells, not the hair.

- If the hay fever is especially bad, you may wish to take your child to an air-conditioned store or theater for a few hours.

- For exposure you can't avoid, or don't want to avoid (e.g., the circus), give an antihistamine 1 hour before and a shower immediately afterward.

- If your child is allergic to ragweed, you may wish to plan a vacation to an area that has little or no ragweed. In essence, only the coastal areas of Washington, Oregon, and California are free of ragweed pollen.

- Moving to another part of the country to avoid pollens is usually not worth the sacrifice, because within 3 years your child will usually develop allergies to plants in the new location.

Related Topics

EAR CONGESTION (see page 535)
ALLERGIES OF THE EYES (see page 522)
SINUS CONGESTION (see page 561)

NOSEBLEED

Symptoms and Characteristics

Nosebleeds (epistaxsis) are very common throughout childhood. They are usually caused by dryness of the nasal lining, plus the normal rubbing and picking that all children do when the nose becomes blocked or itchy. Vigorous nose-blowing can also cause them. All of these behaviors are increased in children with nasal allergies. Many times they begin unexpectedly, even during sleep. If the nosebleed was caused by an injury, turn directly to the guideline on NOSE TRAUMA, page 77.

Call Your Child's Physician

Immediately If

- There are any skin bruises not caused by an injury.
- Your child also has unexplained bleeding from the mouth or gums.
- Your child has fainted or feels dizzy when he or she stands up.
- A large amount of blood has been lost.
- Your child acts or looks very sick.

During Office Hours If

- Your child is under 1 year old.
- Difficult-to-stop nosebleeds are a recurrent problem for your child.
- Your family has a history of easy bleeding.
- You think your child needs to be seen.

Home Care

Lean Forward and Spit Out Any Blood—Have your child sit up and lean forward so he or she does not have to swallow the blood. Have a basin so your child can spit out any blood that drains into the throat. Your child's nose should be blown free of any large clots that interfere with pressure.

Squeeze the Soft Part of the Nose—Then tightly pinch the lower soft part of the nose against the center wall for 10 minutes. Don't release the pressure until 10 minutes are up. If the bleeding continues, you may not be pressing on the right spot. During this time, tell your child to breathe through the mouth. Reassure your child that you can stop the bleeding.

If All Else Fails, Use Vasoconstrictor Nose Drops and Squeeze Again—If the nosebleed hasn't stopped, insert a piece of gauze covered with vasoconstrictor nose drops (e.g., Neosynephrine) into the nostril. If nose drops are not available, put petroleum jelly on a piece of gauze. Squeeze again for 10 minutes. Leave the gauze in for another 10 minutes before removing it. If bleeding persists, call your physician, but continue the pressure in the meantime.

Common Mistakes

- A cold washcloth applied to the forehead, back of the neck, bridge of the nose, or under the upper lip does not help stop nosebleeds.
- Pressing on the bony part of the nose.
- Avoid packing the nose with anything, because when it is removed, bleeding usually recurs.
- Swallowed blood is irritating to the stomach. Don't be surprised or worried if it is vomited up.

Call Your Child's Physician Later If

- The bleeding has not stopped after two 10-minute attempts at pinching the nostrils closed.

- Nosebleeds occur daily even after petroleum jelly and humidification are used.
- Your child develops any of the "Call Your Child's Physician" symptoms.

Prevention of Nosebleeds

- A small amount of petroleum jelly applied twice a day to the center wall (septum) inside the nose is often helpful for relieving dryness and irritation.
- Increasing the humidity in the home by using a humidifier may also be helpful.
- If your child picks his nose a lot, help him give up this habit or at least make him more aware of it. With his permission, have him put a Band-Aid on his index finger each morning as a reminder. Also cut his fingernails weekly.
- Get your child into the habit of putting 2 or 3 drops of warm water in each nostril before blowing a stuffy nose.
- In addition, always avoid aspirin. One aspirin can increase the tendency of the body to bleed easily for up to a week and can make nosebleeds last much longer.
- If your child has nasal allergies, treating them with antihistamines will help break the itching-bleeding cycle. (See HAY FEVER, page 556.)

SINUS CONGESTION

Symptoms and Characteristics

- Sensation of fullness, pressure, or pain on the face overlying a sinus
- Pain can be above the eyebrow, behind the eye, or over the cheekbone.
- Pain is usually just on one side of the face.
- Runny or blocked nose
- A sensation of continuous postnasal drip
- Under 5 years of age, use the COLDS topic instead (page 550).

If your child's symptoms are different, call your physician for help.

Cause—The nose has seven bony, air-filled chambers (sinuses) that help to warm and humidify the air passing by them. Sinus congestion occurs when the sinus openings are blocked and normal sinus secretions accumulate and cause a sensation of pressure and fullness. Sinus congestion occurs mainly with colds and hay fever.

Expected Course—Sinus congestion usually goes away on its own. Without treatment, the sinuses usually open after about a week. The main complication is when bacteria multiply within the blocked sinus. This leads to fever lasting more than 3 days, yellow or green nasal discharge lasting more than 10 days, and increased sinus pain. Sometimes the overlying skin (around the eye or cheek) becomes red or swollen. This type of sinusitis needs antibiotics and occurs in 5 percent of colds. Frequent throat-clearing of postnasal secretions usually leads to a sore throat. Swallowing the sinus secretions is normal and harmless but may cause some nausea. Recent studies have shown that untreated sinus infections can cause a chronic cough (or even wheezing).

Call Your Child's Physician

Immediately If
- Redness or swelling occurs on the cheek, eyelids, or forehead.
- Sinus pain is severe even after treatment.
- Your child acts or looks very sick.

Within 24 Hours If
- A fever is present for more than 3 days.
- Sinus pain persists more than 1 day after your child starts treatment.
- Nasal secretions become yellow or green for more than 3 days in association with sinus congestion.
- The sinus congestion persists for more than 1 week.
- Nasal discharge lasts for more than 14 days.
- Your child is also coughing a lot.
- You think your child needs to be seen.

Home Care

Nasal Washes—Use warm water or saline nose drops followed by suction or nose blowing to wash dried mucus or pus out of the nose. Do nasal washes at least 4 times a day or whenever your child can't breathe through the nose. If the air in your home is dry, run a humidifier.

Decongestant Nose Drops or Spray—If the sinus still seems blocked after the inhalation of warm mist, long-acting vasoconstrictor nose drops or sprays (such as oxymetazoline) can be used. These are non-prescription items; ask your pharmacist to recommend a brand. The usual dose for adolescents is 2 drops or sprays per side twice a day. For younger children use 1 drop or spray. Use them routinely for the first 2 or 3 days of treatment. Then don't repeat them unless the sinus congestion or pain recurs. The nose should first be cleared by sniffing or nasal suction.

The openings to the sinuses are on the outer side of the nasal passages. Point the nasal spray in this direction. To deliver nose drops to this location, they must be put in while your child is lying on a bed with the head tipped back and turned to one side.

The drops or spray must be stopped after 5 days to prevent rebound swelling.

Pain Relief Medicines—Your child will usually need to take acetaminophen or ibuprofen temporarily to relieve pain until the obstructed sinus is opened. The application of ice wrapped in a wet cloth over the sinus for 20 minutes may also help to relieve pain.

Oral Antihistamines—If your child also has hay fever, give him his allergy medicine. If your child is not allergic, avoid oral antihistamines because they can slow down the movement of secretions out of the sinuses.

Contagiousness—Sinus infections are not contagious. Your child can return to school or day care when he or she is feeling better and the fever is gone.

Call Your Child's Physician Later If
- The sinus congestion and fullness persists for more than 1 week.
- You feel your child is getting worse.
- Your child develops any of the "Call Your Child's Physician" symptoms.

Prevention of Sinus Infections
Jumping into the water feet first can cause sinusitis of the frontal sinuses and should be avoided unless the nose is pinched. Swimming does not worsen sinusitis, but deep diving should be avoided unless your child wears nose plugs.

Related Topics

MOUTH AND THROAT

BAD BREATH (Halitosis)

Symptoms and Characteristics
- The exhaled breath has an unpleasant odor.
- The problem can be a recent or long-standing one.
- Bad breath only on awakening is normal and due to poor saliva flow at night.

Causes—Causes are numerous. If your child has one of the following, turn directly to that guideline:

CANKER SORES (see page 565)
COLDS (see page 550)
SINUS CONGESTION (see page 561)
SORE THROAT (see page 570)

- If your child has dental cavities, make a dental appointment.
- If your child is forgetful about brushing her teeth, help her brush more frequently.
- If your child sucks the thumb, a blanket, or other object, the bad breath will resolve when this habit is given up. Over age 4, ask your child's physician about some ways to discourage it before the permanent teeth come in. (See THUMBSUCKING, page 363.)
- Eating pungent foods, such as onions or garlic, can cause bad breath.
- Halitosis is occasionally a marker for disease (such as a sinus infection).

Call Your Child's Physician During Office Hours If
- The cause of your child's bad breath remains unclear.

Home Care

More frequent toothbrushing improves most cases of mild bad breath. Also brush the surface of the tongue. Mouthwashes and chewable breath fresheners are heavily promoted in our society but provide temporary improvement at best. Since some products contain 20 to 30 percent alcohol, they also carry a risk of poisoning in children who swallow them. The complaint of foul breath is unusual in children, and the cause should be uncovered and dealt with directly.

CANKER SORES (Mouth Ulcers)

Symptoms and Characteristics

- Painful, shallow ulcers (sores) of the lining of the mouth
- Gums or inner sides of the lips or cheeks are the usual sites
- No fever

If your child's symptoms are different, call your physician for help.

Similar Condition—If thrush is suspected, save time by turning directly to the guideline for THRUSH, page 141.

Cause—The cause of canker sores is unknown, but some may be due to prolonged contact with food that gets stuck in the teeth. Others may be due to forgotten injuries from toothbrushes, toothpicks, rough foods (e.g., corn chips), hot foods, or self-biting. Herpes simplex causes recurrent fever blisters (on the outside of the lip) but does not cause recurrent canker sores (of the inner mouth).

Expected Course—The white color of canker sores is the normal color of healing tissue in the mouth. This is not pus. They heal up in 1 to 2 weeks. Once begun, no treatment shortens the course. For many people they are a recurrent problem.

Call Your Child's Physician

Immediately If

- Your child could have swallowed an acid or alkali.
- Pain is severe.

Within 24 Hours If
- The gums are red, swollen, and tender.
- A raised yellow or red bump is present on the gums.
- A fever is present.
- Fluid intake is poor.
- The eyelids or genitals have any ulcers.
- You think your child needs to be seen.

During Office Hours If
- Four or more mouth ulcers are present.
- The canker sores began after taking a medicine.
- You have other questions or concerns.

Home Care

Pain Relief—To reduce the pain, swish 1 tablespoon of a liquid antacid in the mouth for several minutes. For a single ulcer, apply an antacid tablet and let it dissolve. This can be repeated 3 or 4 times a day. Give acetaminophen as necessary for pain (especially at bedtime).

Diet—The diet can be changed to reduce the pain. Use a glass instead of a bottle if your child is a baby. Avoid giving your child salty or citrus foods and foods that need much chewing. Change to a soft diet for a few days. Cold drinks and milkshakes are especially good. If brushing the teeth is painful, have your child rinse the mouth with water after meals.

Call Your Child's Physician Later If
- They last for more than 2 weeks.
- You feel your child is getting worse.
- Your child develops any of the "Call Your Child's Physician" symptoms.

Prevention of Canker Sores

Canker sores tend to recur throughout life. Good attention to toothbrushing after meals may prevent some. At a minimum, rinse the mouth with water after eating anything. Be careful with toothpicks and rough foods. Try to identify any offending foods. Was tomato, citrus fruit, peppermint, cinnamon, nuts, or shellfish taken within the previous day? If you find a food that you think may be causing the problem, eliminate it from the diet for 2 weeks and then offer some to see whether it causes a recurrence of the canker sores. If it does, the food should be eliminated from the diet permanently.

COLD SORES (Fever Blisters)

Symptoms and Characteristics

- A cluster of painful 2 to 3 mm blisters on the outer lip
- On one side of the mouth only
- Tingling or burning on the outer lip just before the cold sores appear and at the same place where they previously occurred (i.e., an early sign of recurrent cold sores)

If your child's symptoms are different, call your physician for help.

Cause—Cold sores are caused by the herpes simplex virus (usually Type I). The first bout follows contact with someone else with herpes. Recurrences occur in 10 percent of teens and 20 percent of adults. They carry the virus in a sensory nerve. The virus is reactivated by sunburn, fever, friction, menstrual periods, or physical exhaustion.

Expected Course—The blisters go on to rupture, scab over, and dry up. The whole process takes 10 to 14 days. They do not cause scars. Treatment can shorten the course by several days.

Call Your Child's Physician Within 24 Hours If

- The sores are spreading.
- Any sores occur near the eye.

During Office Hours If

- You want a prescription for an antiviral medicine to take the next time your youngster gets cold sores.

Home Care

Treatment

- If you feel tingling in the usual place but blisters are not yet present, apply an ice cube or ice pack continuously for 30 minutes. This may abort the infection.

- Cover the fever blisters with petroleum jelly to reduce the pain.
- Give acetaminophen or ibuprofen for pain relief (see the dosage tables on pages 238–40).
- Once you get fever blisters, you usually can't shorten the course unless you have anti-herpes pills and start them as soon as any small bumps appear. These require a prescription and some physicians don't approve of them for this purpose. Anti-herpes ointments are not effective.

Call Your Child's Physician Later If
- The sores last more than 2 weeks.
- Your child develops any of the "Call Your Child's Physician" symptoms.

Prevention of Cold Sores

Since fever blisters are often triggered by exposure to intense sunlight, prevent them in the future by using a lip balm containing sunscreen with an SPF of 30. Avoid spreading this germ to the eye, because an infection there can be serious. Therefore, discourage picking or rubbing and wash the hands frequently.

If your teenager is going skiing or to the beach and had frequent herpes flare-ups in the past, despite careful use of sunscreen, talk to your physician. Recent research has found that starting an anti-herpes pill by mouth before such outings can prevent most flare-ups.

Since the condition is contagious, avoid kissing other people during this time. If your child is young and puts everything in his or her mouth, avoid sharing toys with other children for a week. In general, most children under age 6 need to stay away from other children until the sores are dry (4 or 5 days). Although one should be careful about contagion, the child with herpes should not be made to feel like a leper. Fever blisters are not a sexually transmitted disease. By age 6, more than 50 percent of children already have antibodies to the cold sore virus.

GEOGRAPHIC TONGUE

Symptoms and Characteristics
- Tongue develops smooth red patches of various shapes and sizes
- Pattern resembles a map and can change from week to week
- Bare spots are painless; sense of taste is preserved

- Usually occurs in children under 6 years of age
- Tongue returns to normal appearance after a period of months to years

Home Care

The cause of geographic tongue is unknown, but it is not due to a vitamin deficiency. The condition is harmless and no treatment is helpful or necessary. No other disease looks like geographic tongue, but if you are uncertain of the diagnosis, call your child's physician during office hours.

LIP, SWOLLEN

Symptoms and Characteristics

The sudden onset of a swollen lip without an injury is usually due to a local allergic reaction. Symptoms of itching or tingling are also present. The allergic substance can be a food, toothpaste, lipstick, lip balm, or other irritant (such as an evergreen resin) that inadvertently is transferred from the hands.

If one of the following is suspected, save time by turning directly to that guideline:

BITES: INSECT, BEE, OR TICK (see page 19)
COLD SORES (see page 567)
MOUTH TRAUMA (see page 75)
POISONING (see page 55)

Call Your Child's Physician

Immediately If

- Breathing or swallowing is difficult (call 911).
- The area looks like a burn.
- The swelling is tender to the touch.
- A fever is present.
- Your child acts or looks very sick.

Home Care

Wash the lips and face with soap and water to remove any irritating substances. Apply ice to the swelling for 20 minutes out of every hour. If you have an antihistamine in your home, give your child the correct dosage 1 or 2 times. In the future, avoid any substance you are suspicious of.

Call your child's physician later if the swelling becomes worse or it lasts more than 2 days.

SORE THROAT (Pharyngitis)

Symptoms and Characteristics

- Complaint of a sore throat
- In children too young to talk, refusal to eat or crying during feedings
- When examined with a light, throat is bright red

If your child's symptoms are different, call your physician for help.

Causes—Most sore throats are caused by viruses and are part of a cold. About 10 percent of sore throats are due to strep bacteria. A throat culture or rapid strep test are the only ways to tell strep pharyngitis from viral pharyngitis. This identification of strep throat is important because without treatment some rare but serious complications (rheumatic fever or glomerulonephritis) can occur. Early treatment also prevents spread of strep to family and friends. A recent study showed that strep is not transmitted by pets.

Tonsillitis (temporary swelling and redness of the tonsils) is usually present with any throat infection, viral or bacterial. The presence of tonsillitis does not have any special meaning.

Children who sleep with their mouths open often wake in the morning with a dry mouth and sore throat. It clears within an hour of having something to drink. Use a humidifier to help prevent this problem. Children with a postnasal drip from draining sinuses often have a sore throat from frequent throat-clearing or the secretions themselves.

Expected Course—Sore throats with viral illnesses usually last 4 or 5 days. Strep throat responds nicely to penicillin or another antibiotic. After 24 hours on medication, strep is no longer contagious, and your child can return to day care or school if the fever is gone and the child is feeling better.

Call Your Child's Physician

Immediately If

- Your child is drooling, spitting, or having great difficulty swallowing (call 911).

- Breathing is difficult (call 911 if severe).
- The pain is severe.
- Your child can't fully open his mouth.
- Your child acts or looks very sick.

Within 24 Hours If
- A fever is present.
- The sore throat has been present more than 48 hours. (Exception: If the sore throat is mild *and* the main symptom is croup, hoarseness, or a cough, a throat culture is not needed.)
- There are any swollen or tender lymph glands in the neck.
- There is any associated abdominal pain.
- There was any recent contact with a person with strep throat or impetigo.
- Your child has a sunburned-looking rash.
- You see any large yellow or white spots on the tonsils while looking at them with a light.
- You think your child needs to be seen.

Home Care

Local Pain Relief—Children over 8 years of age can gargle with warm salt water (¼ teaspoon salt per glass). Children over 4 years of age can suck on hard candy (butterscotch seems to be a soothing flavor) or lollipops as often as necessary. Children over age 1 can sip warm chicken broth or warm apple juice. Taking frequent sips of fluids is often the best way to bring temporary relief from a sore throat.

Soft Diet—Swollen tonsils can make some foods hard to swallow. Provide your child with a soft diet for a few days if he or she prefers it.

Fever—Acetaminophen or ibuprofen may be given for a few days if your child has a fever over 102°F (39°C) or a great deal of throat discomfort. (For dosage, see the tables on pages 238–40.)

Common Mistakes
- Avoid expensive throat sprays or throat lozenges. Not only are they no more effective than hard candy, many also contain an ingredient (benzocaine) that may cause a drug reaction.

- Avoid using leftover antibiotics from siblings or friends. These should be thrown out because they deteriorate faster than other drugs. Unfortunately, antibiotics only help strep throats. They have no effect on viruses, and they can cause harm. They also make it difficult to find out what is wrong if your child becomes sicker.

Persistent Strep Throat—About 10 percent of children with strep throat don't respond to initial antibiotic treatment. Therefore, if your child continues to have a sore throat or mild fever after treatment is completed, return for a second strep test. If it is positive, your doctor will re-treat your child with a different antibiotic.

Call Your Child's Physician Later If

- The sore throat lasts more than 48 hours (without major improvement).
- You feel your child is getting worse.
- Your child develops any of the "Call Your Child's Physician" symptoms.

Related Topic

CANKER SORES (see page 565)

SWALLOWING DIFFICULTY

Symptoms and Characteristics

Difficulty in swallowing is usually due to a sore throat or mouth ulcers in a child too young to tell us what's happening. However, it can be caused by some serious conditions.

Call 911 If

- Your child is also having difficulty breathing.
- Your child is drooling (or spitting) saliva and unable to swallow anything.
- This could be a reaction to a food, drug, or insect sting.

Call Your Child's Physician

Immediately If

- A bone or other foreign object could be caught in the throat.
- Your child could have swallowed some acid, alkali, or other poison.
- Your child has croup.
- Your child can't fully open his mouth.
- Your child has not urinated in more than 8 hours.
- Your child acts or looks very sick.

Within 24 Hours If

- You do not know the cause of your child's swallowing difficulty.

Related Topics

CANKER SORES (see page 565)
SORE THROAT (see page 570)

TEETHING

Symptoms and Characteristics

Teething is the normal process of new teeth working their way through the gums. "Cutting teeth" is too strong a term. The first teeth normally erupt between 6 and 10 months of age in the lower jaw. Most children have completely painless teething. The only symptoms are increased saliva, drooling, and a desire to chew on things. Teething occasionally causes some mild gum pain, but not enough to interfere with sleep. Your child won't be miserable from teething. When the back teeth (molars) come through (6 to 12 years old), the overlying gum may become bruised and swollen (eruption hematoma). This is harmless and temporary.

Delayed eruption of primary teeth is rarely a problem. If no teeth are present by 12 months of age, discuss it with your child's physician.

Usually the primary (baby) tooth falls out before the corresponding permanent tooth erupts. Occasionally both teeth are temporarily present. As long as the baby tooth is a little loose, everything should go well. Have your child wiggle the baby tooth each day. The permanent tooth will find its way to the correct position once the baby tooth is out. If the primary tooth is still in place after 1 month of rocking, go to your child's dentist.

Home Care

Gum Massage—Find the irritated or swollen gum. Vigorously massage it with your finger for 2 minutes. Do this as often as necessary. If you wish, you may use a piece of ice to massage the gum.

Teething Rings—Your baby's way of massaging the gums is to chew on a smooth, hard object. Teethers or teething rings are helpful. Most children like them cold. Offer a teething ring that has been chilled in the refrigerator, but not frozen in the freezer. A piece of chilled banana may help. Avoid ice or Popsicles, which could cause frostbite of the gums.

Avoid hard foods that your baby might choke on (like raw carrots), but teething biscuits are fine.

Diet—Avoid salty or acidic foods. Your baby probably will enjoy sucking on a bottle nipple, but if that seems to cause pain, use a cup for fluids temporarily.

Medication—If the pain increases, give acetaminophen or ibuprofen orally for 1 day. Since your child will be teething for 2 years, use pain medicines with caution. Special teething gels are unnecessary and probably not beneficial. Many teething gels contain benzocaine, which can cause an allergic reaction. In addition it's unlikely they can numb the gums because they are washed out of the mouth and swallowed within a few minutes. If you still want to use a gel, do not apply it more than 4 times a day.

Common Mistakes

- Since teeth erupt almost continuously from 6 months to 2 years of age, many unrelated illnesses are blamed on teething. Fevers are also common during this time because after 6 months infants lose the natural protection provided by their mother's antibodies.
- Teething does not cause fever, sleep problems, diarrhea, diaper rash, or lowered resistance to any infection. It probably doesn't cause crying. If your child has any of these symptoms, see that guideline. If your baby develops fever while teething, the fever is due to something else, so refer to the list on page 427.

• Don't tie the teething ring around the neck. It could catch on something and strangle your child. Use a clip.

Call Your Child's Physician During Office Hours If
• Your child develops a fever over 101°F (38.3°C).
• Your child develops crying that doesn't appear to have a cause.
• You have other questions or concerns.

TONGUE-TIE

True tongue-tie, or tight tongue, is a very rare condition. The length of the lingual frenum, which is a thin band of tissue under the tongue, varies among individuals. At birth, the tongue is normally short and the band is tight. The tongue grows and the band stretches with use. After 1 year of age any tightness may be considered abnormal only if:
• The tip of the tongue can't be protruded past the teeth or gumline.
• The end of the tongue becomes notched when it is protruded. Without these findings, your child's tongue is normal.

Call Your Child's Physician During Office Hours If
• Breast-feeding is painful.

Treatment
If your child has these findings, mention them during your child's next checkup. Keep in mind that a tongue with less movement than normal does not cause delay or difficulty with speech. Occasionally it can cause sore nipples and painful breast-feeding because the shortened tongue cannot milk the areola. Under these conditions, frenulum release can be very helpful. Otherwise, frenulum release, or clipping of the band under the tongue, is rarely done anymore, because it is usually unnecessary and also carries the small risk of bleeding, infection, and tight scar tissue. It is rarely done before 1 year of age.

TONSIL AND ADENOID SURGERY

Surgical removal of the tonsils and adenoids (known as a T&A) is one of the most common operations performed on children in our country. Only 2 or 3 percent of children have adequate medical indications for this procedure. Although the decision to proceed is a medical one, parents need to be armed with enough facts to prevent unnecessary surgery.

The tonsils are not just some worthless pieces of tissue that block our view of the throat. They have a purpose, producing antibodies that fight nose and throat infections. They confine the infection to the throat, rather than allowing it to spread to the neck or bloodstream. Other beneficial functions of the tonsils and adenoids are under study.

Risks of a T&A

T&A procedures are not without risk. Under ideal conditions, the death rate is 1 child per 250,000 operations. Approximately 4 percent of children bleed on the fifth to eighth postoperative day. A few of these children may require a transfusion or additional surgery. All the children experience throat discomfort for several days. Some children with previously normal speech develop hypernasal speech because the soft palate no longer closes completely. In addition, the operation is expensive.

Erroneous Reasons for a T&A

Some T&A's are performed for the following unwarranted reasons. By all means, don't pressure a surgeon to remove your child's tonsils. A few physicians have difficulty saying no. You can always find someone to perform surgery on your child; in fact, this is the main risk of "doctor-shopping."

"Large Tonsils"—Large tonsils do not mean "bad" tonsils or "infected" tonsils. The tonsils are normally large during childhood (called physiological tonsillar hypertrophy). They can't be "too large" unless they touch each other. The peak size is reached between 8 and 12 years of age. Thereafter, they spontaneously shrink in size each year, as do all of the body's lymph tissues.

Recurrent Colds and Viral Sore Throats—Several studies have shown that T&A's do not decrease the frequency of viral upper respiratory infections. These URIs are unavoidable. Eventually your child develops immunity to these viruses and experiences fewer colds per year.

Recurrent Strep Throats—Newer studies have shown that the frequency of streptococcal infections of the throat do not decrease after the tonsils are removed unless your child experiences 7 or more per year (a rare occurrence). In children with 7 or more proven strep throat infections per year, some physicians will recommend daily penicillin for 6 months instead of a T&A, since penicillin can almost always eradicate the strep bacteria from the tonsils. The strep carrier state (which causes no symptoms, is harmless, and is not contagious) is not an indication for a T&A.

Recurrent Ear Infections—Research has shown that removal of the adenoids will not open the eustachian tube and decrease the frequency of ear infections or fluid in the middle ear. The exceptions are children who also have persistent nasal obstruction and mouth breathing due to large adenoids. Persistent middle-ear fluid may need ventilation tubes inserted in the eardrums.

School Absence—If your child misses school for vague reasons (including sore throats), removing the tonsils will not improve attendance. (See SCHOOL PHOBIA OR AVOIDANCE, page 379.)

Miscellaneous Conditions—A T&A will not help hay fever, asthma, febrile convulsions, or bad breath. There is little in medicine that has not at one time or another been blamed on the tonsils.

Medical Indications for a T&A

Yes, sometimes the tonsils should come out. But the benefits must outweigh the risks. All of the following are valid reasons for an evaluation. If a T&A is indicated, the ear, nose, and throat surgeon will decide if the tonsils, adenoids, or both need removal.

Persistent Mouth Breathing—Mouth breathing during colds or hay fever is common. Continued daily mouth breathing is less common and deserves an evaluation to see if it is due to large adenoids. The open-mouthed appearance results in teasing, and the mouth breathing itself leads to changes in the facial bone structure (including an overbite, which could need orthodontia).

Abnormal Speech—The speech can be muffled by large tonsils or made hyponasal (no nasal resonance) by large adenoids. Although other causes are possible, an evaluation is in order.

Severe Snoring and Obtructive Sleep Apnea—Snoring can have several causes. In severe cases, the loud snoring is associated with retractions (pulling in of the spaces between the ribs) choking, and interruptions of breathing (obstructive sleep apnea) (see SNORING, page 582). If your child has severe snoring, make a 5-minute audiotape and bring it to your physician for a listen.

Heart Failure—Rarely, large tonsils and adenoids interfere so much with breathing that blood oxygen is reduced, and the right side of the heart goes into failure. Children with this serious condition are short of breath, have limited exercise tolerance, and have a rapid pulse.

Persistent Swallowing Difficulties—During a throat infection, the tonsils may temporarily swell enough to cause swallowing problems. Some children refuse meats because they are difficult to swallow. If the problem is persistent and the tonsils are seen to be touching when they are not infected, an evaluation is in order. This problem usually occurs in children with a small mouth to begin with.

Recurrent Abscess (Deep Infection) of the Tonsil—Your child's physician will make this decision.

Recurrent Abscess of a Lymph Node Draining the Tonsil—Your child's physician will make this decision.

Suspected Tumor of the Tonsil—These rare tumors cause one tonsil to be much larger than the other. The tonsil is also quite firm to the touch, and usually enlarged lymph nodes are found on the same side of the neck.

Call Your Child's Physician During Office Hours If

• You think your child has a valid indication for a T&A.

• You have other questions or concerns.

(Remember: Do not give permission for a T&A unless your child has one of the preceding indicators or until you have received a second opinion from another physician.)

TOOTHACHE

Symptoms and Characteristics

If your child complains of a painful tooth, it may just be a temporarily sensitive tooth, but usually it means decay or a cavity is present. One complication of a decaying tooth is a gum boil just below the gumline. The infection in the tooth may also spread to the face (giving a swollen cheek) or the lymph node just under the jawbone. Dental decay must be treated in both the baby and permanent teeth. Unchecked cavities in primary teeth not only cause pain but also can damage the underlying permanent teeth.

Call Your Child's Dentist

Immediately If
- The pain is very severe.
- Fever is present.
- The face is swollen.

During Office Hours If
- The pain has been present for more than 24 hours.
- You can see a brown cavity in the painful tooth.
- There is a red (occasionally yellow) bump at the gumline of the painful tooth.
- You think your child needs to be seen.

Home Care

Flossing—First use dental floss on either side of the painful tooth. The removal of a jammed piece of food may bring quick relief.

Pain Relief Medicines—For now, treat the toothache with ibuprofen or acetaminophen. If the pain lasts for more than 24 hours or becomes severe, call your dentist. An ice pack on the jaw for 20 minutes may also help.

Oil of Cloves for Severe Toothache—If you cannot see a dentist for several days and an open cavity is visible: Clean all food out of the cavity with a toothpick, Water Pik, or water in a syringe. Buy some oil of cloves (80 percent eugenol) at a pharmacy; no prescription is needed. Place a few drops of the oil of cloves into the open pit, keeping in mind that it has no effect if applied to the tooth's surface. If the cavity is large, pack it with a small piece of cotton soaked with oil of cloves. Try to keep the oil of cloves off the tongue, because it stings. The cavity can also be temporarily sealed with melted candle wax. Just rub it in with your fingertip.

Call Your Child's Physician If

• You can't reach your dentist and it's an emergency.

Related Topic

TOOTH DECAY PREVENTION (page 194)

LUNGS (RESPIRATORY)

BREATHING, NOISY

Call Your Child's Physician Immediately If

- Your child has serious and sudden difficulty in breathing. (See also BREATHING DIFFICULTY, SEVERE, page 36.)
- Wheezing is present. (See also WHEEZING, page 594.) Wheezing is a high-pitched purring or whistling sound produced during breathing out (expiration). Most squeaky sounds are wheezes.
- Stridor is present. Stridor is a harsh, raspy, low-pitched sound on breathing in (inspiration) and is associated with a brassy, tight, hoarse cough. (See the guideline on CROUP, page 588.)

Types of Nonemergency Noisy Breathing

Keep in mind that noisy breathing is due to vibrations set up somewhere in the airway (nose, throat, vocal cords, or chest). If your child's noisy breathing is intermittent and doesn't fit any of the following patterns, tape-record it and bring the tape to your physician's office.

Rattling Sounds—Rattling sounds are due to vibrations from mucus pooling in the lower throat. These gurgling sounds can be eliminated by coughing or swallowing. Many parents are needlessly concerned about a rattly chest. (See the guideline on COUGH, page 584.)

Snorting Sounds—Intermittent snorting sounds are due to mucus partially blocking the nasal passages. If the snorting makes your child uncomfortable, the problem can be eliminated by warm water nose drops and nasal suction. (See the guideline on COLDS, page 550.) Increased humidity in the home will also help prevent dried secretions. During the first year of life, many babies normally make nasal sounds off and on during sleep simply because the nasal passages are so narrow. Since the sounds do not interfere with sleep, no treatment is necessary.

Snoring—Snoring is noisy breathing during sleep. Snoring is caused by partial obstruction of the nose or throat during sleep. Most children snore occasionally when they have a cold that partially blocks the nose. About 20 percent of children snore every night. Most of this snoring is benign and doesn't cause any awakening or difficulty breathing. However, about 2 percent of children (10 percent of those with nightly snoring) have severe nasal obstruction, which can cause complications. Most have large tonsils and adenoids, the peak age for this being 2 to 5 years. A few have severe nasal allergies (e.g., due to a cat that sleeps in their bedroom). These children need to be evaluated by their physician. Call for an appointment during regular office hours for any of the following symptoms during snoring:

• Respiratory pauses for more than 15 seconds (obstructive sleep apnea)
• Respiratory pauses followed by gasps or sobs
• Choking or gasping for breath during snoring
• Struggling to breathe with increasingly louder snoring or retractions (pulling in of the spaces between the ribs)
• Bluish lips or face
• Snoring in a child less than 1 year old

CHEST PAIN

Symptoms and Characteristics

Your child may complain of pain in the chest. Most acute chest pain is associated with a hacking cough. Coughing can cause sore muscles in the chest wall, upper abdomen, or diaphragm. Occasionally, chest pain follows strenuous exercise, lifting, or work that involves the upper body. This type of muscle soreness often increases with movement of the shoulders. Heart disease is hardly ever the cause of chest pain in children.

The most common cause of recurrent chest pains in adolescents and adults is precordial catch syndrome. This pain occurs on the left side (often just below the left nipple) and comes on suddenly. The pain feels sharp or knifelike, causing the person to freeze. Usually within 1 minute, the pain is gone. Although the cause is unknown, it may be due to a pinched nerve. Although it may last for years, the precordial catch syndrome is completely harmless. Daily stretching exercises sometimes reduce these lightning pains.

Call Your Child's Physician

Immediately If

- The breathing is difficult or fast (call 911).
- The pain is severe.
- The pain is unexplained *and* has lasted more than 2 hours.
- The pain prevents taking a deep breath.
- Your child also faints or feels dizzy.
- The pain followed a direct blow to the chest.
- Your child acts or looks very sick.

During Office Hours If

- Coughing is also present.
- Fever is present.
- Chest pains are a recurrent problem for your child.
- You think your child needs to be seen.

Home Care

Treatment—Treat the chest wall pains (associated with sore, strained muscles) with acetaminophen or ibuprofen (for dosage, see the tables on pages 238–40). Continue this until 24 hours have passed without pain. You can also relieve muscle spasm by applying a heating pad or warm washcloth to the area. They will probably clear within 3 days. If the pain is due to coughing, begin a cough suppressant medicine while waiting to talk with your physician. (See the guideline on COUGH, page 584.)

Call Your Child's Physician Later If

- The pains last more than 3 days on treatment.
- You feel your child is getting worse.
- Your child develops any of the "Call Your Child's Physician" symptoms.

Related Topic

Cough (see below)

CONGESTION, RESPIRATORY

Congestion means many things to different people. One of the following guidelines will probably meet your needs:

Breathing, Noisy (see page 581)
Colds (see page 550)
Cough (see below)
Ear Congestion (see page 535)
Sinus Congestion (see page 561)

COUGH

Symptoms and Characteristics

- The cough reflex expels air and secretions from the lungs with a sudden explosive noise.
- Cough can be dry and hacky or wet and productive.
- A coughing spasm is more than 5 minutes of continuous coughing.

Similar Conditions—If one of the following is suspected, save time by turning directly to that guideline:

Croup (see page 588)
Wheezing (see page 594)

Causes—Keep in mind that coughing has a purpose: to clear the lungs and protect them from pneumonia.

Most coughs are due to a viral infection of the trachea (windpipe) and bronchi (larger air passages) called acute tracheitis or bronchitis. Most children get this a couple of times a year as part of a cold.

While coughs may be associated with sinus infections, they are not due to postnasal drip. People swallow while they are asleep, so secretions don't pool in the throat.

The role of milk in thickening the secretions is also doubtful, except for the 2 percent of infants with proven milk allergy.

Expected Course—Usually viral bronchitis gives a dry, tickly cough that lasts for 2 to 3 weeks. Sometimes it becomes loose (wet) for a few days, and your child coughs up a lot of phlegm (mucus). This is usually a sign that the end of the illness is near.

Call Your Child's Physician

Immediately If
- A toy, food, or other foreign object could possibly be caught in the windpipe (especially likely if the cough came on suddenly after a choking episode and your child is under 3 years old) (call 911).
- Breathing is difficult (call 911 if severe).
- Your child is less than 1 month old. (Exception: your child coughs 1 or 2 times.)
- The respirations are fast or labored (when your child is not coughing).
- Wheezing is present.
- Your child has passed out with coughing spasms.
- The lips have turned bluish with coughing spasms.
- Coughing spasms occur continuously for more than 1 hour.
- Any blood-tinged sputum has been coughed up.
- Your child acts or looks very sick.

Within 24 Hours If
- A fever has lasted more than 72 hours.
- Your child also has sinus pain.
- Your child also has asthma.
- Your child is 1 to 3 months old *and* the cough has been present for more than 72 hours.
- You think your child needs to be seen.

During Office Hours If
- The cause could be an allergy (like pollen).
- Coughing causes lots of lost sleep.
- The coughing has caused vomiting 3 or more times.
- The coughing has caused bad chest pains.
- The cough has caused your child to miss 3 or more days of school.
- You have other questions or concerns.

Home Care for Cough

Cough Drops—Most coughs in children over age 4 can be controlled by sucking on cough drops freely.

Homemade Cough Syrup—Children over age 1 year can be given ½ to 1 teaspoon of corn syrup instead. (Avoid giving honey to babies under 1 year of age, because of the small risk of botulism for this age group.) Corn syrup can thin the secretions and loosen the cough. For coughing fits, take a warm shower with your child. (Caution: Avoid very hot water or steam, which can cause burns or dangerous high temperatures.)

Warm Liquids for Coughing Spasms—Coughing symptoms are often due to sticky mucus caught on the vocal cords or windpipe. Warm, clear liquids usually relax the airway and loosen up the mucus. Start with warm lemonade, warm apple juice, or warm herbal tea if your child is over 4 months old. Avoid adding any alcohol, because of the aggravation of the cough as the fumes of alcohol are inhaled into the lungs, and also the risk of intoxication from unintentional overdosage. Children over 4 years old can suck on butterscotch hard candy or cough drops to coat the irritated throat.

Cough-Suppressant Medicines—Since the cough reflex protects the lungs, cough-suppressant drugs are given in a dosage to reduce (but not eliminate) coughing. They are indicated only for dry coughs (nonproductive of mucus) that interfere with sleep, school attendance, or work. They also help children who have chest pain from coughing spasms. They should not be given to infants under 12 months of age or for wet productive coughs.

A nonprescription cough suppressant is dextromethorphan (DM). Ask your pharmacist for help in choosing a brand that contains DM without any other active ingredients. See the dosage table for DM on page 239.

Often corn syrup can be given during the day, and DM given at bedtime and during the night.

Humidifiers—Dry air tends to make coughs worse. Dry coughs can be loosened up by encouraging a good fluid intake and using a humidifier in your child's bedroom. Don't add medicine to the water in the humidifier, because it irritates the cough in some children.

Postural Drainage for Coughing Spasms—Some coughing spasms are due to choking on lung mucus that comes up and sticks to the vocal cords. If your child is under 3 years old and coughing up lots of mucus at night, try to improve matters by giving postural drainage at bedtime. Start by having your child breathe in warm mist from a shower, a wet washcloth over the face, or a humidifier. Have your child lie stomach down on your outstretched legs, with the head lower than the rest of the body. Then gently pat your child on the back of the rib cage, working from the lower back to the shoulders. Do this for 10 minutes, and expect some productive coughing.

Vomiting with Coughing Spasms—Refeed your child after this type of vomiting. Offer smaller amounts with each feeding to reduce the chances of repeated vomiting.

Active and Passive Smoking—Since tobacco smoke agitates coughing, don't let anyone smoke around your coughing child. Better yet, try to protect your child from all passive smoking. If one parent smokes in the house, that's equivalent to your child actively smoking 30 to 40 cigarettes per year. Remind the teenager who smokes that his or her cough may last weeks longer than it normally would without smoking.

Exercise—Teenagers will find that required gym and exercise trigger coughing spasms when they have bronchitis. If so, these activities should be avoided temporarily.

Common Mistakes—Antihistamines, decongestants, and fever medicines are found in many cough syrups. These ingredients have no impact on coughs, but they can have side effects. Antihistamines are illogical for productive coughs, because they dry secretions and make them harder to cough up. While the expectorants are safe, they have recently been shown to be ineffective. Stay with the simple remedies mentioned previously, or give DM for severe coughs. Keep in mind that prescription cough medicines (unless they contain codeine) offer no advantage over nonprescription ones.

Milk does not need to be eliminated from the diet, since most sick babies want their formula, and restricting it improves the cough only if the child is allergic to milk. Never stop breast-feeding because of a cough.

Raising the head of the bed is of questionable value, since more coughing is caused by lung mucus than nasal mucus.

Lastly, physicians can usually evaluate coughs and exclude pneumonia without a chest X-ray (so don't expect one).

Call Your Child's Physician Later If
- The cough lasts more than 3 weeks.
- You feel your child is getting worse.
- Your child develops any of the "Call Your Child's Physician" symptoms.

CROUP (Croupy Cough and Stridor)

Symptoms and Characteristics of Croupy Cough
- All children with croup have a distinctive cough that is tight and sounds like a barking seal.
- The voice is usually hoarse.

Symptoms and Characteristics of Stridor
- A harsh, raspy, vibrating sound occurs during inspiration.
- Breathing in is very difficult.
- Stridor only occurs with severe croup.
- Most stridor occurs intermittently with crying or coughing.
- If the stridor occurs continuously, your child has severe respiratory distress.

Similar Conditions—EPIGLOTTITIS (see page 655) is a life-threatening bacterial infection that causes stridor, fever, drooling, and difficulty swallowing. WHEEZING (see page 594) is a high-pitched meowing or whistling sound produced during expiration. If either of these is what your child has, call your physician immediately.

Cause—Croup is an infection of the vocal cords, voice box (larynx), and windpipe (trachea), often caused by the parainfluenza virus. It is usually part of a cold. The hoarseness is due to swelling of the vocal cords. Stridor occurs as the opening between the vocal cords becomes more narrow. Croup occurs yearly and in severe epidemics every other year.

Expected Course—Croup usually lasts for 5 to 6 days and generally gets worse at night. During that time, it can change from mild to severe many times. The worst symptoms are seen in children under 3 years of age.

First Aid for Attacks of Stridor with Croup

If your child suddenly develops stridor or tight breathing, do the following:

Inhalation of Warm Mist—Warm, moist air seems to work best to relax the vocal cords and break the stridor. The simplest way to provide this is to have your child breathe through a warm, wet washcloth placed loosely over the nose and mouth. Another good way, if you have a humidifier (not a steam vaporizer), is to fill it with warm water (a little warmer than body temperature) and have your child put his or her face in the stream of humidity and breathe deeply through an open mouth.

The Foggy Bathroom—In the meantime, have the warm shower running with the bathroom door closed. Once the room is all fogged up, take your child in there for at least 10 minutes. Try to allay fears by cuddling your child and reading a story. Panic and crying make croup worse. If the crying can be stopped, the breathing will be easier.

Cold Air—Cold air sometimes relieves the stridor associated with croup. If it's cold outside, take your child outdoors for for 5 minutes. Why the cold air should break the stridor remains a mystery. Others respond to taking a few deep breaths while being held in front of an open refrigerator.

Results of First Aid—Most children settle down with the above treatments and then sleep peacefully through the night. If the stridor continues in your child, call your physician immediately. If your child turns blue, passes out, or stops breathing, call the rescue squad (911).

Call 911 If

- Breathing is difficult (when your child is not coughing).
- Your child is drooling, spitting, or having great difficulty swallowing. (If your child normally drools, call only if it has increased greatly.)
- Your child has passed out.
- The lips are bluish or dusky.
- A toy or other small foreign object could be caught in the windpipe.
- The croup started suddenly after taking a medicine, eating a food to which your child is allergic, or being stung by an insect.

Call Your Physician (and Also Begin the First Aid for Stridor, Above)

Immediately If

- Your child can't bend the neck forward.
- Your child is constantly uncomfortable.
- Your child has been unable to sleep.
- Coughing spasms occur continuously for over 1 hour.
- The stridor is unresponsive to warm mist.
- There are retractions (tugging in) between the ribs.
- Your child acts or looks very sick.

Within 24 Hours If

- Your child is under 1 year old.
- The attacks of stridor have occurred more than 3 times.
- The fluid intake is poor.
- A fever over 105°F is present.
- A fever lasts more than 3 days.
- You think your child needs to be seen.

Home Care for a Croupy Cough Without Stridor

Mist—Dry air tends to make coughs worse. Keep the child's room humidified. Use a humidifier and have it run 24 hours a day. Don't add any camphor or menthol oils to the water, because they are irritating to the cough in most children. If you don't own a humidifier, hang wet sheets or towels in your child's room. For coughing fits, take a warm shower with your child. (Caution: Avoid very hot water or steam, which could cause burns or dangerously high body temperatures.)

Warm, Clear Fluids for Coughing Spasms—Coughing spasms are often due to sticky mucus caught on the vocal cords. Warm apple juice, lemonade, or herbal tea may help relax the vocal cords and loosen the sticky mucus.

Cough Medicines—Medicines are less helpful than either mist or swallowing warm fluids. Children over 4 years old can be given cough drops for the cough, and children over 1 year old can be given ½ to 1 teaspoon corn syrup. If your child has a fever (over 102°F) you may give him acetaminophen or ibuprofen. (See the dosage tables on pages 238–40.)

Close Observation—While your child is croupy, sleep in the same room temporarily. Consider bringing your child's mattress into your bedroom. If stridor develops, croup can be a dangerous disease.

Avoid Smoke Exposure—Don't let anyone smoke around your child; smoke can make croup worse.

Contagiousness—The viruses that cause croup are quite contagious until the fever is gone or at least until 3 days into the illness. Since spread of this infection can't be prevented, your child can return to school or child care once he feels better.

Call Your Child's Physician Later If
- Croupy cough lasts more than 10 days.
- You feel your child is getting worse.
- Your child develops any of the "Call Your Child's Physician" symptoms.

Related Topics

CHOKING (see page 10)
COUGH (see page 584)

HOARSENESS

Symptoms and Characteristics
- The voice is raspy.
- If hoarseness is severe, your child can do little more than whisper.
- A cough is often associated.

Similar Conditions—If appropriate, turn directly to the following guidelines:

CROUP (CROUPY COUGH AND STRIDOR) (See page 588)
HAY FEVER (See page 556)

Causes—Hoarseness is usually caused by a cold or croup virus (laryngitis) or overuse of the vocal cords (e.g., shouting or screaming). Cheerleaders and avid sports fans are prone.

Expected Course—Hoarseness usually lasts 1 to 2 weeks. Repeated vocal cord abuse can cause thickening of the cords and a slow recovery.

Call Your Child's Physician

Call 911 If

- Breathing is difficult.
- A toy, food, or other foreign object could possibly be caught in the windpipe.
- Your child choked on anything recently.

During Office Hours If

- Your child is under 2 months old.
- You think your child needs to be seen.

Home Care for Hoarseness

Treatment—Have your child gargle with warm water with a little salt added and suck on hard candy or cough drops several times a day. Younger children can sip warm liquids like apple juice. Encourage your child to rest the voice and avoid the vocal strain that comes from yelling and screaming. Your child should talk as little as possible for a few days. If the hoarseness gets really bad, have your child whisper or write notes. Also run a humidifier in your child's bedroom.

Call Your Child's Physician Later If

- The hoarseness lasts more than 2 weeks.
- You feel your child is getting worse.
- Your child develops any of the "Call Your Child's Physician" symptoms.

INFLUENZA (Flu)

Symptoms and Characteristics

Influenza is a viral infection of the nose, throat, trachea, and bronchi. It occurs yearly and in severe epidemics every 3 or 4 years (e.g., Asian influenza). The main symptoms are a stuffy nose, sore throat, and nagging cough. There may be more muscle pain, headache, fever, and chills than with usual colds. Since there are many influenza viruses, and they are constantly changing, we can easily come down with influenza almost yearly. Spread is rapid because the incubation period is only 24 to 36 hours and the virus is very contagious. For most people, influenza is just a bad cold. The dangers of influenza for normal, healthy people (under 65 years of age) are overrated.

Call Your Child's Physician

See the guidelines on fever, cough, colds, sore throat, sinus congestion, earache, and so forth. Ear infections, sinus infections, and pneumonia are the most common complications.

Home Care for Influenza

The treatment of influenza depends on your child's main symptoms and is no different from that suggested for other viral respiratory infections. Bed rest is unnecessary.

Fever or Aches—Use acetaminophen or ibuprofen. (See the tables on pages 238–40 for dosage.) Aspirin should be avoided in children and adolescents with suspected influenza because of the possible link with Reye's syndrome.

Cough or Hoarseness—Cough drops for children over 4 years of age and corn syrup (½ to 1 teaspoon) for children over 1 year old should help. (See the guidelines on COUGH, page 584, or HOARSENESS, page 591.)

Sore Throat—A soft diet will help. For children over age 1, offer sips of warm chicken broth. Children over age 4 can suck on hard candy.

Stuffy Nose—Warm-water or saline nose drops and suction (or nose-blowing) will open most blocked noses. Use nasal washes at least 4 times per day or whenever your child can't breathe through the nose. Saline nose drops are made by adding ½ teaspoon of salt to 1 cup of warm water.

Contagiousness—Spread is rapid because the incubation period is only 24 to 36 hours and the virus is very contagious. Therefore, your child may return to day care or school after the fever is gone and he or she feels up to it.

Antiviral Medicine—All antiviral drugs must be given within 48 hours of the start of influenza symptoms to have an effect. Their benefits are limited: they reduce the duration of symptoms by 1 to 1 ½ days. Most doctors do not use them to treat an existing case of influenza in healthy children, but they do use them for high-risk children. Talk with your health care provider about this.

Prevention and Influenza Vaccine (Flu Shot)

In 2003, the American Academy of Pediatrics recommended that all children age 6 months through 23 months receive the influenza vaccine. Recent research has demonstrated that healthy children younger than 24 months are at as great a risk of influenza complications as are previously recognized high-risk groups. Otherwise the vaccine is optional for healthy children (unless an especially severe form of influenza comes along). One reason is that influenza vaccine gives protection for only 1 or 2 years.

However, children over 6 months of age with the following conditions have a high complication rate from influenza (especially pneumonia) and need yearly influenza boosters each fall. The parents and siblings of high-risk children should also receive the influenza vaccine.

• Lung disease (e.g., asthma, cystic fibrosis, bronchopulmonary dysplasia)
• Heart disease (e.g., congenital heart disease, rheumatic heart disease)
• Muscle disease (e.g., muscular dystrophy)
• Metabolic disease (e.g., diabetes mellitus)
• Renal disease (e.g., nephrotic syndrome)
• Cancer and diseases caused by compromised immune systems
• Diseases requiring long-term aspirin therapy

WHEEZING

Symptoms and Characteristics

Wheezing is a high-pitched purring or whistling sound produced during breathing out (expiration).

Similar Conditions—Some other respiratory sounds can be confused with wheezing. If one of the following is suspected, save time by turning directly to that guideline:

• CROUP (CROUPY COUGH AND STRIDOR) (see page 588) gives a harsh, raspy, vibrating sound on breathing in (inspiration) and is associated with a hoarse, tight cough, like a barking seal.

• Snorting sounds are due to mucus partially blocking the nasal passages. These sounds can be eliminated by warm-water nose drops and nasal suction. (See the guideline on COLDS, page 550.)

• Rattling sounds are due to mucus in the lower throat. These sounds can be eliminated by coughing or swallowing.

Asthma as a Cause of Wheezing—If your child has asthma, maintain close contact with the physician who coordinates your child's treatment program. Try to learn as much about asthma as you can. The most common mistake in treating asthma is delaying the start of asthma medicines. Many children wheeze soon after they get coughs and colds. If this is the case for your child, start the asthma medicine or inhaler at the first sign of any coughing. The best "cough medicines" for a child with asthma are the asthma medicines. Always keep the medicine handy, and take it with you on trips. If your supply runs low, request a refill.

Another mistake is not eliminating asthma triggers. Try to discover and avoid the substances that trigger attacks in your child. Routinely avoid common triggers such as feather pillows and tobacco smoke. Try to keep pets outside, or at least out of your child's room (cats cause more allergic reactions than any other pet). Learn how to dustproof your child's bedroom. Avoid wool rugs. Change the filters on your hot air heating system or air conditioner regularly. If there has been any recent contact with grass, pollen, weeds, or animals that your child might be allergic to, the pollen remaining in the hair and clothing is probably keeping the wheezing going. Have your child shower, wash his hair, and put on clean clothes.

Call Your Child's Physician

If your child definitely has wheezing, call your child's physician immediately. Although asthma (reactive airway disease) is the most common cause of wheezing, there are many causes, and it can be an emergency. Let your physician help you sort out what is going on.

ABDOMEN (GASTROINTESTINAL)

ABDOMINAL PAIN

Symptoms and Characteristics
- Your child complains that his stomach (abdomen) hurts.

Similar Condition—For babies under 3 months old with fussy crying, see CRYING BABY (COLIC), page 253.

Causes—The causes are numerous. Usually it's something simple like overeating, gas pains from too much soda pop, or other types of indigestion. Sometimes it signals the onset of a viral gastroenteritis, and vomiting or diarrhea soon follow. In children and adults, the most common cause of recurrent abdominal pain is stress and worries. They occur in over 10 percent of children. The pain occurs in the pit of the stomach or near the belly button. The pain is low-grade but real. Recurrent stomachaches can have numerous causes and deserve a medical evaluation.

Expected Course—With harmless causes, the pain is usually better or resolved in 2 hours. With gastroenteritis, belly cramps may precede each bout of vomiting or stooling. With serious causes (such as appendicitis) the pain worsens and becomes constant.

Call Your Child's Physician
Immediately If
- The pain is severe (e.g., causes constant crying).
- Your child walks bent over or holding the abdomen.

- Your child is lying down and refuses to walk.
- The pain is constant *and* has lasted more than 2 hours (especially if the pain is on the lower right side, where the appendix is located).
- The pain comes and goes (cramps) *and* lasts more than 12 hours. (Exception: Vomiting or diarrhea is your child's main symptom and the stomachache clears each time your child vomits or passes a stool.)
- Your child is under 1 year old.
- The pain is in the scrotum or testicle.
- Any blood has appeared in the bowel movements.
- Poisoning with a plant, medicine, or chemical is a possibility.
- The abdomen was recently injured.
- Your child looks or acts very sick.
- When you press on your child's abdomen with your hand, the abdomen is quite tender to the touch.

During Office Hours If

- This is a recurrent problem for your child.
- You think your child needs to be seen.

Home Care

Treatment—Have your child lie down and rest until feeling better. A warm washcloth or heating pad on the abdomen may speed recovery. Avoid giving your child solid foods; permit only sips of clear fluids. Keep a vomiting pan handy. Younger children are especially likely to refer to nausea as a "stomachache."

Common Mistakes—Do not give any medicines for stomach cramps unless you have talked with your physician. Painkillers may mask the problem. More importantly, avoid laxatives and enemas. If your child has appendicitis, these medicines could cause the appendix to rupture.

The Worried Stomach—If your child has been evaluated by a physician and the diagnosis is that she has a "worried stomach" (i.e., is getting stomachaches because of emotional upset or worry), try the following to ease the pains:

- Help your child lighten up. Children with recurrent bellyaches tend to be sensitive, serious, conscientious, even model children. This makes them vulnerable to the normal stresses of life, such as changing schools or a recent move. Help your youngster talk about events that trigger his pains, and how he's going to cope with them.

- Make sure that your youngster doesn't miss any school because of stomachaches. These children have a tendency to stay home when the going gets rough.
- Teach him to use relaxation exercises for mild pains. Have him lie down in a quiet place, take deep, slow breaths; and think about something pleasant. Listening to relaxation tapes may help.
- Caution: Your child should have a complete medical checkup before assuming that recurrent stomachaches are due to worrying too much.

Call Your Child's Physician Later If

- The pain is constant *and* no better in 2 hours.
- Call sooner if it rapidly becomes worse.
- Call in 12 hours if it's the kind of pain that comes and goes.
- You feel your child is getting worse.
- Your child develops any of the "Call Your Child's Physician" symptoms.

Related Topics

Pain with:

CONSTIPATION (see page 599)
COUGH (see page 584)
DIARRHEA (see page 603)
MENSTRUAL CRAMPS (see page 630)
URINATION, PAIN WITH (see page 624)
VOMITING (see page 619)

AMOXICILLIN DIARRHEA

Amoxicillin causes diarrhea in 10 percent of children receiving it, depending on the dosage. This is an irritative reaction (i.e., amoxicillin acts like a laxative), not an allergic one. The loose stools begin within a day or two of starting the antibiotic. Amoxicillin diarrhea is usually mild and occasionally moderate in degree. Dehydration and weight loss do not occur. As soon as you finish the course of amoxicillin, the BMs will return to normal.

Home Care

The amoxicillin does not need to be discontinued. The diet does not need to be changed, unless you wish to cut back on foods like bran products, beans, and fresh fruits and vegetables. Yogurt restores healthy bacteria to the GI tract. If your child is over 12 months old, give 2 to 6 ounces of yogurt with active cultures twice a day.

Sometimes the diarrhea causes a diaper rash. Wash the irritated area with water and then protect the skin with a thick layer of petroleum jelly or other ointment. Call your child's physician if you feel the amoxicillin needs to be changed.

CONSTIPATION

Symptoms and Characteristics

- Painful passage of stools. The best sign of constipation is the occurrence of pain or discomfort with the passage of a bowel movement.
- Inability to pass stools. These children feel a desperate urge to have a BM, have discomfort in the anal area, but are unable to pass a BM after straining and pushing for more than 10 minutes.
- Infrequent movements. Going 3 or more days without a BM can be considered constipation, even though this may cause no pain in some patients and even be normal for a few. Exception: After the first month or so of life, many breast-fed babies have normal, large, soft BMs at infrequent intervals (up to 7 days can be normal). These infrequent normal stools are passed without pain or excessive straining.

Common Misconceptions in Defining Constipation—Large BMs or hard BMs unaccompanied by any pain or discomfort are usually normal variations. Some people normally have hard BMs each day without any pain. Children who eat large quantities of food normally pass large BMs. Babies less than 6 months of age commonly grunt, push, strain, draw up the legs, and become flushed in the face during passage of bowel movements. However, they don't cry. These behaviors are normal and should remind us that it takes some time for the bowels and rectum to become coordinated. Also, it is difficult to have a bowel movement while lying down. Help your straining baby by holding the knees against the chest to simulate squatting (the natural position for pushing out a BM). In fact, some straining with BMs is normal at any age.

Causes—Constipation is usually due to a diet deficient in fiber (found in fruits, vegetables, and whole-grain foods). Fiber is not digested and makes stools larger, softer, and easier to pass. Eating or drinking too many milk products also causes constipation. Another common cause is repeated postponement of the urge to go because of embarrassment about school toilets, public toilets, or long waiting times for the home bathroom. The memory of painful stools can make younger children hold back. If constipation begins during toilet training, the parent is usually applying too much pressure. (See the guideline on TOILET-TRAINING YOUR CHILD: THE BASICS, page 286.)

Expected Course—Constipation usually is easy to relieve with dietary changes. After your child is better, be sure to keep him or her on a high-fiber diet so that it doesn't happen again. On some occasions, the trauma to the anal canal causes an anal fissure (a small tear). This is confirmed by finding small amounts of bright-red blood on the toilet tissue or the stool surface. Anal fissures heal quickly, usually in 1 or 2 days.

Call Your Child's Physician

Immediately If
- Your child is in severe pain.
- Pain is constant *and* has persisted for more than 2 hours.

During Office Hours If
- Your child is less than 2 months old.
- Four or more days have passed without a BM.
- Your child is soiling (leaking BMs).
- You are giving suppositories or enemas.
- The anal area has any tears (fissures) that are deep or won't heal.
- Anal fissures have bled more than twice.
- Toilet training is in progress *and* there is any resistance (see page 290).
- Constipation is a recurrent problem for your child.
- You think your child needs to be seen.

Home Care

Diet Treatment for Babies Under 1 Year Old—For babies over 2 months old on only formula or breast milk, add fruit juices (like apple or pear) twice a day. Try prune juice as a next step. Switching to soy formula may also give looser stools. If your baby is over 4 months old, add baby foods with high fiber content—peas, beans, bananas, prunes, pears, plums, or cereal—twice a day. (Note: If necessary, strained peas or oatmeal cereal can be added to the formula of younger babies.) All strained fruits and vegetables are helpful for constipation (this includes strained apples and bananas). Corn syrup is not very helpful for constipation and the American Academy of Pediatrics is opposed to using it before 1 year of age.

Diet Treatment for Children Over 1 Year Old

- Increase fruits/vegetables. Have your child eat fruits and vegetables at least 3 times a day. Peas, beans, bananas, and apples are especially good because they are palatable and high in fiber. (Disregard the myth that bananas are constipating. High-fiber foods are beneficial for both constipation and diarrhea.) Other good choices are prunes, raisins, peaches, pears, apricots, cauliflower, broccoli, and cabbage. (Warning: Avoid any foods your child can't easily chew.)

- Increase bran. Bran is an excellent natural laxative, since it has high fiber content. Have your child eat bran daily in one of the "natural" cereals, bran flakes, bran muffins, shredded wheat, graham crackers, oatmeal, high-fiber cookies, brown rice, or whole-wheat bread. Popcorn is a high-fiber food for children over age 4.

- Decrease constipating foods. Cow's milk, ice cream, cheese, and yogurt are constipating and should be kept to moderate amounts (3 servings per day).

- Increase water. Be sure your child drinks plenty of water.

- Increase the amount of fruit juices your child drinks. The best ones are high in sorbitol (pear, prune, plum). Orange juice is not as helpful as others.

- A natural product that can be mixed with foods (such as orange juice or applesauce) is unprocessed (unmilled) bran, available in most health food stores. The starting dosage is ½ to 1 teaspoon twice daily, depending on age. Try this for one week and then as necessary.

Stool Softeners—If a change in diet doesn't relieve the constipation, give a stool softener with dinner every night for one week. Stool softeners are not habit-forming. They work 8 to 12 hours after they are taken. Examples of stool softeners that you can buy at your drugstore without a prescription are milk of magnesia, Metamucil, Citrucel, and mineral oil. Give ½ to 1 tablespoon daily.

Sitting on the Toilet—Encourage your child to establish a regular bowel pattern by sitting on the toilet for 10 minutes after meals, especially breakfast. Some children and adults repeatedly get blocked up if they don't look after this habit. If mornings are hurried at your house, try to get up earlier so your child has time to sit on the toilet. If your child is resisting toilet training by holding back, temporarily discontinue the training and put him back in diapers. For infants who hold back, they will often release the BM while sitting in warm bathwater.

Treatment for Anal Fissure—Streaks or flecks of blood noted on the surface of the stool or toilet tissue indicate that your child probably has an anal fissure. Anal fissures can be prevented with the diet changes already discussed and are treated with 20-minute sitz baths in warm salt water 3 times a day, followed by 1 percent hydrocortisone cream (no prescription needed). If the pain is severe, apply 2½ percent Xylocaine ointment (no prescription needed) 4 times a day for a few days to numb the area.

Common Mistakes—Don't use any suppositories or enemas without your physician's advice. These can cause irritation of the anus, resulting in pain and stool-holding. Do not use strong laxatives by mouth without consulting your physician, because they can cause cramps. Keep in mind that constipation will probably become a recurrent problem if the dietary changes aren't continued.

Relieving Rectal Pain—If your child has rectal pain needing immediate attention, one of the following will usually provide quick relief:

- Sitting in a warm bath to relax the muscle around the anus (anal sphincter)
- Giving your child a glycerin suppository (through the anus)
- Gently putting a lubricated thermometer or cotton-tipped applicator in the anus for 10 seconds to stimulate the rectal muscle

If your child is still having problems with constipation after trying the treatment guidelines above, talk to your health care provider about using an enema.

Call Your Child's Physician Later If
- Your child does not have a BM after 3 days on a nonconstipating diet.

• BMs continue to cause pain.

• Your child develops any of the "Call Your Child's Physician" symptoms.

Related Topic

STOOLS, BLOOD IN (See page 616)

DIARRHEA

Symptoms and Characteristics

Diarrhea is the sudden increase in the frequency and looseness of bowel movements. Mild diarrhea is the passage of a few loose or mushy stools. Moderate and severe diarrhea give many watery stools. The best indicator of the severity of the diarrhea is its frequency. Watery stools that occur hourly is definitely severe diarrhea. Keeping your child on nothing but clear fluids for more than 2 days also can cause green, watery BMs ("starvation stools").

The main complication of diarrhea is dehydration from excessive loss of body fluids. Symptoms are a dry mouth, the absence of tears, a reduction in urine production (e.g., none in 8 hours), and a darker, concentrated urine. The main goal of diarrhea treatment is to prevent dehydration.

Causes—Diarrhea is usually caused by a viral infection of the lining of the intestines (gastroenteritis). Occasionally it is caused by bacteria or parasites. Occasionally it's due to excessive fruit juices or to a food allergy. If only 1 or 2 loose stools are passed, the cause often turns out to be something unusual your child ate (indigestion). Remember that diarrhea is the body's way of purging itself of harmful organisms until it can build up immunity to them.

Normal Stools in Infants—Newborns have frequent BMs that can be mistaken for diarrhea. Breast-fed babies during the first 2 months pass from 4 stools per day to 1 after each feeding. The stools are normally liquid. Formula-fed babies pass 1 to 8 stools per day during the first week, then 1 to 4 per day until 2 months of age. After 2 months of age, most infants (regardless of type of feeding) pass 1 or 2 stools per day (or 1 every other day) and no longer appear to have diarrhea.

Expected Course—Viral diarrhea stools usually last from several days to 2 weeks, regardless of the type of treatment. Diarrhea is usually most severe on days 1 and 2. The main goal of therapy is to prevent dehydration by giving enough oral fluids to keep up with the fluids lost in the diarrhea. Don't expect a quick return to solid stools. Since 1 loose stool can mean nothing, don't start dietary changes until there have been at least 2.

Similar Condition—If your child has vomited more than twice, turn directly to the guideline on VOMITING, page 619. The treatment of vomiting takes priority over the treatment of diarrhea, until your child has gone 8 hours without vomiting. A good approach to vomiting is "1 swallow at a time every 5 minutes." (See instructions on page 621.)

Call Your Child's Physician

Immediately If
- Your child is less than 1 month old and definitely has diarrhea. (Caution: Normal stools of breast-fed infants can look like diarrhea—see page 603.)
- Your child has not urinated in more than 8 hours.
- Crying produces no tears.
- The inside of the mouth is dry rather than moist.
- Any blood appears in the diarrhea.
- Severe abdominal cramps are present.
- More than 8 diarrhea stools have occurred in the last 8 hours.
- The diarrhea is watery *and* your child also vomits clear fluids repeatedly.
- Your child feels dizzy with standing.
- Your child acts or looks very sick (e.g., loses interest in people and surroundings).

Within 24 Hours If
- The diarrhea has caused loss of bowel control in a toilet-trained child.
- Your child was exposed to someone with bacterial diarrhea (especially in foreign travel).
- Abdominal cramps come and go for more than 12 hours.
- A fever has been present for more than 72 hours.
- Your child is on any medicines that could cause diarrhea.
- You think your child needs to be seen.

During Office Hours If
- Mucus or pus is present in the stools.
- Diarrhea is a recurrent problem for your child.
- You have other questions or concerns.

Home Care

Dietary changes are the mainstay of home treatment for diarrhea. The optimal diet depends on your child's age and the severity of the diarrhea. There are 4 basic scenarios—go directly to the part that pertains to your child.

Special Diet for Diarrhea

1. Mild diarrhea in a child of any age
- Continue a regular diet with a few simple changes.
- Continue full-strength formula or milk.
- Avoid all fruit juices. They make diarrhea worse.
- Avoid raw fruits and vegetables, beans, spicy foods, and any other foods that cause loose stools.

2. Bottle-fed infants and frequent, watery diarrhea
- If your child has severe diarrhea, buy Pedialyte or Infalyte (oral glucose-electrolyte solutions) at your pharmacy or supermarket. (These special solutions are not needed for diarrhea unless it's severe.) Give as much of the special liquid as your baby wants (give at least 10 ml every hour for every pound your child weighs). Diarrhea makes children thirsty, and your job is to satisfy that thirst and prevent dehydration. Never restrict fluids when your child has diarrhea.

  Until you get one of these special solutions, continue giving your baby full-strength formula in unlimited amounts. Avoid giving your baby Jell-O/water mixtures or sports drinks because they have inadequate sodium content. Fruit juice will also make the diarrhea worse.

  If you aren't able to get an oral glucose-electrolyte solution, ask your doctor about making a homemade solution as follows: Mix ½ cup of dry infant rice cereal with 2 cups (16 oz) of water and ¼ level teaspoon of salt. Be very careful not to add too much salt (reason: risk of salt poisoning).

  Continue giving your baby Pedialyte or Infalyte for at least 4 to 6 hours. After that, switch back to formula if your baby becomes hungry, the diarrhea becomes less watery, and the child is making lots of urine.

Returning to Formula—After being given clear fluids for 4 to 6 hours, your baby will be hungry, so begin her regular formula. If the diarrhea continues to be severe, switch to a soy formula. If you give cow's-milk formula and the diarrhea doesn't improve after 3 days, change to a lactose-free formula (milk-based lactose-free or a soy formula). Often there is less diarrhea with soy formulas than with cow's milk formulas because the soy formulas don't contain milk sugar (lactose). If you need to start soy formula, plan to keep your baby on the soy formula until the diarrhea is gone for 3 days.

Continuing Solids—Foods that contain a lot of starch are more easily digested than other foods during diarrhea. If your baby is over 4 months old, continue her solid foods if she wants to eat them. Good choices are the following starchy foods: any cereal, mashed potatoes, applesauce, strained bananas, strained carrots, and other high-fiber foods.

3. Breast-fed infants with frequent, watery diarrhea

Definition of Diarrhea—No matter how it looks, the stool of the breast-fed infant must be considered normal unless it contains mucus or blood or develops a bad odor. In fact, breast-fed babies can normally pass some green stools or stools with a water ring around them. Frequency of movements is also not much help. As previously stated, during the first 2 or 3 months of life, the breast-fed baby may normally have as many stools as one after each feeding. The presence of something in the mother's diet that causes rapid passage should always be considered in these babies (e.g., coffee, cola, or teas). Diarrhea can be diagnosed if your baby's stools abruptly increase in number. Additional clues are if your baby feeds poorly, acts sick, or develops a fever.

Treatment—If your breast-fed baby has diarrhea, treatment is straightforward. Continue breast-feeding, but at more frequent intervals. Breast-feeding should never be discontinued because of diarrhea. If urine production is decreased, offer Infalyte or Pedialyte between breast-feedings for 4 to 6 hours. Breast-feeding may have to be temporarily discontinued if your baby requires intravenous fluids for severe diarrhea and dehydration. Pump your breasts to maintain milk flow until nursing can be restarted (usually within 12 hours).

4. Older Children (Over 1 Year Old) with Frequent, Watery Diarrhea

- The choice of solids is the key factor—starchy foods are absorbed best. Give cereals (especially rice cereal), oatmeal, bread, crackers, rice, noodles, mashed potatoes, carrots, applesauce, strained bananas, etc. Pretzels or saltine crackers can help meet your child's sodium needs. On the second day of diarrhea, soft-boiled eggs and yogurt are easy to digest and provide some protein.
- For fluids, use water (if solids are being consumed) or half-strength Gatorade. If your child refuses solids, give your child milk (or formula) rather than water.
- Avoid all fruit juices; they usually make diarrhea worse.
- Optional: Avoid milk for 2 or 3 days if it makes the diarrhea worse. (Reason: lactose is not as easily absorbed as complex carbohydrates.) Active culture yogurt is fine.
- Infalyte or Pedialyte is rarely needed, unless diarrhea is very watery and urine production is decreased.

Common Mistakes in Treating Diarrhea

- Using boiled skim milk or any concentrated solution can cause serious complications for babies with diarrhea, because these liquids contain too much salt.
- Kool-Aid, soda pop, or rice water should not be used as the only food because they contain little or no salt.
- Fruit juices (especially apple and grape) should be avoided because they are too concentrated and make the diarrhea worse. Using apple juice to treat diarrhea is the most common cause of "green squirts of diarrhea."
- By 24 hours at the latest, add formula or solids to the diet, because your baby needs more calories than clear fluids alone can provide. If not, he will become hungry and miserable and will lose weight. Keeping him only on clear fluids for more than 2 days can cause watery BMs ("starvation stools").
- The most dangerous myth is that the intestine should be "put to rest"; restricting fluids can cause dehydration.
- Keep in mind that there is no effective, safe drug for diarrhea and that extra water and diet therapy work best.

Diaper Rash from Diarrhea—The skin near your baby's anus can become "burned" from digestive enzymes and other chemicals found in the diarrhea stools. Wash the skin after each BM and then protect it with a thick layer of petroleum jelly or other protective ointment. This protective shield is especially needed during the night and during naps. Changing the diaper quickly after BMs also helps.

Overflow Diarrhea in a Child Not Toilet-Trained—For children in cloth diapers, diarrhea can be a mess. Despite treatment, loose stools usually continue for a week. Place a cotton washcloth or a 6-inch piece of cut-up towel inside the diaper to trap some of the more watery stool. Use disposable superabsorbable diapers temporarily to cut down on cleanup time. Use the ones with snug leg bands or cover the other type with a pair of plastic pants. Wash your child under running water in the bathtub. Someday your child will be toilet-trained.

Call Your Child's Physician Later If

- Any signs of dehydration occur (no urine in more than 8 hours, very dry mouth, no tears).
- The diarrhea does not improve after 48 hours on the special diet.
- Mild diarrhea lasts more than 2 weeks.
- You feel your child is getting worse.
- Your child develops any of the "Call Your Child's Physician" symptoms.

Prevention of Diarrhea

Diarrhea is very contagious. Hand-washing after diaper changing or using the toilet is crucial for keeping everyone in the family from getting diarrhea. Some of the more serious diarrhea caused by bacteria can be prevented if one takes precautions preparing poultry and ground beef, cleaning aquariums, and touching turtles or reptiles.

FOREIGN BODY, SWALLOWED

Symptoms and Characteristics

Most swallowed nonfood solid items are coins. Smaller coins (dimes or pennies) usually pass with ease. Larger coins (and rarely the smaller ones) can get hung up at a narrow segment of the esophagus. Dangerous objects are pointed ones such as nails, needles, and toothpicks.

Swallowed glass, on the other hand, usually passes harmlessly. A new threat to children are the button batteries found in watches, calculators, and cameras. These contain acid or alkali, which can erode the lining of the intestines.

Call Your Child's Physician

Immediately If

- Your child is choking or coughing severely (call 911). (Also, turn directly to the guideline on CHOKING, page 10.)
- There is difficulty breathing (call 911).
- There is any increased salivation, drooling, gagging, or difficulty swallowing (call 911).
- There is any discomfort in the throat or chest.
- Your child eats slowly and cautiously.
- There is any abdominal pain or vomiting.
- The object was sharp.
- The object was longer than 1 inch.
- The object was larger than a penny.
- The object was a small button battery.
- You're not sure what your child swallowed.
- The object could be poisonous.
- You think your child needs to be seen.

Within 24 Hours

In all other children who have probably swallowed a foreign body. The medical evaluation of this situation is somewhat controversial. Rarely, a foreign body can become stuck in the esophagus and yet not cause any symptoms. If the swallowed object was metal, a chest X-ray may be needed to be certain the foreign body has reached the stomach (even if the object is a small coin). Another approach is to obtain an X-ray if the object hasn't passed within 72 hours.

Home Care

Diagnostic Trial of Eating—If no symptoms (e.g., difficulty swallowing or pain in the throat) are present, give your child some water to drink. If this causes no symptoms such as gagging or pain, your child should eat some bread or other soft solid food. If this goes smoothly, the object is probably in the stomach. Swallowed foreign bodies almost always make it to the stomach, travel through the intestines, and are passed in a normal bowel movement in 2 or 3 days. There is nothing you can do to hurry it along.

Checking Bowel Movements—Normally, for small, smooth objects, bowel movements do not need to be checked. However, for sharp, long (larger than 1 inch), or valuable objects, the bowel movements should be collected by having your child wear a diaper or defecate on newspapers. Cut the BMs up with a knife or strain them through a piece of screen until the object is retrieved.

Call Your Child's Physician Later If

- The stools are being checked *and* the foreign body hasn't passed in 7 days.
- Abdominal pain, vomiting, or bloody stools develop in the next 2 weeks.

Prevention of Swallowed Foreign Bodies

Young children who put everything in their mouths must be protected from small objects they might inadvertently swallow. Check your floors periodically for coins, buttons, jewelry, small toys, pins, staples, and the like. Dispose of button batteries carefully. Avoid pierced earrings in children under 4 years of age. Store your sewing boxes up high.

GAS, EXCESSIVE

Symptoms and Characteristics

A normal but embarrassing part of the human condition is to pass bowel gas (flatus) on a daily basis. Most people also belch or burp up stomach gas occasionally. In fact, the average adult on a regular diet passes gas 10 to 20 times a day. This amounts to approximately 1 quart of gas per day. Gas should not be considered excessive unless it occurs at more than twice the normal frequency.

Causes—The main causes of normal gas are swallowed air, gas-producing foods, and certain diseases that interfere with sugar absorption. Every baby is somewhat "gassy" because of swallowing air during sucking. This process is increased by sucking on a clogged nipple, a nipple with too small an opening, a bottle that does not have milk in it, a pacifier, the thumb, or a blanket. Babies also swallow air during crying. Children at a later age swallow air with gum-chewing. Children with nasal allergies swallow air if they are "sniffers." Some children have a nervous habit of frequent swallowing. The carbonation in soft drinks releases gas in the stomach. Stomach gas is more likely to pass into the intestines if a child is lying down. Gas (unlike food) can pass through the gastrointestinal tract in 20 minutes.

Some foods (such as beans) are made up of complex carbohydrates that are not completely digested in the small bowel. These foods are converted into gas by bacteria in the large bowel. Eating lots of beans can increase gas production tenfold.

The most common medical condition that causes increased gas production is milk intolerance. The enzyme (lactase) that normally digests milk sugar (lactose) progressively decreases in amount between ages 4 and 20 years in large segments of our population. Those most affected people are Asians, blacks, and Eastern Europeans. The undigested lactose is converted into hydrogen by the bacteria in the large bowel. The amount of gas produced depends upon the amount of milk ingested. The main symptoms are bloating, abdominal cramps, diarrhea, and increased passage of gas.

Gas can be temporarily increased with bouts of infectious diarrhea. Gas can also build up behind constipation and be released in large amounts. Bowel gas is usually odorless. Bowel gas can develop an offensive odor during a bout of infectious diarrhea or in children on a high meat diet.

Call Your Child's Physician During Office Hours If

- You think your child has excessive gas and you don't know the cause.
- Your child is losing weight.
- You have other questions or concerns.

Home Care

In general, the passage of gas causes no symptoms. By age 5 or 6 most children can be taught to release gas in a quiet and socially acceptable manner. Gas does not need to be released by inserting anything in the rectum.

Air swallowing can be reduced by eliminating some of the previously mentioned habits (e.g., pacifier habit).

A reduced intake of beans and carbonated beverages will decrease gas production in all children.

If you feel your child has a milk intolerance (especially if your family history is positive), reduce milk intake to 2 glasses a day. Milk does not need to be completely eliminated in most people with lactose intolerance. The supplemental enzyme lactase (in drops or pill form) can also be taken with milk products. Yogurt is easily digested and can be continued. If you suspect milk intolerance and symptoms persist after dietary change, consult your child's physician about current recommendations for this disorder.

Related Topic

DIARRHEA (see page 603)

HICCUPS

Symptoms and Characteristics

Hiccups are strange gulping sounds made by involuntary, sudden contractions (spasms) of the diaphragm, which draws in a quick gasp of air against closed vocal cords. They may be uncomfortable in older children. They often accompany indigestion or an overly full stomach (from overeating) that presses against the diaphragm. Drinking excessive carbonated beverages (sodas) is a common cause of recurrent hiccups. In small infants, hiccups are normal.

Home Care

Treatment—Give 1 teaspoon of dry granulated sugar and have your child swallow it quickly. If this doesn't work the first time, repeat it 3 times at 2-minute intervals. Babies can be given a swallow of sugar water. Also, lying down usually helps, possibly because this position relaxes the abdominal wall.

If this doesn't work and your child is very uncomfortable, gag your child 1 or 2 times by pushing down the back of the tongue with the handle of a spoon or toothbrush. Other children are helped by rubbing the uvula or soft palate with a cotton swab, or by pulling the tongue outward with the fingers.

Call Your Child's Physician Later If
- The hiccups last more than 3 hours (the usual time needed to empty the stomach) and your child is uncomfortable.

NAUSEA

Symptoms and Characteristics

Nausea is an urge to vomit or a general uneasiness in the stomach. Nausea is often caused by a stomach virus and accompanied by vomiting. If so, turn directly to the guideline for VOMITING, page 619. Nausea can also be due to indigestion or fear. If nausea is your child's only symptom, it's rarely caused by anything serious.

Home Care

Treatment—Temporarily, serve your child clear fluids. Avoid medicines such as ibuprofen, which can irritate the stomach.

Call Your Child's Physician Later If
- New symptoms develop that worry you.
- Your teenager could be pregnant.
- The nausea lasts more than 1 week.

Related Topics

MOTION SICKNESS (see page 519)
VOMITING (see page 619)

PINWORMS

Symptoms and Characteristics

A pinworm is a white, very thin worm, about ¼ inch long, that moves. If it doesn't wiggle it's probably lint or a thread. Pinworms are usually seen in the anal and buttocks area, especially at night or early in the morning. Occasionally one is found on the surface of a bowel movement. They infect the anal area and large intestine. More than 10 percent of children have them. They do not cause any serious health problems, but they can cause considerable itching and irritation of the anal area and buttocks. Occasionally in girls, vaginal itching becomes a symptom. If the skin around the anus is red and tender, it is probably a strep infection, so call your child's physician during office hours.

Home Care When Pinworm Is Seen

Anti-pinworm Medicine—The drugs for killing pinworms all require a prescription. If you have definitely seen a pinworm, call your child's physician during office hours for a prescription. The following information may also help you.

Treatment of Other Family Members—Children are usually infected by children outside the family. If anyone else in your family has anal symptoms or anyone sleeps with your child, call your physician during office hours for instructions. Physicians do not agree on whether to treat everyone in the family or only those with symptoms. If any of your child's friends have similar symptoms, be sure to tell their parents to get them tested.

Call Your Child's Physician During Office Hours If

- The skin around the anus becomes red or tender (strep bacteria have a special affinity for this site).
- The anal itching is not resolved within a week after treatment.
- You have other questions or concerns.

Home Care for Suspicious Symptoms Without Pinworm Being Seen

Suspicious Symptoms—If your child has itching or irritation of the anal area, it could mean pinworms. Keep in mind that many children get itching here solely from washing their anal area too frequently or vigorously with soap. The anal area can also become red and sore from diarrhea or local strep infections.

Check your child for pinworms as follows: First, look for a ¼-inch white, threadlike worm that moves. Examine the area around the anus, using a flashlight. Do this a few hours after your child goes to bed and first thing in the morning for 2 consecutive nights. If no adult pinworm is seen, do a Scotch-tape test for pinworm eggs.

Instructions for Scotch-Tape Test—Pick up glass slides or a special pinworm lab packet at your physician's office (2 for each child) and mark your child's name on the slide. Touch a piece of clear Scotch tape (with the sticky side down) to the skin on both sides of the anus. Do this in the morning soon after your child has awakened, and definitely before any bath or shower. Do it 2 mornings in a row. Apply the piece of tape to the slide. If slides are unavailable, the transparent tape that has touched the skin can be applied to a second piece of tape. Bring the slides in for examination with a microscope. Your physician will call with the results. If pinworm eggs are seen, a medicine will be prescribed. (See PINWORM IS SEEN, on page 614, for details on home treatment.)

Home Care for Pinworm Exposure or Contact

If your child had recent contact with a child with pinworms but has no symptoms, your child probably won't get them. Pinworms are harmless and are never present very long without causing some anal itching. The swallowed egg will not mature into an adult pinworm for 3 to 4 weeks.

Prevention of Pinworms

Infection is caused by swallowing pinworm eggs. Your child can get pinworms no matter how carefully you keep the kids and your house clean. The following hygiene measures, however, can help to reduce the chances of reinfection of your child or new infections in other people. Pets don't carry pinworms.

- Have your child scrub hands and fingernails thoroughly before each meal and after each use of the toilet. Keep the fingernails cut short, because eggs can collect here. Thumbsucking and nail-biting should be discouraged.
- Don't eat food that has fallen on the floor.
- Vacuum or wet-mop your child's entire room once a week, because any eggs scattered on the floor are infectious for 1 to 2 weeks.
- Machine-washing at hot temperature will kill any eggs present in clothing or bedding.

STOOLS, BLOOD IN

Symptoms and Characteristics

Blood in the stools (bowel movements) is usually bright red. Rarely, blood comes out tar-black if it is from bleeding in the stomach. Swallowed blood also will look this way, so your child may have a tarry stool within 24 hours after a severe nosebleed.

Similar Condition—If your child has eaten anything red in the last 24 hours, turn first to the guideline for STOOLS, UNUSUAL COLOR OF, page 618. Most red stools are not due to blood.

Call Your Child's Physician

Immediately If

- Bright-red blood is mixed throughout the stool.
- There is a large amount of bright-red blood.
- The toilet water turns red.
- There has been a tar-black stool.
- Diarrhea is also present.
- Any blood has been vomited.
- A stomachache is also present.
- Your child faints or feels dizzy with standing.
- There are any skin bruises not caused by an injury.
- Your child acts or looks very sick.

During Office Hours If

- The cause of bleeding is unknown. If you suspect an anal fissure, however, see below. More than 90 percent of children with blood in their stools have an anal fissure as the cause.

Be sure to bring a sample of the blood in your child's stool with you to the physician's office for testing.

ANAL FISSURE

Symptoms and Characteristics

An anal fissure is a shallow tear or crack in the skin at the opening of the anus. More than 90 percent of children with blood in their stools have an anal fissure. Your child probably has an anal fissure if the following findings are present:

- The blood is bright red.
- The blood is only a few streaks or flecks.
- The blood is on the surface of the stool or on the toilet tissue after wiping.
- Your child passed a large or hard bowel movement just before the bleeding started.
- You may see a shallow tear at the opening of the anus when the buttocks are spread apart, usually at 6 or 12 o'clock. A tear cannot always be seen.
- Touching the tear causes mild pain.

If your child's symptoms are different, call your physician for help.

Cause—Trauma to the anal canal during constipation is the usual cause of anal fissures.

Expected Course—Bleeding from an anal fissure stops on its own in a few minutes.

Call Your Child's Physician

Within 24 Hours If

- The bleeding increases in amount.
- The bleeding occurs more than 2 times (especially if it's painless).
- You think your child needs to be seen.

Home Care

Warm Saline Baths—Give your child warm baths for 20 minutes, 3 times a day. Have him sit in a basin or tub of warm water with about 2 ounces of table salt or baking soda added. Don't use any soap on the irritated area. Then gently dry the anal area.

Ointments—If it seems irritated, you can apply 1 percent hydrocortisone ointment (nonprescription). If the pain is severe, apply 2½ percent Xylocaine ointment (no prescription needed) a few times to numb the area.

Diet—The most important aspect of treatment is to keep your child on a nonconstipating diet. Increase the intake of fiber with more fresh fruits and vegetables, beans, and bran products. Reduce the amount of milk products your child eats or drinks. Occasionally a stool softener (such as mineral oil) is needed temporarily.

Call Your Child's Physician Later If

- The anal fissure is not completely healed after 3 days of treatment.
- You feel your child is getting worse.

Related Topics

STOOLS, BLOOD IN (see page 616)
CONSTIPATION (see page 599)

STOOLS, UNUSUAL COLOR OF

Unusual colors of the stool (some color other than brown) are almost always due to food color or food additives. In children with diarrhea, the passage time is very rapid and stools often come out the same color as the Kool-Aid or Jell-O that went in. Stool color relates more to what is eaten than to any disease.

Unusual Stool Colors and Common Causes

- Red: blood, red Jell-O, red Kool-Aid, red cereals, tomato juice or soup, cranberries, beets, red medicines
- Black: blood from the stomach, iron supplements, bismuth (e.g., Pepto-Bismol), licorice, Oreo cookies, cigarette ashes, charcoal, grape juice
- Green: green Jell-O, iron supplements, spinach, diarrhea (due to rapid passage of normal bile), breast-feeding (especially during the first 2 months of life)
- Yellow-white: aluminum hydroxide (antacids), excessive milk, hepatitis

Call Your Child's Physician

- If stools are red without an explanation, see the guideline on STOOLS, BLOOD IN, page 616.
- If tar-black without an explanation, also see the guideline on STOOLS, BLOOD IN, page 616.
- For other unusual colors, eliminate the suspect food. If the color continues for more than 72 hours without an explanation, call your child's physician during office hours. Be prepared to bring a stool sample with you.

VOMITING

Symptoms and Characteristics

Vomiting (throwing up) is the forceful emptying of a large portion of the stomach's contents through the mouth. Nausea and abdominal discomfort usually precede each bout of vomiting. The mechanism is strong stomach contractions against a closed stomach outlet.

By contrast, reflux is the effortless spitting up of 1 or 2 mouthfuls of stomach contents, which is commonly seen in babies under 1 year of age.

Similar Conditions—If appropriate, turn directly to the following guidelines:

COUGH (when vomiting is strictly triggered by coughing spells) (see page 584)
MOTION SICKNESS (see page 519)
SPITTING UP (REFLUX) (see page 138)

Causes—Most vomiting is caused by a viral infection of the lining of the stomach (viral gastritis) or by food poisoning. Usually the viral type is associated with DIARRHEA (see page 603). Vomiting that persists for more than 24 hours as an isolated symptom without any diarrhea can have a serious cause. Vomiting is a protective mechanism to keep harmful substances out of the intestines.

Expected Course—The vomiting usually stops in 6 to 24 hours. Changes in the diet can prevent excessive vomiting and dehydration. If your child also has diarrhea, it will usually continue for many days.

Call Your Child's Physician

Immediately If

- Your child is difficult to awaken (call 911).
- Your child is confused or delirious.
- Your child is less than 1 month old (exception: reflux).
- Your child has not urinated in more than 8 hours.
- Crying produces no tears.
- The inside of the mouth is dry rather than moist.
- Any blood appears in the vomited material *and* it's not from a recent nosebleed.
- Abdominal pain has persisted for more than 2 hours.
- Your child's abdomen is very swollen.
- Your child has vomited clear fluids 3 or more times *and* has passed 3 or more diarrhea stools.
- The head was recently injured (with vomiting 2 or more times).
- The abdomen was recently injured.
- A foreign object could have been swallowed and caught in the esophagus.
- Your child acts or looks very sick (e.g., loses interest in people and surroundings).

Within 24 Hours If

- Your child has been vomiting for more than 12 hours if under 6 months old, 24 hours if 6 months to 2 years old, or 48 hours if over 2 years old.
- Your child is on any medicine that could cause vomiting.
- You think your child needs to be seen.

During Office Hours If

- Vomiting is a recurrent problem for your child.
- You have other questions or concerns.

Home Care for Vomiting

Special Diet for Bottle-Fed Infants (Less than 1 Year Old)

- Offer Infalyte or Pedialyte for 8 hours (no solids).
- For vomiting once, offer half-strength formula.
- For vomiting 2 or more times, offer Infalyte or Pedialyte.

- Give small amounts (1 teaspoon [5ml]) every 5 minutes by spoon or syringe.
- After 4 hours without vomiting, increase the amount.
- After 8 hours without vomiting, return to formula.
- For infants more than 4 months old, also return to cereal, strained bananas, etc.
- A normal diet can be restarted in 24 to 48 hours.

Special Diet for Breast-Fed Infants

- Reduce the amount per feeding.
- Provide breast milk in smaller amounts. Your goal is to avoid filling the stomach.
- If the child vomits twice, nurse on only 1 side every 1 to 2 hours.
- If the child vomits more than 2 times, nurse for 4 to 5 minutes every 30 to 60 minutes.
- If vomiting continues, switch to Pedialyte for 4 hours. Offer 1 teaspoon (5 ml) every 5 minutes by spoon or syringe.
- After 8 hours without vomiting, return to regular breast-feeding.

Special Diet for Older Children (More Than 1 Year Old)

- Offer clear fluids in small amounts for 8 hours (no solids).
- Water or ice chips are best for vomiting without diarrhea because water is directly absorbed across the stomach wall.
- Other options: half-strength flat lemon-lime soda or Popsicles. Stir soda until the fizz is gone because the bubbles can inflate the stomach.
- Give small amounts (1 tbsp [15 ml]) every 5 minutes.
- After 4 hours without vomiting, double the amount.
- For severe vomiting, rest the stomach completely for 1 hour, then start over with smaller amounts.
- For older children (more than 1 year old) add bland foods after 8 hours without vomiting.
- Stay on bland, starchy foods (any complex carbohydrates) for 24 hours. Start with saltine crackers, white bread, dry cereals, rice, mashed potatoes, etc.
- A normal diet can be resumed in 24 to 48 hours.

Sleep

Help your child go to sleep. Sleep often empties the stomach and relieves the need to vomit. Your child doesn't have to drink anything for a few hours if he feels nauseated, wants to sleep, and doesn't also have diarrhea.

Medicines—Discontinue all nonessential medicines for 8 hours. Oral medicines can irritate the stomach (especially ibuprofen) and make vomiting worse. If your child has a fever over 103°F, consider using acetaminophen suppositories (no prescription necessary). Call your physician if your child needs to be taking a prescription medicine such as an antibiotic.

Common Mistakes—A common error is to give as much clear fluid at one time as the child wants, rather than gradually increasing the amounts. This almost always leads to continued vomiting. Another error is to force the child to drink when he or she doesn't want anything.

Keep in mind that there is no effective drug for vomiting.

Various suppositories have caused serious reactions; in addition, they alleviate only vomiting related to anesthesia, poisoning, or motion sickness—but not the type caused by an irritated stomach lining. Diet therapy is the answer. Vomiting alone without diarrhea rarely causes dehydration.

Call Your Child's Physician Later If

- Your child develops watery diarrhea *and* repeatedly vomits clear fluids.
- The vomiting continues for more than 12 hours if your child is under 6 months old, 24 hours if between 6 and 24 months, or 48 hours if over 2 years.
- Any signs of dehydration occur (no urine in over 8 hours, very dry mouth, no tears).
- Your child develops any of the "Call Your Child's Physician" symptoms.

VOMITING OF BLOOD

Blood in the vomited material can be bright red or the dark-brown color of coffee grounds, if it has been acted on by stomach acid.

Call Your Child's Physician Immediately

- In every case.
- Exception: If your child swallowed blood from a cut in the mouth or a nosebleed in the preceding 4 to 6 hours, don't call. One episode of vomited blood under these circumstances is presumably due to swallowed blood and is unimportant.
- If you are asked to come in, bring a sample of the bloody material with you so it can be tested.

BLADDER (URINARY)

URINATION, PAIN WITH

Symptoms and Characteristics
- Discomfort with passing urine
- Burning or stinging with passing urine
- Urgency (can't wait) and frequency (passing small amounts) are occasionally associated.
- In children too young to talk, child begins to cry regularly when passing urine.

If your child's symptoms are different, call your physician for help.

Causes—The most common cause of mild pain or burning with urination in young girls is an irritation and redness of the vulva (vulvitis) and opening of the urethra (urethritis). The irritation is usually caused by bubble bath, shampoo, or soap that was left on the genital area. This soap urethritis occurs almost exclusively prior to puberty. At that age, the lining of the vulva is very thin and sensitive. Circumcised boys are also susceptible to urethral irritation from soap. Since 5 percent of young girls get urinary tract infections (UTIs), one must always consider this diagnosis. A UTI is a bacterial infection of the bladder (cystitis) and sometimes the kidneys (pyelonephritis).

Expected Course of Soap Urethritis—With warm-water soaks, the pain and burning usually clear in 12 hours.

Call Your Child's Physician

Immediately If
- The pain with urination is severe.

- Your child has a fever or chills.
- Any abdominal or back pain is present.
- Your child can't pass urine.
- The urine is bloody or cola-colored.
- Your child acts or looks very sick.

Within 24 Hours If

- There is any frequency, urgency, or straining with urination.
- There is a recent onset of day or night wetting.
- Your child is a male.
- Your child is female *and* she had previous urinary tract infections.
- She has any vaginal discharge.
- You think your child needs to be seen.

Home Care

Warm Baking Soda/Water Soaks—Have your child soak her bottom in a basin or bathtub of warm water for 20 minutes. Put 4 tablespoons of baking soda in the water. (Baking soda is much better than vinegar for young girls who have not entered puberty.) Be sure she spreads her legs and allows the water to cleanse the genital area. No soap should be used. Repeat this every 4 hours while she is awake for 1 day. This will remove any soap, concentrated urine, or other irritants from the genital area. It will also promote healing. With soaks the burning will usually clear in 24 hours. Thereafter, cleanse genital area once daily with warm water and without soap.

Avoid Soap, Shampoo, or Bubble Bath to the Vulva Area—See PREVENTION OF SOAP URETHRITIS IN YOUNG GIRLS for details (page 626).

Instructions for Collecting a Midstream, Clean-Catch Urine Specimen at Home—If you are told to bring a urine sample with you, try to collect the first one in the morning. Use a sterile jar. Wash off the genital area several times with cotton balls and warm water. Have your child then sit on the toilet seat with her legs spread widely so that the labia (skin folds of the vagina) don't touch. Have her start to urinate into the toilet, and then place the clean container directly in line with the urine stream. Remove it after you have collected a few ounces but before she stops. Catch urine from the middle of the stream, as the first or last drops that come out of the bladder may be contaminated with bacteria. Store the urine in the refrigerator until you take it to the physician's office. Bring it in on ice.

Call Your Child's Physician Later If
- The pain and burning continue more than 24 hours after a warm baking soda/water soak. (You will probably need to bring a urine specimen with you.)
- Your child develops any of the "Call Your Child's Physician" symptoms.

Prevention of Soap Urethritis in Young Girls
- Don't use bubble bath before puberty; it's extremely irritating.
- Don't put any soaps into the bath water. Don't let a bar of soap float around in the bathtub. If you are going to shampoo your child's hair, do this at the end of the bath.
- Wash the genital area with water, not soap. (The tissue inside the vaginal lips is very sensitive to soap.) If this washing causes any pain, you need to do it differently.
- Keep bath time less than 15 minutes. Have your child urinate immediately after baths.
- If this doesn't help, switch to showers.
- Teach your daughter to wipe herself correctly from front to back, especially after a bowel movement.
- Try not to let your child get constipated. (If she does, see the guideline for CONSTIPATION, page 599.)
- Encourage her to drink adequate fluids each day to keep the urine light-colored. This will increase the amount of urine she makes, and the extra urine "washes out" the kidneys and bladder.
- Encourage her to empty the bladder at least every 3 to 4 hours during the day and not to "hold back." (If she avoids public restrooms, help her overcome this reluctance.) If this doesn't help, have her empty her bladder every 2 hours.
- Have her wear loose cotton underpants. Polyester or nylon underpants, tights, and panty hose don't allow the skin to breathe. Discourage wearing underpants during the night.
- These precautions also reduce the frequency of bladder infections.

URINE, BLOOD IN

Symptoms and Characteristics

Blood in the urine can make it pink, red, brown, tea-, or cola-colored. There are some harmless causes for these colors—beets, for instance. Keep in mind that dark-yellow (amber) urine is usually due to being a little dehydrated from poor fluid intake, sweating, and/or fever.

If blood in the urine is suspected, your child needs to have the urine checked. Collect a specimen of the bloody urine in a clean container and keep it in the refrigerator until you go to your physician's office. If your child is in diapers, bring along the diaper with the pink or red spot on it.

Call Your Child's Physician

Immediately If

- A headache is present.
- The eyelids are puffy.
- Fever is present.
- The eyes or skin is yellow (jaundice).
- Your child is urinating much less than usual.
- Pain is present in the back or side.
- The back has recently been injured.
- Your child acts or looks very sick.

Within 24 Hours If

- All other children with suspected blood in the urine need medical consultation. If your child is a young male and the opening at the tip of the penis appears to have a crack in it that is bleeding, apply petrolatum while waiting.

URINE, STRONG ODOR

Symptoms and Characteristics

The urine has a pungent, often unpleasant odor of recent onset. The color of the urine is usually darker than normal at these times.

Similar Conditions—A dark-yellow urine may contain bilirubin; check the whites of the eyes for a yellow color (i.e., jaundice). Urinary tract infections cause a foul-smelling urine. Blood in the urine can cause pink, red, or cola-colored urine.

If one of the following is suspected, save time by turning directly to that guideline:

JAUNDICE (see page 497)
URINATION, PAIN WITH (see page 624)
URINE, BLOOD IN (see page 627)

Causes—Most strong-smelling urine is produced when your child is mildly dehydrated. Exercise, a fever, hot weather, or a hot room can lead to slight dehydration. Children in cloth diapers can acquire a strong odor of ammonia if the bacteria in the stool have time to break down the urine. Certain drugs (e.g., penicillin and amoxicillin) are excreted in the urine and cause an unusual odor. Certain foods (e.g., asparagus) or a high-protein diet can lead to strong-smelling urine.

Call Your Child's Physician During Office Hours If

- The unusual odor has been present since birth.
- The unusual odor lasts more than 24 hours without explanation.
- You have other questions or concerns.

Home Care

Increase your child's water intake during warm weather or fevers. Reduce your youngster's protein intake (remember that milk is largely a protein). Refer to the guideline on DIAPER RASH, page 133, if the odor is ammonia. By and large, most of these odors are not caused by anything harmful.

GENITALS

FOREIGN BODY IN VAGINA

Symptoms and Characteristics

During normal exploration of the body, young girls may put a foreign object in their vagina. Common ones are toilet tissue, a crayon, or a bead. The objects must be removed to prevent a vaginal infection. Often they are not discovered until after the girl is brought in for a bad-smelling vaginal discharge.

Prevention—The most common foreign body in young girls is toilet tissue. Teach your daughter to pat her vulva dry after going to the bathroom rather than rubbing it with tissue. Rubbing causes balls of tissue to break off and become lodged in the vagina.

Call Your Child's Physician

Immediately If

- The object was sharp.
- There is any bleeding.
- The object is causing any pain or discomfort.
- The object has been in the vagina for less than a day.
- You are concerned about sexual abuse.

Within 24 Hours If

All other children need medical consultation within 24 hours. In the meantime, leave the object alone lest it be pushed in farther.

MENSTRUAL CRAMPS (Dysmenorrhea)

Symptoms and Characteristics
- Cramps during the first 1 or 2 days of a period
- Pain in lower mid-abdomen
- Pain may radiate to the lower back or both thighs
- Associated symptoms of nausea, vomiting, diarrhea, or dizziness in some girls

If your child's symptoms are different, call your physician for help.

Cause—Menstrual cramps (dysmenorrhea) are experienced by more than 50 percent of girls and women during menstrual periods. Therefore, cramps are not abnormal. They are caused by strong contractions (even spasms) of the muscles in the womb (uterus) as it tries to expel menstrual blood. Menstrual periods usually are not painful during the first 1 to 2 years after menarche. However, once ovulation (the release of an egg from the ovary) begins, the level of progesterone and other hormones in the bloodstream increases and leads to stronger contractions and some cramps.

Expected Course—Cramps last 2 or 3 days and usually occur with each menstrual period. Current drugs usually can reduce the pain to a mild level. The cramps may be reduced after the first pregnancy and childbirth, probably due to the stretching of the opening of the womb (cervical os). Other women gain some improvement by age 25.

Call Your Child's Physician

Immediately If
- The pain is so bad that your daughter is unable to walk normally.
- She also has an unexplained fever.
- She acts or looks very sick.

During Office Hours If
- Any school is missed because of menstrual cramps.
- Vaginal discharge was also present before the period.
- Any pain occurs with urination or bowel movements.
- The pain is located on one side only.

- Any pain persists beyond the third day of flow.
- You think your child needs to be seen.

Home Care

Pain Relief—Ibuprofen is an excellent drug for menstrual cramps. It not only decreases the pain but also decreases contractions of the uterus. You do not need a prescription to get ibuprofen in 200 mg tablets.

The teen can take 2 tablets 4 times a day. Always give 3 tablets (600 mg) as the first dose if your teen weighs more than 100 pounds. Start the drug as soon as there is any menstrual flow, or even the day before, if possible. Don't wait until the menstrual cramps begin. Ibuprofen should make the child feel well enough not to miss anything important.

If you don't have ibuprofen, the child can take acetaminophen until you can get ibuprofen.

Heat—A heating pad or warm washcloth applied to the area of pain may be helpful. A 20-minute warm bath twice a day may also reduce the pain.

Aggravating Factors—If your daughter is tired or upset, the pain will feel more severe. Have her try to avoid getting exhausted or too little sleep during menstrual periods. If she has troubles or worries, encourage her to talk to someone about them.

Full Activity During Menstrual Cramps—Your daughter does not need to miss any school, work, or social activities because of menstrual cramps. If the pains are limiting her activities even though she is using ibuprofen, ask your child's physician about stronger prescription medication.

Common Mistakes—A common mistake is to go to bed when the cramps are bad. However, people who are busy usually notice their pain less. There are absolutely no restrictions on your child's activities. She can go to school, take gym, swim, take a shower or bath, wash her hair, go outside in bad weather, date, etc., during her menstrual periods.

Prevention of Toxic Shock Syndrome—Over 80 percent of cases of this life-threatening disease occur in girls during a menstrual period. Most cases occur in girls who use a tampon overnight. This condition can usually be prevented if tampons are changed every 3 to 4 hours during the day and external pads are used during sleep.

Call Your Child's Physician Later If

- Ibuprofen does not provide adequate pain relief. (Note: Talk with your teen's doctor about using naproxen for severe menstrual cramps.)
- The pain lasts more than 3 days.
- Your child develops any of the "Call Your Child's Physician" symptoms.

SWELLING, GROIN OR SCROTUM

Symptoms and Characteristics

This guideline covers a swelling, bulge, or lump in the scrotum or groin in males.

Similar Conditions—If one of the following is present, save time by turning directly to that guideline:

GENITAL TRAUMA (See page 71)
LYMPH NODES (OR GLANDS), SWOLLEN (See page 498)

Causes—A hydrocele is a painless collection of clear fluid above the testicle, present at birth. (See HOME CARE OF A HYDROCELE, below.) Unlike the other conditions, both sides are commonly involved.

An inguinal hernia may be diagnosed at birth or later.

A lymph node in the groin can swell up following a rash or infection of the leg on that side. While all the other conditions cause swelling of the scrotal sac, the enlarged node is found in the groin crease.

Two emergency conditions that begin with scrotal swelling and severe pain are torsion (rotation) of the testicle, and an infected testicle (orchitis). Don't assume it's just a pulled groin muscle.

Call Your Child's Physician

Immediately If

- The area is tender to the touch.
- The area is painful.
- The scrotum is swollen (exception: hydrocele diagnosed at birth).

Home Care of a Hydrocele

Hydroceles are present in about 10 percent of normal newborn males. If your child's physician has made this diagnosis, the following information may be helpful. A hydrocele is usually caused by the pressure on the abdomen during delivery, which pushes clear fluid downward through the channel that surrounds the spermatic cord and blood vessels to the testicle. A hydrocele may take 6 to 12 months to clear completely. It is harmless, but can be rechecked during regular visits.

If the swelling frequently changes in size (especially becoming larger with crying), a hernia may also be present, and you should call your physician during office hours for an appointment. If you suspect a hernia and it becomes stuck and causes crying, call your physician now.

VAGINAL IRRITATION OR ITCHING

Symptoms and Characteristics
- Genital area pain, burning, or itching
- No pain or burning with urination

If your child's symptoms are different, call your physician for help.

Similar Conditions—If pain accompanies urination, save time by turning directly to the guideline on URINATION, PAIN WITH, page 624.

If your child also has itching of the anus and buttocks, see the guideline on PINWORMS, page 613.

Causes—Most vaginal itching or discomfort is due to a soap irritation of the vulva or outer vagina. The usual irritants are bubble bath, shampoo, or soap left on the genital area. Occasionally it is due to poor hygiene. This soap vulvitis occurs almost exclusively prior to puberty. If the vagina becomes infected, a vaginal discharge will be noted.

Expected Course of Soap Vulvitis—It responds within 1 to 2 days with proper treatment.

Call Your Child's Physician
Immediately If
- An unexplained fever is present.
- There is severe abdominal pain.
- Sexual abuse could be the cause.

During Office Hours If

- There is any vaginal discharge.
- You think your child needs to be seen.

Home Care

Baking Soda/Warm Water Soaks—Have your daughter soak her bottom in a basin or bathtub of warm water for 20 minutes. Add 4 tablespoons of baking soda per tub of warm water. (Note: Baking soda is better than vinegar soaks for the younger age group.) Be sure she spreads her legs and allows the water to cleanse the genital area. No soap should be used. Help her dry herself completely afterward. Repeat this in 2 hours and again in 12 hours. This will remove any soap, concentrated urine, or other chemicals from the genital area. Thereafter, cleanse the genital area once a day with warm water on a washcloth.

Hydrocortisone Cream—Apply 1 percent hydrocortisone cream (no prescription needed) 2 times a day to the genital area for 2 or 3 days.

Call Your Child's Physician Later If

- The pain and itching are not cleared within 48 hours on treatment.
- Your child develops any of the "Call Your Child's Physician" symptoms.

Prevention of Soap Vulvitis

- Don't use bubble bath or put any other soaps into the bathwater. Don't let a bar of soap float around in the bathtub. If you are going to shampoo your child's hair, do this at the end of the bath.
- Wash the genital area with warm water, not soap. If this process causes any pain, you need to do it differently.
- Your child should wear cotton underpants. Polyester or nylon underpants, tights, and panty hose don't allow the skin to breathe. Discourage wearing underpants during the night.
- Teach your daughter to wipe herself correctly from front to back, especially after a bowel movement.

BONES, JOINTS, AND MUSCLES

BACKACHE, ACUTE

Symptoms and Characteristics

- Your child complains of back pain.
- Usually the mid- or lower back is involved.
- The pain is worsened by bending.
- The muscles on one side of the spine are tender and in spasm.
- Acute backache mainly occurs in adolescents.

Causes—Backaches are usually a symptom of a strain of some of the 200 muscles in the back that allow us to stand upright (i.e., a pulled muscle). Often the triggering event is carrying something too heavy, lifting from an awkward position, bending too far backward or sideways, or prolonged digging in the garden (overexertion of back muscles).

Expected Course—The pain and discomfort usually resolve in 1 to 2 weeks. Recurrences are common.

Call Your Child's Physician

Immediately If

- The pain is severe.
- Your child can't walk.
- The back pain shoots into the buttock or back of the thigh.
- Numbness occurs in the legs or feet.
- The backache followed an accident or injury.
- A fever is present.

- Passing urine causes pain or burning.
- The urine contains blood.
- Your child acts or looks very sick.

During Office Hours If
- Your child is under 5 years old.
- Your child doesn't walk normally.
- The pain interferes with sleep.
- The cause of the pain is unknown.
- Back pain is a recurrent problem for your child.
- You think your child needs to be seen.

Home Care

Pain-Relief Medicines—Give acetaminophen or ibuprofen (for dosage, see the tables on pages 238–40). Continue this until 24 hours have passed without any pain. This is the most important part of the therapy, because back pain causes muscle spasm, and these medicines can greatly reduce both the spasm and the pain.

Local Cold—During the first 2 days, massage the sore muscles with a cold pack or ice pack for 20 minutes 4 times per day. (Caution: Avoid frostbite.)

Local Heat—After 2 days, apply a heating pad or hot water bottle to the most painful area to relieve muscle spasm. Do this whenever the pain flares up. Don't allow your child to go to sleep on a heating pad, because it can cause burns.

Sleeping Position—The most comfortable sleeping position is usually on the side with a pillow between the knees. If your child sleeps on the back, it may help to place a pillow under the knees. Avoid sleeping on the abdomen. The mattress should be firm or reinforced with a board.

Activity—Complete bed rest is unnecessary. Have your child avoid lifting, jumping, horseback riding, motorcycle riding, and vigorous exercise until he or she is completely well.

Call Your Child's Physician Later If
- The pain is no better in 72 hours.
- The pain is still present after 2 weeks.
- You feel your child is getting worse.

Prevention of Backaches

The only way to prevent future backaches is to keep the back muscles in excellent physical condition. This will require 5 minutes of back and abdominal exercises per day, possibly for the rest of your child's life. Helpful strengthening exercises are sit-ups, 6-inch leg raises, flattening the back against the floor, and chest and leg lifts while on the abdomen. Also perform stretching exercises. The strengthening exercises should be avoided when your child is having active back pain, but the stretching exercises should be continued. Remind your child to lift objects with the leg muscles and not by bending or twisting the back.

LIMB PAIN

Symptoms and Characteristics

- Your child complains of pains in the arms or legs.
- Your child does not have a limp.
- The pain is not due to a known injury.

Similar Conditions—If appropriate, turn directly to the following guidelines:

LIMP (see page 638)
BONE, JOINT, AND MUSCLE TRAUMA (see page 663)

Causes—There are 2 main causes of mild limb pain. *Brief* pains (1 to 15 minutes) are usually due to muscle spasms or cramps. Foot or calf muscle cramps are especially common at night. Cramps become more frequent in children with poor calcium intake. *Continuous* acute pains (lasting hours to a day) are usually due to overstrenuous activities or forgotten muscle injuries. Both of these normal pains have been erroneously referred to as "growing pains" (although they have nothing to do with growth). Mild muscle aches also occur with many viral illnesses.

Call Your Child's Physician

Immediately If

- The limb pain is severe (e.g., causes constant crying).
- A joint is swollen.
- A joint can't be moved fully.
- Your child acts or looks very sick.

Within 24 Hours If
- A fever is present (especially if the pain is located at one site).
- You think your child needs to be seen.

During Office Hours If
- The pain interferes with sleep.
- Limb pain is a recurrent problem for your child.
- You have other questions.

Home Care

Treatment for Muscle Cramps—Muscle cramps in the feet or calf muscles occur in a third of children. During attacks, stretch the foot and toes upward as far as they will go to break the spasm. Massaging the painful muscle can also help.

Future attacks may be prevented by daily stretching exercises of the heel tendons (Achilles tendon). (Lean forward at the ankles with the knees straight.) A glass of water at bedtime may prevent some of these night cramps, as will adequate fluids during sports. Also be sure your child is consuming adequate calcium.

Treatment for Acute Strained Muscles—Massage the sore muscles with ice for 20 minutes several times on the first 2 days. Give acetaminophen, or ibuprofen for pain relief. (For dosage, see the tables on page 238–40.)

If stiffness persists after 48 hours, have your child relax in a hot bath for 20 minutes twice a day, and gently exercise the involved part underwater.

Call Your Child's Physician Later If
- The pain lasts more than 3 days on treatment.
- You feel your child is getting worse.
- Your child develops any of the "Call Your Child's Physician" symptoms.

LIMP

Symptoms and Characteristics

A limp is a painful type of walking (gait) in which the child tries to avoid putting much weight on one leg or hurries off it when walking. Some children flat-out refuse to stand or walk at all. Most of these children have limb pain but may be too young to express this in words. The most common cause of an unexplained limp in young children is a minor injury from jumping off furniture.

Call Your Child's Physician

Immediately If
- A severe limp followed a recent injury.
- Your child won't walk at all.
- A fever is present.
- A joint is swollen.
- A joint can't be moved fully.

During Office Hours If
- The limp has no obvious cause. (First consider a simple cause such as tight new shoes, a sliver in the foot, a plantar wart, or an intramuscular injection within the previous 24 hours.)
- A slight limp (due to an injury) lasts more than 72 hours (as with a pulled muscle, bruised bone, stubbed toe, or scraped knee).

NECK PAIN, ACUTE

Symptoms and Characteristics
- Your child complains of pain in the back of the neck or upper back.
- Pain in the front of the neck usually is due to a sore throat or swollen lymph node.
- The head is often cocked to one side.
- Often the neck muscles are tender to the touch.

Similar Condition—LYMPH NODES (OR GLANDS), SWOLLEN (see page 498)

Causes—Acute neck pain (wryneck) is usually caused by sleeping in an awkward posture, painting a ceiling, reading in bed, or prolonged typing.

Serious spinal cord injury can occur with diving accidents, trampoline accidents, or other accidents involving the neck. Children who have suffered such an accident should not be moved until a neck brace or spine board has been applied.

A stiff neck (in which your child can't bend forward and touch the chin to the chest) is an early symptom of meningitis. (Fever should also be present.)

Expected Course—A strained neck isn't serious and usually lasts 5 to 7 days.

Call Your Child's Physician

Immediately If

- The pain was caused by an injury. Call a rescue squad (911) and don't move your child.
- Numbness or tingling is present in the arms or upper back.
- The pain is severe.
- Your child cannot touch his chin to the center of his chest.
- A fever is present.
- Your child looks or acts very sick.

During Office Hours If

- Your child is under 5 years old.
- The pain interferes with sleep.
- Neck pain is a recurrent problem for your child.
- You think your child needs to be seen.

Home Care

Pain-Relief Medicines—Give acetaminophen or ibuprofen until your child has gone 24 hours without any pain. (For dosage, see the tables on pages 238–40.) This is the most important part of therapy, because neck pain causes muscle spasm, and these medicines can interrupt this cycle.

Local Cold—During the first 2 days, massage the sore muscles with a cold pack or ice pack for 20 minutes 4 times per day. (Caution: Avoid frostbite.)

Local Heat—After 2 days, apply a heating pad, hot water bottle, or hot shower spray to the most painful area to relieve muscle spasm. Do this whenever the pain flares up.

Sleeping Position—Instead of a pillow at night, your child may prefer a folded towel wrapped around the neck. This homemade collar will keep the head from moving too much during sleep. (A foam cervical collar with a Velcro closure can be obtained at a pharmacy.) Avoid sleeping on the abdomen.

Exercises—Your child should avoid any neck exercises until completely well.

Call Your Child's Physician Later If
- The pain is no better in 72 hours.
- The pain is still present after 1 week.
- You feel your child is getting worse.

Prevention of Neck Pain

If your child has had more than one neckache, usually the child has an activity or habit that overstresses the neck muscles or bones (cervical spine). Such activities are working with the neck turned or bent backward, carrying heavy objects on the head, carrying heavy objects with one arm (instead of both arms), standing on the head, contact sports, or even friendly wrestling. Avoid these triggers. Also improve the tone of the neck muscles with 2 or 3 minutes of gentle stretching exercises per day. Helpful neck exercises are touching the chin to each shoulder, touching the ear to the shoulder, and moving the head forward and backward. Don't apply any resistance during these stretching exercises.

VII. Glossary

A GLOSSARY OF CHILDREN'S DISEASES REQUIRING PHYSICIAN CONSULTATION

All of these conditions require a physician's input for diagnosis or treatment. Therefore, they are purposely not covered in this book. Your education on how to manage them should come from your child's physician and his or her associates.

If your child is born with or develops a chronic (long-term or lifetime) disease, to best serve your child you will need to learn almost as much about symptoms and treatment as your physician. To gain such a knowledge base, you can turn to local parent support groups or a national organization, as well as medical specialists. In many cases, a parents' handbook on your child's disease is available. The Internet also has much to offer. If your child is hospitalized, you have the right to ask the staff questions, and they will usually be able to schedule a meeting with you once a day for this purpose.

This chapter is divided into three parts: chronic diseases or conditions, severe acute illnesses usually requiring admission to the hospital, and acute illnesses usually treatable at home but requiring diagnosis by a physician or lab test.

CHRONIC DISEASES OR CONDITIONS

Acquired immune deficiency syndrome (AIDS): A life-threatening disease due to markedly reduced lymphocytes and immunity. Pediatric cases are rare except for the offspring of affected mothers or children who have required multiple transfusions (hemophiliacs, for instance). Currently 1 in 240 Americans is infected with HIV (the virus that causes AIDS). AIDS causes more deaths worldwide (3 million annually) than any other infectious disease.

Adrenogenital syndrome: An inherited disease present at birth in which the infant has accelerated sexual development and an inability to produce steroids. Females with this disease may resemble male newborns (ambiguous genitals).

Amblyopia: Decreased vision or blindness.

Anorexia nervosa: In adolescents, excessive weight loss (more than 20 percent below ideal weight) and denial of being underweight. Over 90 percent of those with this condition are female. Psychotherapy is essential.

Asthma: An abnormal condition of the lungs where the small airways (bronchioles) easily go into spasm and become narrow. The main symptoms are wheezing and a tight cough. The main triggers for asthma attacks are viral respiratory infections, exercise, inhaled allergens, and inhaled irritants. Occurs in 10 percent of children.

Astigmatism: Distorted vision due to variations in refractive power on different parts of the cornea.

Attention-deficit/hyperactivity disorder (ADHD): An inherited condition that causes poor attention span and difficulty completing tasks. Other symptoms are increased distractibility and poor impulse control. Occurs in 6 percent of children.

Biliary atresia: Blockage of the bile ducts at birth leading to severe liver damage. Sometimes treatable with surgery.

Bronchopulmonary dysplasia (BPD): Lung damage that occurs in some prematures who needed mechanical ventilation for survival. Portable oxygen administration may be needed over the first 1 or 2 years until lung improvement occurs.

Bulimia: In adolescents, periodic food binging followed by self-induced vomiting or laxative-induced diarrhea to prevent weight gain. The weight, however, is usually kept in the normal range. Psychotherapy is essential.

Cerebral palsy: A nonprogressive motor disability due to brain injury that usually occurs before birth. The most common type is spastic diplegia (weakness and tightness of both legs).

Chorea: Abnormal and unexpected muscle jerks. The location of the chorea can vary. Sydenham's chorea is a type seen following rheumatic fever.

Chronic fatigue syndrome: A disease with symptoms of extreme fatigue and sleepiness, muscle weakness, muscle and joint pain, confusion, memory loss, and eye pain lasting 6 months or longer. Most cases are due to a virus, but not infectious mono. Some cases are caused by depression or by Lyme disease.

Cleft lip and/or palate: The incomplete closure of the lip and/or roof of the mouth. Can occur in various combinations. A birth defect of unknown cause. Requires surgical repair and speech therapy.

Clubfoot: A fixed (inflexible) deformity of the foot (usually downward and inward) present at birth. Requires repeated casts or surgical correction.

Congenital heart disease: A birth defect of the heart that is usually not inherited. The defects are of many types. Surgery is frequently required.

Cow's-milk allergy: An allergy to cow's-milk protein resulting in the onset of diarrhea (often bloody) during the first 8 weeks of life. Responds to a non-cow's-milk formula. Occurs in 1 to 2 percent of newborns and resolves spontaneously by 1 year of age in most children.

Craniosynostosis: An early closure of the sutures (growth lines) of the skull. Surgery is required if multiple sutures are involved, and should be done before 6 months of age.

Cryptorchidism: An undescended testicle that remains in the abdomen. Needs to be surgically brought down into the scrotal sac by 1 year of age.

Cystic fibrosis: An inherited disease causing very thick mucus that blocks the lungs and pancreas. The main symptoms are recurrent pneumonia, diarrhea, and poor weight gain.

Diabetes insipidus: The inability to concentrate the urine, making the child predisposed to dehydration. Symptoms of increased drinking (polydipsia) and urination (polyuria). The causes are several.

Diabetes mellitus: The inability of the pancreas to produce insulin, leading to high blood sugar and sugar in the urine. The main symptoms are increased drinking and eating, excessive urination, and weight loss. The child needs daily insulin injections.

Down syndrome: Newborns with Down syndrome are mentally retarded, floppy, and have a characteristic facial appearance. They are commonly the offspring of older mothers. Caused by an extra chromosome (trisomy 21). Can be diagnosed during pregnancy by amniocentesis.

Epilepsy: A recurrent seizure disorder. The types and causes are many. In grand mal epilepsy the child falls and the entire body jerks for several minutes. In petit mal epilepsy (staring spells) a child loses consciousness and stops what he or she is doing for 5 to 15 seconds, but doesn't fall down.

Exercise-induced bronchospasm: Attacks, lasting 20 to 30 minutes, of coughing and wheezing after (but sometimes during) exercise. Running in cold air is the main offender. Occurs in 10 to 20 percent of people (90 percent of those with asthma). Prevented by taking an inhaled asthma medicine before exercise.

Fetal alcohol syndrome: Birth defects due to maternal alcohol intake in excess of 1 drink per day during pregnancy. The most common abnormalities are small eyes, a small head, low birth weight, and delayed development.

Fragile X syndrome: In males, an abnormal X chromosome. Accounts for 25 percent of mental retardation in males. Features include a long face, large jaw, large testes, and scars from hand-biting.

Galactosemia: An inherited enzyme defect that causes vomiting, diarrhea, liver damage, and mental retardation. Detection by newborn screening permits treatment with a galactose-free diet. Galactose is one of the sugars in milk.

Gastroesophageal reflux: The regurgitation or vomiting of food because the junction of the esophagus (food tube) and stomach doesn't close completely. The mild form is present in 50 percent of newborns and resolves by 1 year of age. The severe form can cause poor weight gain or vomited blood due to acid irritation of the end of the esophagus. This form requires special medicines.

Hemophilia: An inherited bleeding tendency due to the inability to produce certain clotting factors. Mainly occurs in males.

Hip, congenital dislocation: Being born with the hip out of the socket. A brace is needed for 3 months to correct the problem. Early diagnosis is important to prevent permanent damage.

Hydrocephalus: Blockage of spinal fluid flow out of the brain, resulting in a large head if not treated early. Treatment is a surgical shunt to drain the fluid to the abdomen.

Hydronephrosis: An enlarged kidney due to obstruction of its drainage system. More severe forms require surgical correction.

Hyperopia: Farsightedness. Close objects are difficult to see.

Hypertension: High blood pressure. The causes are many in children. In adolescents, the cause is usually genetic (i.e., essential hypertension).

Hypospadias: A birth defect in which the urethra opens onto the shaft of the penis rather than the end. Surgical correction is usually required.

Hypothyroidism: An underactive thyroid gland. When this condition occurs in newborns, it can cause very slow growth and development. Treated with thyroid medicine. Diagnosis before 6 weeks of age is important.

Inborn errors of metabolism: Genetic diseases that involve the absence of a particular enzyme the body requires. Examples are phenylketonuria and galactosemia.

Irritable colon of childhood: The most common cause of chronic diarrhea in infants. The loose, mushy stools do not interfere with normal weight gain. The cause is unknown but the condition spontaneously resolves at 2½ to 3 years of age.

Klinefelter's syndrome: In males, an extra X chromosome (i.e., XXY). Features include tall stature, borderline intelligence, breast development, small testes, and sterility.

Lactose intolerance: An inherited reduction in lactase, the enzyme needed to break down lactose in milk. Milk intake causes loose stools and gas. The condition usually has an onset at 5 to 10 years of age. Unlike milk protein allergy, lactose intolerance is not seen in infants.

Learning disabilities: Specific learning limitations (e.g., in mathematics or reading) in children of normal intelligence and motivation. Usually inherited. Illiteracy (the inability to read and write adequately to function in our society) is often due to untreated severe reading disability. Most schools have special programs to help these children.

Leukemia: A cancer of the white blood cells. The most common cancer of childhood. With modern treatment, over 80 percent of children in the United States are cured.

Malabsorption: An intestinal condition that interferes with the absorption of fat, protein, or sugar. Symptoms are severe diarrhea and weight loss. The causes are legion.

Mental retardation: An intelligence quotient (IQ) less than 70. Children with an IQ over 50 can often learn to function independently. The causes are many.

Microcephaly: Small head size due to below-average brain growth. Extremely small heads are associated with mental retardation.

Migraine headaches: A headache that is incapacitating, throbbing, and on one side of the head. Nausea and vomiting are often present. Over 70 percent have a family history of similar headaches.

Minimal brain dysfunction (MBD): In the 1960s, MBD was considered the main cause of attention deficit hyperactivity disorder, dyslexia, and other learning disabilities. Most physicians have discarded this simplistic, unfounded, and harmful label.

Muscular dystrophy: An inherited disease of progressive muscle weakness. Onset at age 2 to 6. Mainly occurs in males.

Myopia: Nearsightedness. Distant objects are difficult to see.

Neuroblastoma: A cancer of the nervous tissue, usually starting in the adrenal glands, located above the kidneys. It can also arise in the neck, chest, or spinal chord.

Neurofibromatosis: A dominant genetic disorder characterized by 5 or more coffee-colored spots and benign tumors of the nerve sheaths (neurofibromas) or nerves (neuromas). Nervous system complications can occur.

Orthostatic proteinuria: Increased amounts of protein are released into the urine when standing but not when lying down. A harmless condition usually found in adolescent males.

Osgood-Schlatter disease: A disease causing knee pain just below the kneecap on a small normal bump called the tibial tubercle. Occurs in adolescents and lasts 1½ to 2 years. No permanent harm.

Pectus excavatum: A pulled-in or sunken breastbone (sternum). The mild form is common and causes no symptoms. The severe form of this congenital defect rarely may interfere with heart function during exercise and requires surgery.

Peptic ulcer: An ulcer of the stomach or duodenum that causes upper abdominal pain, vomiting, or bleeding.

Phenylketonuria (PKU): An inherited enzyme defect that causes mental retardation, a light complexion, and seizures. Detection by newborn screening permits early treatment with a low-phenylalanine formula, followed by a restricted diet.

Polio: An infection of the spinal cord with serious complications like muscle paralysis and inability to breathe. The polio vaccine has eliminated polio from the United States, Europe, Latin America, and the Caribbean. The rates in Asia and Africa have been reduced.

Polydactyly: Extra fingers or toes present at birth. The extra digit is usually adjacent to the little finger or toe. Dominant type of inheritance, meaning that 50 percent of an affected person's offspring will have it as well. Surgical removal for cosmetic reasons is fairly simple.

Prematurity or preterm: Birth of a newborn prior to 37 weeks gestation. Usually weighs less than 2,500 grams (5½ pounds). Occurs in 7 percent of births. The smaller the baby, the higher the complication rate. Neonatal intensive care units have drastically improved survival rates and reduced complications.

Recurrent abdominal pains (RAP): Recurrent stomachaches occur in 10 percent of children. While the causes are legion, over 90 percent have a nonphysical basis (e.g., stress and worry).

Retrolental fibroplasia: Damage to the retina that occurs in the smallest premature infants (less than 1,500 grams) with high oxygen therapy requirements. The name comes from overgrowth of fibrous tissue behind the lens. The result is reduced vision or blindness.

Rett syndrome: A type of mental retardation that occurs only in girls. These children start out normal but lose intellectual and motor function between 6 and 18 months of age. The most characteristic symptom is repeated wringing of the hands.

Rheumatic fever: A rare complication of an untreated strep throat. The symptoms are migrating joint pains and fever. The heart is involved over half the time and can sustain permanent damage of the valves.

Rheumatoid arthritis: An arthritis that usually involves large joints on both sides of the body. Morning stiffness is common. Joint damage is occasionally seen.

Scoliosis: A sideways curving of the spine. Usually begins at age 10. Predominantly in girls. Screened for in most schools. Bracing is needed if the curve exceeds 20 degrees.

Serous otitis media: Fluid in the middle ear due to blocked eustachian tubes. A problem of young children, sometimes requiring the insertion of ventilation (tympanostomy) tubes for 1 or 2 years. Also called middle-ear effusion.

Sickle-cell anemia: An inherited type of anemia where the normally round red blood cells periodically become sickle-shaped and block off small blood vessels, causing severe pain. Also interferes with growth. Mainly occurs in blacks at a frequency of 1 in 500.

Sickle-cell trait: Children with sickle-cell trait carry 1 gene for sickle-cell anemia. It takes 2 genes to develop the disease. No symptoms of anemia. Present in 10 percent of healthy blacks.

Spina bifida: A birth defect of the spinal column and cord that causes paralysis below the level of involvement, as well as poor bladder-bowel control. Also called meningomyelocele. One of the preventable causes is low folic acid intake in pregnant women.

Strabismus: A birth defect of the eye muscles causing crossed eyes (i.e., inward or outward turning of 1 or both eyes). Usually requires surgery. More than 90 percent of children suspected of having this actually have pseudostrabismus due to a broad nasal bridge or folds of tissue (epicanthal folds) over the inner parts of the eye. These decrease the visible sclera (white part) on the inside of the eyes and give an optical illusion of turning in.

Tay-Sachs disease: An inherited disease in which the brain degenerates. Onset at 3 to 6 months of age. Findings are blindness, arrested development, and seizures. Mainly occurs in East European Jews.

Tourette's syndrome: Frequent facial muscle jerks (tics) present for over 1 year. Associated irrepressible sounds (such as grunting or profanity) are common. Onset at 2 to 6 years of age. Inherited in 50 percent of cases.

Turner's syndrome: In females, a missing X chromosome (i.e., X instead of XX). Features include short stature, abnormal ovaries, lack of sexual development, and infertility. The intelligence is normal.

Ulcerative colitis: Inflammation of the lining of the large bowel, which causes intermittent or continuous loose stools and cramps. Usually the stools contain mucus, pus, or blood.

Von Willebrand's disease: An inherited bleeding tendency due to problems with both platelets and clotting factor 8. Symptoms include severe nosebleeds, excessive menstrual flow, and increased bruising with trauma. Not as severe as hemophilia.

Wilson's disease: An inherited disease in which the liver can't excrete copper. The onset is after age 10, with jaundice, tremors, and deterioration in school performance.

ACUTE ILLNESSES USUALLY REQUIRING ADMISSION TO THE HOSPITAL

Apnea: An episode of cessation of breathing for 15 seconds or more, often associated with cyanosis (a bluish color of the lips). Apnea usually occurs in infants under 6 months of age. The causes are many and usually serious.

Appendicitis: A blockage and infection of the appendix. The appendix is a blind pouch the size of your little finger that comes off the cecum (first part of the large bowel). Appendicitis gives constant pain in the right lower abdomen and requires surgical intervention.

Botulism: The most serious type of food poisoning. First symptoms are double vision, slurred speech, and swallowing problems. The cause is a toxin produced by bacteria in improperly canned food. Contaminated food looks and tastes normal. During the first year of life, botulism germs can be acquired from swallowing dust or normal honey. Progressive weakness (of suck, cry, and neck muscles) and constipation are the main symptoms in these babies.

Cellulitis: A spreading bacterial infection of the skin, often following a wound infection.

Cerebellar ataxia, acute: The abrupt onset of an unsteady gait, shaky hands, and slurred speech. Due to a viral infection of the cerebellum (balance center of the brain). Resolves in 4 to 8 weeks.

Child abuse: The mistreatment of children by adult caretakers (less commonly by strangers). The two most common types are physical abuse (inflicted injuries) and sexual abuse.

Cholecystitis: An infection of the gall bladder, often occurring because the gall bladder is blocked by gallstones. Surgical intervention is usually necessary.

Conversion reaction: The sudden onset of a physical disability (e.g., paralysis or blindness) on an emotional basis. Commonly the youngster shows lack of concern (indifference) for the symptom. Also called a hysterical reaction. Requires psychotherapy.

Diphtheria: A serious bacterial infection of the throat with complications of suffocation, heart disease, and paralysis. Preventable with DTaP immunizations.

Diplopia: Double vision. Caused by drug reactions, botulism, eye muscle or brain disease.

Encephalitis: An infection of the brain caused by various viruses. Also called sleeping sickness.

Endocarditis: An infection of the valves and lining of the heart.

Epiglottitis: A life-threatening infection of the tissues above the vocal cords. The cause usually is the *Hemophilus influenzae* bacterium. The epiglottis is the flap of tissue that normally covers the opening of the windpipe during swallowing and keeps food and drink off the larynx.

Failure to thrive: A malnourished, underweight condition usually occurring during the first year of life. While the causes are many, in our country over half the cases are due to underfeeding (i.e., child neglect).

Guillain-Barré syndrome: An acute progressive symmetrical paralysis that starts in the feet and moves up the body over several days. Usually follows a viral infection. Some children develop respiratory paralysis and need to be placed on a ventilator temporarily.

Hematemesis: Vomiting up blood. The causes are many.

Hemolytic-uremic syndrome: A combination of anemia from red blood cell breakdown (hemolysis) and kidney failure. Often preceded by bloody diarrhea. Caused by a bacteria called *E. coli* O157 that is commonly found in undercooked hamburgers.

Hemoptysis: Coughing up blood. The causes are many.

Hemorrhagic disease of the newborn: A bleeding disorder that occurs on day 2 to day 7 of life. The bleeding usually occurs into the intestines, skin, or circumcision site. Due to vitamin K deficiency and preventable by routine vitamin K administration at birth. This problem is making a resurgence with home deliveries and breast-feeding.

Idiopathic thrombocytopenic purpura (ITP): The most common bleeding disorder of childhood. Due to a temporary depletion of platelets (which are needed for clotting) following various viral infections.

Intussusception: Obstruction of the bowel due to a telescoping of one segment of intestine into an adjacent one. Cases diagnosed early may become unstuck with a barium enema, but some require surgery. Usually occurs in children less than 2 years old.

Kawasaki disease: A disease of young children characterized by a red rash, red eyes, red mouth, enlarged nodes, and a fever lasting over 5 days. The cause is unknown. Over 20 percent of the children who get it develop heart disease. Early treatment with intravenous immune globulin can prevent some coronary artery disease. Also called mucocutaneous lymph node syndrome.

Malaria: A parasite transmitted by mosquitoes. The main symptom is 3- to 6-hour bouts of fever and shaking chills every 2 or 3 days. Also causes anemia, convulsions, and coma. Affects over 300 million people worldwide and kills over 1 million annually. Tropical Africa suffers 90 percent of the cases. Sleeping under an insecticide-treated mosquito net is the most effective method to prevent malaria. Could be eradicated if adequate funds were provided. (Note: Doesn't occur in the United States.)

Mastoiditis: A bacterial infection of the air cells in the bone behind the ear. A complication of an untreated ear infection. Often requires surgery.

Melena: The passage of tar-colored blood in the stool. Blood darkens only if it comes from the stomach or upper intestines.

Meningitis: An infection of the meninges or thin membranes surrounding the brain and spinal cord. Most serious cases are caused by bacteria. Called aseptic meningitis when due to a virus.

Nephritis: Kidney disease where blood is passed in the urine. The causes are many, but strep throat is one of the more common forerunners. Can become chronic.

Nephrosis: Kidney disease where protein is passed in the urine, leading to swelling (edema) of the face and feet. Often becomes chronic.

Omphalitis: An infection of the navel or belly button. Can be serious in the first month of life.

Osteomyelitis: A bacterial infection of bone.

Papilledema: Swelling of the optic disc in the back of the eye. Reflects increased pressure inside the head. Various causes, usually serious.

Pelvic inflammatory disease (PID): A bacterial infection of the Fallopian tubes—often due to gonorrhea or chlamydia. Also called salpingitis.

Pericarditis: An infection of the sac that covers the heart.

Peritonitis: An infection of the lining of the abdomen. Usually caused by a ruptured appendix.

Pertussis: A serious bacterial infection of the windpipe and lungs. Also called whooping cough because coughing spasms often end with a high-pitched whoop. Preventable with DTaP immunizations.

Pneumothorax: A blowout of the lung leading to the escape of air into the space between the lung and the chest wall. Symptoms are chest pain and difficulty breathing.

Pulmonary embolism: A blood clot carried through the bloodstream to the lungs. Causes severe chest pain and difficulty breathing.

Pyloric stenosis: An obstruction of the stomach outlet occurring in the first 3 to 8 weeks of life. Causes projectile vomiting and requires surgery.

Reye's syndrome: Abrupt swelling of the brain, presenting with confusion, sleepiness, and persistent vomiting. Liver destruction also occurs. Although the cause is unknown, it sometimes follows chicken pox or influenza, especially when they are treated with aspirin. The disease is now very rare, following the abandonment of aspirin therapy for fever in children and teens.

Rocky Mountain spotted fever: A life-threatening disease caused by a rickettsia that is carried by ticks. The symptoms include a purple-red rash of the extremities, fever, headache, and delirium. It responds to antibiotics.

Scalded skin syndrome: A bright-red, painful rash in which the skin peels off in sheets like a burn. The rash is caused by a toxin released by staph bacteria, often residing in the nose. The outcome is good.

Septicemia: A bacterial infection of the bloodstream in which the bacteria are actually multiplying there. Also called sepsis.

Subdural hematoma: A blood clot on the surface of the brain, usually due to direct trauma. Violently shaking a child by the shoulders so the head is snapped forward and back can also cause this life-threatening condition.

Sudden infant death syndrome (SIDS): The sudden unexplained death of a healthy infant under 12 months of age during sleep. The incidence is 1.4 per 1,000 live births. The peak age is 2 to 4 months. Sleeping on the back has reduced the SIDS rate by 40 percent. The cause of the remaining cases is unknown.

Testicular torsion: An unexplained twisting of a testicle that shuts off its blood supply and requires emergency surgical release. Presents with testicular pain and scrotal swelling.

Tetanus: A serious bacterial wound infection that progresses from local muscle spasms to total body rigidity and seizures. Preventable by DTaP immunizations and tetanus boosters.

Thrombophlebitis: An infection of the lining of a vein, often the deep veins of the calf muscles.

Tonsillar abscess: An abscess deep within the tonsil that causes a severe sore throat, muffled voice, inability to open the mouth fully, and drooling. Requires surgical drainage.

Toxic shock syndrome: Symptoms include shock, fever, diarrhea, and a bright-pink (scarlet-fever-like) rash. Caused by a toxin produced by a hidden staph infection. One common source of staph overgrowth is a tampon left in the vagina overnight.

Typhoid fever: A severe form of bacterial diarrhea (often bloody) that can lead to a bloodstream infection or intestinal complications. Treatable with antibiotics.

ACUTE ILLNESSES USUALLY TREATABLE AT HOME BUT REQUIRING A PHYSICIAN FOR DIAGNOSIS

Amenorrhea: The absence of menstrual periods. When regular periods stop, the most common causes are dieting, stress, or pregnancy.

Anaphylactoid purpura: A disease consisting of unexplained rash of the buttocks, hands, and feet (100 percent), joint pains (70 percent), abdominal pain (30 percent), and blood in the urine (50 percent). The cause is unknown. Also called Henoch-Schonlein purpura.

Anemia: A low red blood cell count. While the causes are many, iron deficiency ranks first. A blood sample is needed to diagnose anemia.

Arthritis: Inflammation of a joint leading to pain, swelling, and limited motion. The causes are many.

Ascaris: A roundworm that causes intestinal infections. The main symptom is abdominal pain. In our country, mainly occurs in the Southeast.

Bell's palsy: An abrupt onset of weakness of the facial muscles on one side. Often associated with an ear infection, in which the seventh (facial) nerve is damaged while traveling through the infected area. Usually clears in 1 to 4 weeks. Early treatment with steroids may be helpful.

Bronchiolitis: An infection of the bronchioles (small air passages) occurring in the first 2 years of life. The main symptoms are wheezing, rapid breathing, cough, runny nose, and fever. Caused by the respiratory syncytial virus.

Cat scratch fever: A swollen lymph node caused by the scratch of a young cat. Usually lasts several months. A bacterium called *Bartonella henselae* has been identified as the infectious agent.

Chlamydia: A germ that causes urethral or vaginal infections. Spread by sexual contact. Can also cause eye infections or pneumonia in newborns by contact at birth.

Chondromalacia of the patella: A roughening of the underside of the kneecap causing knee pain in adolescents. Often due to excessive deep knee bends or running upstairs. Helped by rest and quadriceps-strengthening exercises.

Cold panniculitis: A lump of frozen fat tissue. Usually occurs in the fatty cheeks of infants less than 1 year of age. Due to prolonged contact with ice, Popsicles, cold metal, or cold weather. The lump can last 2 weeks, and occasionally the overlying skin turns red.

Creeping eruption: A localized itchy rash consisting of a wavy red line. Caused by a tunneling young hookworm, from skin contact with dog or cat excrement. Common along the Atlantic coast. Lasts 1 to 2 months without treatment.

Ganglion: A cyst (smooth circular swelling filled with thick fluid) usually occurring on the back of the wrist. These outpouchings of the joint capsule probably result from trauma. Most eventually disappear. Surgery is necessary only if they become very large or painful.

Giardia: A small parasite that causes diarrhea. Without treatment, the diarrhea can last for months.

Goiter: An enlarged thyroid gland, found in the front of the neck. The causes are many.

Gonorrhea: A bacterium that can cause genital infections. Spread by sexual contact. Eye infections of newborns are usually prevented by routine application of silver nitrate or antibiotic eyedrops.

Granuloma annulare: Rings of little bumps, usually found at the ankle. The overlying skin looks normal. The cause is unknown. Clears spontaneously in 2 years.

Gynecomastia: The development of breast tissue in a boy. Usually mild (just breast buds) and a temporary normal condition of 14- to 16-year-old boys. Can be caused by an endocrine problem. Not to be confused with fat deposits in this area, commonly seen in overweight boys.

Heart murmur: A swishing noise heard over the heart. Due to turbulence in blood flow as it goes through the heart. While a murmur can be caused by heart disease, 99 percent are normal sounds (innocent or functional heart murmurs). Your physician can tell the difference. More than 50 percent of normal children have innocent murmurs.

Hematuria: Blood in the urine. The causes are many.

Hepatitis: A viral infection of the liver leading to jaundice (yellow eyes and skin), light-colored bowel movements, and dark-colored urine.

Hernia, inguinal: A bulging in the groin due to a hole in the abdominal wall. Requires surgery.

Herpes stomatitis: A viral infection causing multiple small, painful ulcers of the gums and lining of the mouth. Associated fever. Usually occurs in young children and doesn't recur (unlike fever blisters).

Hot tub folliculitis: Bumpy, pink rash of the trunk occurring within 3 days of being in a spa that has an inadequate sanitizer level (bromine or chlorine). Caused by superficial infection of hair follicles by pseudomonas bacteria. Resolves in 1 to 2 weeks without treatment.

Hyperventilation: Rapid, deep-breathing attacks due to fear or anxiety. The symptoms include a sensation of smothering, dizziness, and tingling of the mouth and fingers. Occasionally proceeds to fainting. Quickly relieved by breathing into a paper bag or deliberately slowing down to 1 breath every 5 seconds.

Hypoglycemia: Low blood sugar with symptoms of hunger, headache, trembling, and sweating. May proceed to convulsions. Commonly overdiagnosed in our country.

Infectious mononucleosis: A viral infection with fever, sore throat, swollen lymph nodes, and an enlarged spleen. Symptoms last 1 to 4 weeks.

Keloids: Overgrowth of scar tissue at sites of surgery or trauma. Some people have a tendency to produce raised scars. Plastic surgery can help.

Kyphosis: An exaggerated posterior curvature of the upper back and shoulders. Usually normal.

Labial adhesions: A fusion of the 2 labia minora by a thin membrane. Caused by irritation of the labia from soaps or a mild infection, followed by healing together. The vaginal opening becomes partially or completely covered over, but the girl is still able to pee. Once adhesions have started, the labia are not easy to keep separated. Fortunately, the labia separate spontaneously with the onset of puberty and stay that way.

Lordosis: An exaggerated anterior curvature of the spine at the lower back. Usually normal.

Menorrhagia: Excessive or prolonged menstrual periods, often leading to anemia.

Mittelschmerz: Sharp lower abdominal pain on one side that occurs in menstruating girls and women midway through their cycle. Lasts 1 to 2 days. Caused by a small amount of blood or fluid contacting the abdominal lining when the egg is released from the ovary.

Molluscum contagiosum: Small ⅛-inch, skin-colored, waxy-looking bumps with indentations in the center. They contain a hard core. Caused by a virus and last 1 to 2 years, as with warts.

Pityriasis rosea: A rash of the chest, abdomen, and back characterized by matching oval-shaped red spots on both sides of the body. Lasts 4 to 8 weeks. Often preceded by a large scaly patch (herald patch) that resembles ringworm. Harmless and not contagious.

Pneumonia: An infection of the lungs. Generally not contagious.

Popliteal cyst: A smooth, firm swelling behind the knee. Over 75 percent disappear spontaneously in 1 to 2 years. Also called Baker's cyst. Surgery unnecessary unless it becomes painful or very large.

Pyelonephritis: A kidney infection.

Scabies: A very itchy skin rash consisting of small red bumps, pimples, and tunnels. Caused by a mite (small insect) that burrows under the skin to lay eggs. Very contagious.

Sexually transmitted diseases: Infections of the male and female genital tracts. Also called venereal diseases. Chlamydia has passed gonorrhea as the most common organism.

Shigella: A bacterium that causes severe diarrhea, often bloody. Treatable with antibiotics.

Spider nevus: A blood-vessel abnormality of the skin which looks like a spider. When the red spot in the center is pressed with a pen, all the small radiating blood vessels or spokes disappear. Occurs normally from age 6 to 12 in 50 percent of children. Clears spontaneously with puberty. Rarely associated with liver disease.

Strawberry hemangioma: A raised bright-red benign tumor that begins in the first month, grows rapidly during the first year, then slowly shrinks down until it disappears at ages 5 to 10. Surgery is almost always unnecessary.

Strep throat: A throat infection caused by streptococcus bacteria. Requires a throat culture or rapid strep test for diagnosis. Responds to oral antibiotics.

Striae: Stretch marks on the skin occurring in areas of rapid weight gain (e.g., the thighs), rapid muscle expansion (e.g., the shoulders of weight lifters), or on the abdomen during pregnancy. Usually temporary.

Subluxation of the radial head: A partial dislocation of one of the bones of the forearm (the radius) at the elbow. Due to being suddenly lifted or pulled by the hand. An infant with this injury will not use the arm and keeps the hand turned down. Easily remedied by your child's physician.

Swimmer's itch: A widespread itchy, bumpy red rash caused by a snail parasite (schistosome) that penetrates the human skin by mistake. While the parasite quickly dies, it causes a reaction for 1 to 2 weeks. Onset following exposure in freshwater lakes. Partially prevented by toweling off immediately on emerging from the water.

Trench mouth: A bacterial infection causing red, swollen, ulcerated gums and bad breath. Responds to dental hygiene and antibiotics. Not contagious.

Trichinosis: A disease due to a small roundworm sometimes found in pork. Transmitted by undercooking the meat. The symptoms of fever, swollen face, and muscle pain begin 1 week later.

Trichomonas: An amoeba-like organism that can cause vaginal infections and discharge.

Tuberculosis (TB): A bacterial disease of the lungs that can go on for years if not treated. Symptoms include cough, fever, and weight loss. Becoming more frequent in the United States due to increased numbers of HIV-positive people, homeless people, and immigrants.

Urethritis: An infection of the urethra, or tube that drains urine from the bladder to the body's surface.

Urinary tract infection (UTI): An infection of the bladder (cystitis) or kidneys (pyelonephritis).

Vaginitis: An infection of the vagina. At least 6 causes, but not always sexually transmitted (e.g., monilial vaginitis).

Vitiligo: A patchy loss of skin pigment giving milk-white splotches of skin. Inherited as a dominant trait. While occurring in all races, it is a major cosmetic stress for dark-skinned people. Current treatment gives unsatisfactory improvement.

INDEX

National Association for Sick Child
Daycare, 412
National Education Association, 318
National Poison Control Center, 3–4, 49,
55, 58
Nausea, 26, 242, 379, 613. *See also* Motion
sickness
Neck: acute pain in, 639–41; and
appearance of infants, 110; boils on,
473; and infant skin care and bathing,
111; injuries to, 4, 6, 8, 41, 47, 64;
pain in, 73; stiff, 8, 43, 46, 250, 429,
447
Needham, G. R., 24
Neurologic diseases, 225
Newborns. *See* Infants
Night terrors, 278–80. *See also*
Nightmares; Sleepwalking
Nightmares, 263, 275, 277–78, 401
Nipples: and formula-feeding, 159; size of
hole in, 202; sore, 152–53, 156;
supply of, 119; and thrush, 142
Nose: and appearance of infants, 104,
110–11; bleeding from, 77, 559–61;
foreign body in, 555–56; home
care for, 77; and infections, 77,
221–22, 223; runny, 381, 412,
454, 458, 552; stuffy or blocked,
552–53, 593; trauma to, 77. *See also*
Colds
Nudity, 373, 402
Nystatin, 142

Obesity, 165, 178, 183, 190, 203. *See also*
Weight
Oral temperature, 434, 435–36
Osteoporosis, 178–79, 180, 181
Over-the-counter drugs: aspirin as
dangerous, 57; in home medicine
chest, 248–50; iron as dangerous,
57; overuse of, 240, 241, 243;
refusal to take, 246; side effects of,
241, 242

Pacifiers: benefits of, 367–68; bottles or
breasts as, 161, 163, 193, 258–59,
264; and colic, 255; and
discontinuing breast- and bottle-
feeding, 166, 167; excessive use of,
368; and gas, 610, 611; and going to
doctor's office, 356; and injury
prevention, 215; introduction of,
367; and overeating, 202; purpose of,
121; and safety, 369; and sleep, 258,
266, 270, 368–69; and spitting up,
139; stopping use of, 369; and
thrush, 142; and thumbsucking, 366,
367–68; types of, 121, 143, 367; and
weaning, 163–64; when to offer, 368
Pain: and emergency symptoms, 7; and
non-life-threatening emergencies, 5;
treatment for, 76, 500, 533, 541,
546, 563, 571, 579. *See also type of
pain or specific disorder*
Pale skin, 501
Paralysis, 27, 28
Parents: and crying babies, 256; guilt of,
328, 330, 346, 357, 408, 414, 415;
periodic breaks for, 387; rights of,
331, 356; single, 415–16; skills of,
95–96; sleeping in bed with, 259,
264, 268, 269, 271, 272, 274,
275–77, 414, 416
Parents Anonymous, 320
Peers: misbehavior toward, 350–52; and
nail-biting, 405; and school phobia,
382; tutoring by, 393
Penis, 71, 106, 114, 134. *See also*
Circumcision; Foreskin
Permethrin, 22, 25
Pertussis, 225. *See also* Whooping cough
Pets, 16–18, 224, 352–53, 413, 485
Phenobarbital, 257
Phenylketonuria, 96
Phlegm: yellow, 242, 243
Phototherapy, 136
Picky eaters, 175–78, 183

Time-outs: and age, 320, 323; benefits of, 320; as boring, 325; choosing place for, 321; coming out early from, 326; delivering of, 316; as discipline technique, 310, 312, 319, 320–27, 348–62; effectiveness of, 320; escaping from, 325, 327; how to administer, 321–22; and hurting other children, 342; keeping child in, 323; length of, 321–22, 325; as not working, 324–26; and positive reinforcement, 317; practicing, 324; refusing to stay in, 323, 327; releasing child from, 322; temporary, 314. *See also specific type of misbehavior*

Tinactin, 472, 479

Tinea versicolor, 487–88

TLC (tender loving care): and breath-holding, 371; and colic, 254–55; and crying, 257; and discipline, 317, 324; and masturbation, 375; and pacifiers, 368; and red or pinkeye, 528; and sleep problems, 258, 260, 262, 264, 266, 267, 278; and spoiled children, 328; and temper tantrums, 334, 336

Toddlers: and sleep problems, 261–63; stubbornness of, 331–33; and suffocation, 59

Toes, 68–71, 107, 508–9

Tofranil, 57

Toilet-training: accidents during, 288–89; and bare-bottom technique, 289; and child care, 292; and clothes, 292, 298; and constipation, 298–99; and daytime wetting/urination, 290–99; definition of, 286; and diapers, 292, 297; and discipline, 312, 360–61; discipline concerning, 289, 290, 292; and encopresis, 290–99; incentives concerning, 203, 288, 289, 291–94; 297; inertial, 289–90; and introduction of underpants, 289; method for, 288–89; and potty

chairs, 287, 290, 292, 297; and power struggle, 295, 296; problems with, 286–308; and readiness, 286; and reminders, 296; resistance to, 290–93; and responsibility of child, 291, 295–96; and sex education, 373. *See also* Bedwetting; Bowel movements; Encopresis

Toilets: and preventing infections, 223

Tongue, 75, 76, 141, 444, 457, 568–69

Tongue-tie, 105, 575

Tonsils, 75–76, 237, 576–78

Toothaches, 194, 381, 578–80

Tourniquets, 34

Toxic rashes, 443, 445

Toys: bottles as, 164, 193; breaking or throwing, 355; and developmental stimulation, 212; and injury prevention, 215; sharing, 351–52; and sleep problems, 262, 266, 270, 276, 282, 283; and taking toys from others, 351; and toilet-training, 290

Training cups, 121

Trauma: and life-threatening emergencies, 4. *See also type of trauma*

Travel, 158, 268, 368, 514, 520, 533, 536

Tuberculosis, 233

Umbilical cord, 111, 112–13, 119, 143–45

Umbilical hernia, 146

Unconsciousness, 4, 6, 12, 13, 41, 44, 54, 72, 73, 370. *See also* Coma

Undressing games, 373

Urinary tract infections, 111, 114, 234, 250

Urination: and appetite, 438; and breast-feeding, 151, 155; burning or pain during, 292, 299, 302, 306, 429, 624–26; calling physician about, 624–25, 626, 627; and chicken pox, 448; and child care/school, 301; and drinking excessive fluids, 306;

frequency of, 299–302; odor of, 627–28; and punishment, 300, 301; and scarlet fever, 464; and sleep, 285, 286–308; as weak and dribbly, 306; and wetting during daytime, 306. *See also* Bedwetting; Toilet-training; Urine

Urine: and appearance of normal infants, 106; blood in, 71, 627; and circumcision, 115; and diaper rash, 133; and foreskin care and problems, 117, 118; and genital trauma, 71; and jaundice, 137; red or cola-colored, 464; stream of, 106, 117, 118

Vaccinations. *See* Immunizations/ vaccinations; *type of vaccination*
Vagina, 105–6, 111, 629, 633–34
Vasomotor rhinitis, 551
Venereal diseases, 234
Venomous fish reactions, 26–27
Ventilation tubes surgery, 547–49
Video games, 399–401
Violence, 396, 397–98, 399, 400–402
Viral infections, 241, 243, 428, 430, 442, 444, 456, 462
Vision. *See* Eyes
Vitamin A, 154, 183, 471
Vitamin B, 183
Vitamin C, 154, 183
Vitamin D, 154, 171, 183
Vitamin K, 96
Vitamins and minerals, 96, 154, 160–61, 171, 173, 177–78, 182–83, 200, 206, 237
Vomiting: and antibiotics, 241, 242; of blood, 622–23; and breath-holding, 371; calling physician about, 620, 623; causes of, 619; common mistakes concerned with, 622; and dehydration, 8; and delirium, 46; diet for, 620–21; and drugs in home medicine chest, 249; and emergency

symptoms, 8; expected course of, 619; and formula-feeding, 158; home care for, 620–22; and medicines, 240, 246, 247, 622; and picky eaters, 176, 177; and school phobia, 381; similar conditions to, 619; and sleep, 262, 622; and spitting up, 138; and subtle symptoms of sick infants, 130; symptoms and characteristics of, 619; viral, 233. *See also specific disorder*

Walking, 7, 211, 214, 220–21, 447. *See also* Motor skills
Warts, 233, 510–11
Washing/bathing: and chicken pox, 447, 448; and discipline, 360–61; and dry skin, 450; equipment and supplies for, 118; and fifth disease, 454; and heat rash, 456; and hives, 457; of infants, 111–13; and preventing infections, 223; and sex education, 372, 373; and smoking, 231
Water: and baby-bottle tooth decay, 194; and breast-feeding, 152; contaminated, 223; and formula-feeding, 159; and healthy diet, 182; and preventing infections, 223; and weight, 206. *See also* Fluids
Weaning, 155, 162–67, 194
Weight: and appetite, 171, 172, 178; and breast-feeding, 150, 151, 155; and cholesterol, 187–88; and crying, 256; and exercise, 187–88, 204, 205, 207–8; and feeding, 100; and formula-feeding, 158; as health problem, 178, 204; and healthy diet, 178; how to help older children and teenagers lose, 204–8; ideal, 188, 203; of infants, 100, 149–50; and infections, 235, 236; and jaundice, 138; losing, 203–8; over-, 178, 188, 203–8; and overeating, 204; and